Immunodeficiency: Therapy, Mechanism and Model

Immunodeficiency: Therapy, Mechanism and Model

Edited by **Gabriel Murray**

Callisto Reference

New York

Published by Callisto Reference,
106 Park Avenue, Suite 200,
New York, NY 10016, USA
www.callistoreference.com

Immunodeficiency: Therapy, Mechanism and Model
Edited by Gabriel Murray

International Standard Book Number: 978-1-63239-428-6 (Hardback)

Printed in China.

Contents

	Preface	**IX**
Section 1	**Immunodeficiency - Immunotherapy**	**1**
Chapter 1	**Immunoglobulin Treatment of Immunodeficient Patients** Yıldız Camcıoğlu	**3**
Chapter 2	**Stem Cell Transplantation for Primary Immunodeficiency** Mary A. Slatter and Andrew R. Gennery	**27**
Chapter 3	**"Wrapped Up" Vaccines in the Context of HIV-1 Immunotherapy** Winni De Haes, Charlotte Pollard, Guido Vanham and Joanna Rejman	**51**
Chapter 4	**Is Anticancer Vaccine Possible: Experimental Application of Produced mRNA Transfected Dendritic Cells Derived from Enriched CD34+ Blood Progenitor Cells** Paula Lazarova, Gunnar Kvalheim and Krassimir Metodiev	**101**
Section 2	**Immunodeficiency - Mechanisms and Pathophysiology**	**113**
Chapter 5	**Fungal Infections in Immunosuppressed Patients** Luis Enrique Jerez Puebla	**115**
Chapter 6	**Pattern of Clinical Presentations in Immunocompromised Patient** Umezurike Hughes Okafor	**143**

Chapter 7	**Chemokine Receptors as Therapeutic Targets in HIV Infection** Cleo G. Anastassopoulou	**157**
Chapter 8	**Selective Antibody Deficiency with Normal Immunoglobulins** Ricardo U. Sorensen, Tammy Harvey and Lily E. Leiva	**191**
Chapter 9	**Emerging Role of MicroRNAs in the Pathophysiology of Immune System** Marco Rossi, Pierosandro Tagliaferri and Pierfrancesco Tassone	**207**
Section 3	**Immunodeficiency - HIV, Human Model**	**219**
Chapter 10	**Coreceptor Usage in HIV Infection** Kerina Duri	**221**
Chapter 11	**HIV-Infected Patients and Potential Impact on Thrombotic Events** Hortensia Álvarez Díaz, Ana Mariño Callejo and José Francisco García Rodríguez	**245**
Chapter 12	**The Role of Liver Transplantation in HIV Positive Patients** Deepak Joshi and Kosh Agarwal	**259**
Chapter 13	**Hodgkin's Lymphoma and Human Immunodeficiency Virus Infection** Moosa Patel	**275**
Chapter 14	**What I Knew was What I Learnt on the Street! Irish Drug Using Sex Workers Accounts of How They Contracted HIV and Hepatitis C** Teresa Whitaker, Paul Ryan and Gemma Cox	**289**
Section 4	**Immunodeficiency - HIV, Feline Model**	**309**
Chapter 15	**Feline Immunodeficiency** Fabiana Alves and Jenner Karlisson Pimenta dos Reis	**311**

Chapter 16 **Simian-Human Immunodeficiency Viruses and Their Impact on Non-Human Primate Models for AIDS** 329
Lara E. Pereira, Priya Srinivasan and James M. Smith

Chapter 17 **Feline Immunodeficiency Virus (FIV) Infection in Cats: A Possible Cause of Renal Pathological Changes** 375
Natasa Tozon, Mauro Pistello and Alessandro Poli

Permissions

List of Contributors

Preface

This book was inspired by the evolution of our times; to answer the curiosity of inquisitive minds. Many developments have occurred across the globe in the recent past which has transformed the progress in the field.

The therapy, mechanism as well as model of immunodeficiency are described in this all-inclusive book. It sheds light on one of the most common medical issues, which, unfortunately is still being researched on. Various medical issues are connected in a straight or indirect way to a particular alteration of the immune system. Therefore, they result in varied pathologic circumstances. Human defense mechanism is complex and different, but is many times defeated by infections, tumor processes, organ, tissue and cell transplantation, allergy, autoimmune processes, as well as various impacts by the environment. This book, jotted down by globally recognized scientists, discusses in detail the questions of what, why, how, when and where the immune system falls weak, what scientific results are exhibited and what are the techniques to cure and prevent immunodeficiency cases. This book will be beneficial to the learners and practitioners of medicine and biology, and will also be knowledgeable to immunologists, microbiologists, virologists, chemotherapists, oncologists, hematologists, transplantologists and pathologists.

This book was developed from a mere concept to drafts to chapters and finally compiled together as a complete text to benefit the readers across all nations. To ensure the quality of the content we instilled two significant steps in our procedure. The first was to appoint an editorial team that would verify the data and statistics provided in the book and also select the most appropriate and valuable contributions from the plentiful contributions we received from authors worldwide. The next step was to appoint an expert of the topic as the Editor-in-Chief, who would head the project and finally make the necessary amendments and modifications to make the text reader-friendly. I was then commissioned to examine all the material to present the topics in the most comprehensible and productive format.

I would like to take this opportunity to thank all the contributing authors who were supportive enough to contribute their time and knowledge to this project. I also wish to convey my regards to my family who have been extremely supportive during the entire project.

Editor

Section 1

Immunodeficiency – Immunotherapy

Chapter 1

Immunoglobulin Treatment of Immunodeficient Patients

Yıldız Camcıoğlu

Additional information is available at the end of the chapter

1. Introduction

There is a large number of immunodeficient patients requiring lifelong IgG replacement. This review is focused on currently available Intravenous Immunoglobulin (IVIG) preparations, manufacturing procedures, dose arrangements, mechanisms of actions, benefits of antibody replacement treatment and careful administration of IVIG considering, numerous side effects. Subcutaneous IgG (SCIG) treatment has gained ground in recent years as an alternative to IVIG. Data show that the efficacy of SCIG in preventing infections is proportional to the steady-state levels achieved and similar to that of IVIG.

Intravenous immunoglobulin (IVIG) is mainly indicated as replacement therapy for patients with primary and selected secondary immunodeficiency diseases characterized by absent or deficient antibody production. Antibody deficiencies are a heterogeneous group of diseases mainly consisting of primary immunodeficiency diseases (PID) [1-4]. Primary antibody deficiencies (PAD) can be divided into four main subgroups: X-linked agammaglobulinaemia, class-switch recombination defects (hyper-IgM syndromes (HIGM), hypogammaglobulinaemia (particularly common variable immunodeficiency (CIVD) and selective immunoglobulin deficiencies (selective IgA deficiency). Over the past 20 years, 18 genetic defects have been defined as leading causes of PAD, but no gene defects were identified in patients with hypogammaglobulinaemia and selective immunoglobulin deficiencies, because of the variability of the affected stages of B cell differentiation and maturation, and the onset time of clinical symptoms like childhood or adulthood with increased susceptibility to mainly bacterial infections [5,6].

Substitution of immunoglobulin G (IgG) is the efficient and standard treatment for many years [7-11]. Immunoglobulins pooled from thousands of healthy donors contain a wide range of antibody specificities. These immunoglobulin preparations also have anti-inflammatory and immunomodulatory effects in addition to their use as replacement therapy [12,13]. The benefits in diseases such as childhood thrombocytopenia and Kawasaki disease refractory to or intolerant of conventional treatment have been well established [14,15]. It has been 30 years since therapeutic contribution of intravenous immunoglobulin (IVIG) administration has been proven by scientists, an increasing number of immune-mediated diseases have been treated with intravenous immunoglobulin rather than corticosteroids and cytoxic drugs. IVIG has become the therapy of choice in autoimmune diseases, severe asthma, neurological diseases, transplantation, sepsis, septic shock, toxic shock syndromes and dermatologic disorders [15,16]. The recommendation of IVIG treatment in other diseases than those approved by FDA is based on limited data or some of these diseases do not have any alternative treatment regimen to compare with [16]. However, IVIG administration in the treatment of many diseases is raising the possibility of product shortages and increasing costs. Thus, concerning the shortages of products, cost and adverse reactions, definite indications for IVIG treatment are essential [12,13,16,17]. The aim of immunoglobulin therapy should be to protect the patients from frequent and severe infections finally resulting in organ damage. Advances in human immunology, has led to identify responsible genes for PID, thereby particular groups of defects are associated with susceptibility to specific types of infection [18]. Improved diagnostic precision is likely to increase more specialized management strategies of patients with PID, some of which are only supported by expert consultation. However, there are no sufficient number of studies in PID, to optimize the quality and uniformity of management of PID.

2. History and recent development (IVIG)

Cohn et al produced the first human immunoglobulin IgG product in1946 and it was referred as immune serum globulin (ISG)[19]. This first commercial human ISG solution tended to form aggregates during storage, therefore it was delivered via the intramuscular or subcutaneous route. After diagnosing his first patient with agammaglobulinemia in 1952, Bruton began to treat his patients by subcutaneous replacement therapy with ISG [20]. After a short time, intramuscular ISG treatment became available for all patients, but the amount of Ig used for treatment was limited and not effective enough to reduce recurrent infections and the adverse effects were also high due to IgG aggregates [21]. These disadvantages were abolished by Cohn fraction II that had been developed in 1960's by Barandum and his colleagues in collaboration with Swiss Red Cross [9,21]. The first IVIG was produced by pepsin digestion (enzymatic method: pepsin or trypsin) to reduce anticomplement activity, but this process cleaved the immunoglobulin molecule into two parts, resulting in fragments of the fc portion and Fab. Several manifacturers produced chemically modified IVIGs containing minimal anti-complement activity and no IgG fragments. Reduced bacterial opsonic activities and shortened circulating half-lives were demonstated in some antibodies of enzyme-digested or chemically modified IVIG preparations. Non-denaturating processes such as precipitation with polyethylene glycol (PEG), ion exchange chromatography, diafiltration and stabilisation of IgG at low pH, do not modify the IgG molecule and the half-life of IgG is generally 22-25 days [21].

Intravenous immunoglobulin (IVIG) preparations contain 16% human serum immunoglobulin and more than 95% IgG, scanty amount of IgA, IgM and other serum proteins. IgA and IgM do not have any therapeutic effects due to their short half-life and small amount [22,23]. Prognosis of patients with deficient IgG production has thoroughly improved after replacement therapy with IVIG [24]. Since 1980, it has been the most striking therapeutic agent due to its unproposed anti-inflammatory and immunomodulatory effects and used to treat a wide variety of pathologies including vasculitis, HIV infection, autoimmune diseases and immune-mediated neurological diseases [12,14,15, 25-28]. Currently, subcutaneous immunoglobulin infusions administered by a special pump has become an alternative to IVIG treatment. It has been demonstrated that this product is safe and has some clinical advantages over intravenous preparations. It has been recommended especially for selected patients with primary immunodeficiencies [29,30].

3. IVIG production

IVIG preparations are derived from plasma of a huge number of human blood donors or paid plasmapheresis donors. Since IVIG preparations are blood-derived products having the risk of transmission of infectious transfusional diseases, viral safety needs to be considered [13,21,23]. The safety of IVIG products depends on donors, validated manufacturing processes and various virus clearance steps as listed below:

a. recruitment of the donor
b. donation screening
c. use of validated manufacturing processes
d. effective viral inactivation/removal procedures

To produce a single product lot, sufficient number of donor recruitment and screening of viral markers (HBs-Ag, HIV-p24 antigen, antibodies to syphilis, HIV-1,HIV-2, HCV, HAV) are necessary to prevent the transmission of viruses [21].

FDA (Center for Biologics Evaluations and Research) and Plasma Protein Therapeutics Association recommended the number of donors to be minimum 15.000, but not more than 60.000. Manifacturing processes implemended in commercial IVIG preparations are the classical Cohn fractionations treated with solvent detergent, caprylate, acid or pepsin to inactivate pathogens [31-33].

Immunoglobulin, produced by cold ethanol fractionation method may contain trace amounts of contaminants such as prekallikrein activator, prekallikrein, activated coagulation factors, complement proteins, IgM, IgA, plasmin and plasminogen. Currently many manufacturers began to use purification with anion exchange (DEAE) chromatography adjusted to cold ethanol fractionations in order to obtain safe products.

Treatment at pH4 with trace amounts of pepsin is also validated by some manifacturers. Both, alcohol fractionation and acid treatment procedures eliminate other proteins and inactivate dangerous live viruses such as HIV, Hepatitis B, HCV.

Improved quality standards for plasma products and new blood borne pathogens such as SARS forced the scientists to develop and integrate new specific viral inactivation methods. RNA virus with lipid envelope, DNA virus with lipid envelope and non-lipid enveloped virusus must all removed by viral inactivation procedures. The heat and chemical treatment processes are able to remove and/or inactive blood-borne pathogens:

a. Pasteurisation: Based on heating to 60°C in an aqueous solution for 10 hours in the presence of stabilizers.
b. Solvent/Detergent: The solvent/detergent consists of an organic solvent (ether, 0.3% tri-n-butylphosphate (TNBT) and 0.2% detergent (Tween 80, sodium cholate or triton-100). The process lasts for 6 hours and destroys infectivity of lipid-enveloped viruses.
c. Nanofiltration: This procedure is effective to remove small non-enveloped (B19V, HAV) viruses.
d. Low pH-incubation: This incubation at elevated temperatures completely removes lipid-enveloped viruses like HIV, HBV/HCV).

Transmission of Prion diseases such as Creutzfeldt–Jakob disease (CJD) or variant CJD by administration of blood products is also possible, since the incubation period of the disease is too long leading to difficulties in risk determination. Because of this possibility, donors who have spent more than 6 months in the United Kingdom from 1986 to the present are not allowed to donate blood or plasma in the United States and Europe [21]. Some researchers demonstrated that depth filtration step that is common in all IVIG production procedures and nanofiltration removed hamster scrapie protein reactivity. The Finish Red Cross Blood Transfusion Service (FRC BTS' Helsinki, Finland) had developed a liquid 5% IVIG product (IVIG-L) in which a nanofiltration step was incorporated into the production process [34]. Van der Meer JWM et al. evaluated efficacy and safety of that nanofiltered liquid IVIG product and showed that IVIG-L was efficacious and pharmacokinetic properties were comparable to other IVIG preparations. In addition relatively low level of adverse reactions and the absence of seroconversion were observed. Thus, this liquid form product is considered to be safe and well tolerable. Over the past years, improved manifacturing processes and integrated specific viral inactivation steps have increased the safety and quality of IVIG products (Table 1). Commercially available products represent recent advancements in IVIG product formulation, but potential transmission of emerging pathogens can still not be ruled out completely.

Currently licensed IVIG preparations are supplied either in lyophilized powder or premixed solution, contains 95% IgG at a concentration of 16.5% (165 mg/ml), all the IgG subclasses, multiple IgG allotypes (Gm and Km), minimal anti-complement activity, broad spectrum of antibodies against viruses and bacteria, and no difference in therapeutic efficacy. Half-life of immunoglobulins is approximately 21-25 days. The osmolarity varies between 253 mOsm/L for a 5% IgG product to1250 mOsm/L for a 10% product. The final sterile product contains varying amounts of sodium, glycine, polyethylene glycol, D-mannitol, D-sorbitol, sucrose, glucose or maltose, glycerol as the stabilizer, and thiomersal as the preservative and has a pH of 6.8 (Table 2).

Virus inactivation/removal procedure	Product
Solvent-detergent inactivation	Gammagard S/D Gammagard liquid Flebogamma 5% DIF Octagam
Heat inactivation(10h at 60 C)	Vivaglobulin Flebogamma 5% Flebogamma 5% DIF
Removal by nanofiltration	Gammagard liquid Carimune NF Privigen
pH4 incubation (in process)	Flebogamma 5% DIF Octagam Privigen
Low pH incubation in final container(21 day)	Gamunex
Low pH incubation at elevated temperature in final container	Gammagard liquid
Pepsin treatment	Carimune NF
Caprylic acid virus inactivation	Gamunex

Table 1. Dedicated virus inactivation procedures used in IVIG production [22]

Product	Manufactu-rer	Dosage form	Sodium Content mEq/mL	Stabilizing agent /PH	Antimicrobial processes	IgA µg/mL	Osmolarity mOsm/kg
Octagam	Octapharma	5 %Liquid	0.03	Maltose PH 5.1-6	Cold ethanol fractionation Solvent-detergent	100	310-380
Gamimune N	Bayer	10%Liquid	Trace	Glycine pH4.25	Dialfiltration, Ultrafiltration Solvent-detergent	Trace	274
Carimune NF liquid	CSL Behring AG	3, 6 ,9,12% lyophilized	<20	sucrose 1.67 per gram protein PH 5.3	Kistler&Nitchman Fractiotion, trace Pepsin, pH 4.0 Nanofiltration	720	192-1074
Gammagard 5% S/D	Baxter	5% lyophilized powder	0.145	2% glucose PH 6.8	Ultrasantrifuge, Ion exchange chromotography, Solvent-detergent	<2.2.	636
Gammagard 10% S/D	Baxter	10% lyophilized powder	0.145	4% glucose PH 6.8	Ultrasantrifuge, Ion exchange, chromotography, Solvent-detergent	270	1250
Gammagard S/D10% (KIOVIG)	Baxter	10% liquid	none	glycine PH 4.85	Cohn-Oncley fractionation, Ion exchange chromotography, Nanofiltration, Solvent-detergent, pH 4 filtration	37	240-300

Product	Manufacturer	Dosage form	Sodium Content mEq/mL	Stabilizing agent /PH	Antimicrobial processes	IgA µg/mL	Osmolarity mOsm/kg
Flebogamma DIF	Grifols	5% , 10% Liquid	<0.032	D-sorbitol PH 5.0-6.0	Cold alcohol fractionation, PEG, Ion exchange, chromotography, PH4 treatment, Solvent-detergent, double sequential nanofiltration	5%: < 50 10%: < 100	240-370
Venoglobulin S	Alpha	5 % 10% Liquid		Albumin (human) D-sorbitol	PEG, Ion exchange Chromotography, Solvent-detergent,	24	
Gammar-PIV	Centeon, L.L.C., Kankakee	lyophilized	0.085	Albumin (human) Sucrose PH 6.8	Cold ethanol fractionation, heat10 hours 60°C	25	258
Iveegam	Immuno US	lyophilized 5%	0.05	Glucose, NaCl	Polyetilene glycol/trypsin	5	>240
Endobulin	Baxter Immuno France	lyophilized	3mg	Glucose, Polyetylene glycol(PEG),	Solvent-detergent		
IgVena	Sclavo	Liquid		Maltose	Solvent-detergent pH 4 filtration	100	
Privigen	CSL Behring AG	Liquid	Trace amount	None	Octanoic acid fractionation, CH9 filtration, pH 4.0 incubation, Depth filtration, Chromotography, Nanofiltration ,	≤25	Isotonic (320)
Gamunex- C	Talecris Biotherape-utics	Liquid	Trace amount	None	Cohn-Oncley fractionation, caprylate precipitation, Sepharose chromatography, Cloth and depth filtration Final container pH 4.25 ±0.25incubation	46	258
Omr-IgG-am	Omrix Biopharmaceuticals Ltd	Liquid		50 mg/mL; 100 mg/mL maltose	Cold ethanol fractionation, S/D, 24 h @ pH 4, pH 5.5 ± 0.4,		

Table 2. Commercial IVIG Products and properties (Data from Immune Deficiency Foundation, October 2011 and reference [17, 22])

All the available IVIG preparations approved by FDA and EMEA should at least have the following features:

- Sterile >4000[5000-10000]donors

- >20 days of half life
- >90 % monomeric IgG
- Effective IgG subclasses, a profile similar to that of human plasma
- Complete Fc functions, complement fixation, opsonophagocytosis
- No pyrogenic and vasoactive agents (kinin or plasmin), protein aggregates
- Low adverse effects
- Trace IgA concentration
- Stabile in solution
- Low price

4. Mechanism of action

Human immunoglobulin is obtained from a large number of donors and exceeding 2.000 donors is preferred. IVIG contains large spectrum of antibody specificities such as antibodies to foreign (non-self) antigens, to self-antigens (natural autoantibodies) and to other antibodies (idiotypic antibodies which represents antibody repertoire of each donor [35]. That is the reason of the differences between immunoglobulin batches [13,21,35]. The mechanism of activity of the substituted IgG is easily understood for immunodeficiency disorders considering common pathogen-specific IgG antibodies are replaced by those from the donor pool [35]. Thereby, regular intravenous immunoglobulin therapy reduces the incidence of infection in these patients compared to their infection rates before IVIG treatment [7-13]. Immunomodulatory effect of IVIG therapy depends on several mechanisms. Proposed early immunomodulatory effects of IVIG infusion are shown below [35-37]:

- Modulation of production and release of proinflammatory cytokines and cytokine antagonists
- Functional blockade of Fc receptor on splenic macrophages
- Neutralization of circulating autoantibodies
- Neutralization of superantigens
- Inhibition of complement-mediated damage
- Changes in solubility and rate of clearance of immune complexes

On the other hand, IVIG infusion downregulates IVIG-reactive B cell clones in long-term. Serum IL-6, IL-8, IL-1Ra and TNFalpha concentrations were increased in patients with primary immunodeficiencies following IVIG infusion, without any difference in serum IL-beta, IFNgamma or IL-2 levels. Understanding these immunomodulatory effects of IVIG is essential to define IVIG indications in autoimmune disorders [35-37]. In severe infections regarding increased catabolism of IgG, IVIG can be added to antibiotic treatments [16, 17].

The concentration of IgG is very important for its pro-inflammatory or anti-inflammatory properties. Low-dose IVIG has proinflammatory properties, but high dose IVIG has anti-inflammatory effects. The proinflammatory properties are dependent on complement activation or binding of the Fc fragment of IgG to IgGspecific (FcγR) on effector cells of the innate immunity leading to receptor clustering, activation of intracellular signaling pathways and finally to cell activation. The anti-inflammatory effect of IgG is still not clear, but IgG is known to inhibit the differentiation and maturation of human dendritic cells (DCs), expression of co-stimulatory molecules like CD80 and CD86, both leading to lower self antigen processing and presentation [8]. Fc and F(ab')$_2$ fragments of IgG molecule are both able to suppress of DCs. Antibodies with the intrinsic capacity to recognize foreign antigens or common pathogen-specific IgG antibodies are replaced by those from the donor pool [35].

At a lower dose, administered generally to patients with immunodeficiencies, however, IVIG exerts a contrasting effect. DCs of patients with common variable immune deficiency (CVID) differentiated in the presence of IVIG and presented with an up-regulated expression of CD1a and the co-stimulatory molecules CD80, CD86 and CD40 [38,39]. Defective functions of DCs have been associated with predisposition to several pathological conditions. CVID patients display high susceptibility to recurrent infections and autoimmune diseases that could be due in part to impaired DC functions [38,39].

Advantages of IVIG administration are the following:

- Painless administration
- Absence of proteolysis of the product
- No sterile abscess
- Rapid onset of action
- Easy administration of large doses

Unfortunately, there are also some disadvantages of IVIG administrations:

- High cost
- Requirement for a venous access
- Long duration of the infusion
- 5-15% adverse events
- Severe adverse reactions such as anaphlaxis

5. IVIG preparations

In recent years, manufactures aim to develop products that provide a high-yield, safe, well tolerated and stable concentrates of polyclonal IgG. Each new intravenous immunoglobulin product has to be tested for its biochemical characterization done by standart methods focusing on purity, integrity and functionality. Efficacy must be shown by opsonization, protein A affinity chromatography and mouse protection tests. Pharmacokinetics of the product, the influence of product on vital functions, acute toxicity, anaphylactoid potential, thrombogenicity should be evaluated in rats, dogs or a rabbit models. Development of new methods for fractionation, combining processes and integrating three dedicated virus clearance steps provided fulfilling the clinical requirements for intravenous administration of second-generation intravenous immunoglobulins products (Table 2) [21].

The US Food and Drug Administration (FDA) standardized clinical trials with IVIG in patients with primary immunodeficiencies. FDA has proposed to measure the rate of serious bacterial infections during regular infusions of investigational IVIG for 12 months to avoid seasonal variations. Serious bacterial infection term has to be well defined, thus bacteremia/sepsis, bacterial meningitis, osteomyelitis/septic arthritis, bacterial pneumonia, and visceral abscess were defined as serious infections [8].

The guidelines for clinical Investigation of human normal Immunoglobulin for Intravenous administration of the European Medicines Agency (EMA/CHMP/BPWP/94033/2007 rev.2) and FDA recommended that an immunoglobulin product is effective if treated patients experience less than 1.0 serious infection per year [21,34]. A new IVIG product must have 'intact IgG' which means pharmacokinetic properties of Immunoglobulin G is similar to endogeneous IgG and available other immunoglobulin preparations.

6. Indications of IVIG treatment

IVIG, has been licensed by FDA for only 6 clinical indications [8,22,23]:

1. Treatment of primary immunodeficiencies
2. Prevention of bacterial infections in patients with hypogammaglobulinemia and recurrent bacterial infections caused by B-cell chronic lymphocytic leukemia
3. Prevention of coronary artery aneurysms in Kawasaki disease
4. Prevention of infections, pneumonitis, and acute graft-versus-host disease (GVHD) after bone marrow transplantation
5. Reduction of serious and minor bacterial infections, to decrease the frequency of hospitalisation in children with HIV
6. Increase of platelet counts in idiopathic thrombocytopenic purpura to prevent or control bleeding

IVIG therapy has been evaluated in a number of clinical conditions mentioned above and categorization of evidence, basis of recommendation and strength of recommendation have been established (Table 3 and Table 4) [16].

Categorization of evidence and basis of recommendation
Ia From meta-analysis of randomized controlled studies
Ib From at least one randomized controlled study
IIa From at least one controlled study without randomization
IIb From at least one one other type of quasiexperimental study
III From nonexperimental descriptive studies such as comparative, correlation or case control studies
IV From expert committee reports or opinions or clinical experience of respected authorities or both
Strenght of recommendation
A Based on category I evidence
B Based on category II evidence or extrapolated from category I evidence
C Based on category III evidence or extrapolated from category I or II evidence
D Based on category IV evidence or extrapolated from category I, II or III evidence

Table 3. Categorization of evidence and basis of recommendation and strength of recommendation [17]

Benefits	Diseases	Evidence	Strenght of

		category	recommendation
Definitely beneficial	Primary immune defects with absent B cells Primary immune defects with hypogammaglobulinemia and impaired specific antibody production	IIb IIb	B B
Probably beneficial	Chronic lymhpocytic leukemia with reduced IgG and history of infection Prevention of bacterial infection in HIV infected children Primary immune defects with normogammaglobulinemia and impaired specific antibody production	Ib Ib III	A A C
Might provide benefit	Prevention of neonatal sepsis	Ia	A
Unlikely to be beneficial	Isolated IgA deficiency Isolated IgG4 deficiency	IV IV	D D

Table 4. Recommendation of IVIG in primary and secondary immunodeficiencies [17]

7. Treatment of primary immunodeficiencies

Primary antibody deficiencies [25], account for approximately 65-50% of primary immunodeficiencies (PID) [3,40]. Due to defects in critical stages of B cell development, B cells areabsent/reduced and B cell functions are impaired in patients with PAD [41]. B cell defects are a heterogeneous group of disorders consisting of patients presenting a wide variety of clinical conditions ranging from asymptomatic to severe and recurrent infections. Patients with selective IgA and IgG subclass deficiencies are often asymptomatic, while children with agammaglobulinemia present encapsulated bacterial infections initiating at 6 months of age. Reduced immunoglobulin concentrations and lack of antibody response against protein antigens (diphtheria, tetanus toxoids) or polysaccharide antigens (pneumococcal polysaccharide) are well defined in patients with agammaglobulinemia or hypogammaglobulinemia [40-42]. Although these patients have frequent or recurrent bacterial infections, they could not mount IgG antibody responses against antigens and this condition is a clear indication for immunoglobulin replacement therapy (Table 5) [21, 42].

Therefore, the aim of replacement therapy is to avoid acute infections, respiratory complications such as bronchiectasis, gastrointestinal complications, to improve quality of life and to increase life expectancy of patients [17, 22]. The delay in diagnosis of primary immunodeficiencies remains a significant problem, as a consequence of delay recurrent pneumonias results in structural lung damage such as bronchiectasis, pulmonary hypertension and finally cor pulmonale [10].

1. Antibody deficiencies	
	X -linked Agammaglobulinemia(XLA)
	Common variable immunodeficiency(CVID)
	Hyper IgM syndrome
	Transient hypogammaglobulinemia of infancy(selected cases)
	IgG subclass deficiency± Selected IgA deficiency (selected cases)
	Impaired specific sntibody production with normal plasma immunoglobulin evel
2. Combined immunodeficiencies	
	All type of severe combined immunodeficiencies(SCID)
3. Other well-defined immunodeficiency syndromes	
	Wiskott –Aldrich syndrome
	DNA repair defects; Ataxia-telangiectasia, Nijmegen breakage syndrome
	Di George Anomaly
	Primary CD4 deficiency
	ICF syndrome
4. Diseases of immune dysregulation	
	X-linked lymphoproliferative syndrome (XLP)

Table 5. Primary Immunodeficiencies benefit IVIG treatment

Evaluation of IVIG use in patients lacking immunoglobulin has demonstrated reduction of acute and chronic bacterial infections frequency, pneumonia, days of antibiotic usage, days of fever and hospital admission [16]. Retrospective studies in patients with XLA revealed that severity and number of infections are decreased depending on IVIG dose. Serious bacterial illnesses and enteroviral meningoancephalitis were prevented when maintained IgG levels were above 800mg/dL [16,21,42,43].

Barıs S et al. evaluated the efficacy of IVIG treatment (500 mg/kg every 3 weeks) in 29 children diagnosed with CVID. During therapy, median serum IgG levels increased from 410 to 900 mg/dL. The mean number of respiratory infections per patient per year decreased significantly from 10.2 to 2.5. The annual number and length of hospital stays decreased significantly from 1.36 to 0.21 and 16.35 to 6.33 days per patient, respectively. The mean annual number of antibiotics used decreased significantly from 8.27 to 2.50 per patient. Twelve patients had developed bronchiectasis before initiation of IVIG [44].

Intravenous immunoglobulin therapy has to be started without any delay in patients with CVID predisposed to chronic lung diseases. Appropriate replacement therapy in these patients, reduced the incidence of pneumonia and prevent progression of lung involvement [17, 42-47].

A 5-year multicenter prospective study on 201 patients with CVID and 101 patients with XLA was conducted to identify the effects of long-term immunoglobulin treatment and the IgG trough level to be maintained over time required to minimise infection risk. Overall, 21% of the patients with CVID and 24% of patients with XLA remained infection free during the study. Pneumonia episodes had been reduced. Patients with pneumonia did not have significant lower IgG trough levels than patients without pneumonia, with the exception of patients whose IgG trough levels were persistently <400 mg/dL. In addition, in XLA co-morbidity risk factor identified for pneumonia was the presence of bronchiectasis [10,23].

Studies have shown that 10 years survival of CVID patients receiving IVIG treatment was 78%; while expected survival in the general population at ten year was 97% [28].

Patients with severe combined immunodeficiency(SCID) syndromes are also agammaglobulinemic and have significant inability to produce antibody against antigens. Hematopoietic stem cell transplantation is choise of therapy for these patients, but functional B-cell reconstitution often fail following marrow engraftment and these patients could not produce antibodies. Regular replacement therapy with IVIG is indicated for these patients.

Hyper IgM syndromes are usually defined with reduced levels of IgG and IgA, but high or normal IgM. These patients have normal B cell counts, but defective class switching do not allow to generate specific antibodies, thus these children experience frequent infections like agammaglobulinemic individuals. Adequate replacement of IVIG has been shown to reduce the incidence of pneumonia from 7.6% to 1.4% per year and patients did not have meningitis [10, 25, 48].

Selective antibody deficiencies or normogammaglobulinemia with impaired specific antibody production are group of disorders characterized by impaired production of specific antibody with normal serum IgG levels. Evidence of recurrent infection and absent or reduced specific antibody production against polysaccharide antigens after vaccination, are requirements for IVIG therapy. Therapy can be stopped after clinical improvement and the immune response of patient should be re-evaluated at least 5 months later. Usually antibody response to antigens, improve in growing children, but in conditions of unresponsiveness to antigens, restart to IVIG treatment is appropriate due to recurrence of infections.

Immunoglobulin treatment is not commonly recommended to patients with selective IgA deficiency unless poor specific antibody or IgG2 subclass deficiency exists [21].

Replacement therapy is also recommended in patients with combined immune deficiencies, other well-defined immunodeficiency syndromes and X-linked lymphoproliferative syndrome (XLP)(Table 5).

8. Choosing a commercial brand for IVIG therapy

There are several factors required for selection of an IVIG brand:

1. To obtain enough information about the IVIG product: lyophilized powder or premixed solution, amount of sodium, IgG and IgA, stabilizing sugar, preservative, viral inactivation methods, concentration, osmolarity
2. Safety and tolerability
3. Price

Regarding lyophilized or liquid forms, sugar content, amount of IgA (varies between <0.4 μg/mL and 720 μg/mL), used antimicrobial processes and stabilizing agent, an appropriate commercial immunoglobulin preparation should be selected for treatment of immunodeficient patients(Table 1). The patients with diabetes may have high blood glucose levels due to maltose-containing products therefore they have to adjust doses of insulin [5, 8, 21, 23, 49].

Patients with selective IgA deficiency carry the risk of anaphylaxis due to production of anti-IgA antibodies. Selective IgA deficient patients having high anti-IgA (>1/1000) titers should not be treated with IVIG or a IgA-free immunoglobulin product should be chosen for the treatment [8, 21, 50, 51]. Since IVIG administration is a life-saving therapy, the treatment should be supported by scientific clinical evidence regardless the economic impact of therapy [52]. Therefore considering scarcity of resource for IVIG, its judicious use must be promoted for the diseases FDA approved.

9. Dose

The common recommended dose of IVIG treatment for antibody replacement is between 0.3 and 0.6 g/kg, administered every 2 to 4 weeks via the intravenous route. The first dose of IVIG infusion usually results more frequently in adverse reactions compared to the following second or third doses. Thus, the first IVIG infusion to a patient with antibody deficiency must be given slowly as a 5% solution, starting with a rate of 0.5 to 1.0 mg/kg per minute. Patient should be monitored closely for any adverse reactions during infusion. If the patient tolerates well, the infusion rate may be increased to 1.5 to 2.5 mg/kg per minute after 15 to 30 minutes. The maximal infusion rate is 4 mg/kg per minute. Infusion of an IVIG product should last 2 to 4 hours. For subsequent infusions IVIG concentrations of 10% and 12% can be used, with rates 4 mg/kg per minute. The aim of IVIG therapy in patients with PID is to maintain serum IgG levels between 350 mg/dl and 500 mg/dl [7,10,16,17,25,42,43,45,48,51].

Since, there is large variation in individual IgG elimination rates, periodic measurement of serum IgG concentration is critical to monitor the adequacy of replacement during therapy.

10. Adverse effects of IVIG

There are two main risks of immunoglobulin treatment: Infusion related adverse effects and transmission of blood–borne viruses [5,7,22,23]. Incidence of adverse reactions, have been found 44% in more than 1.000 patients with PID, in a study done by Immune Deficiency Foundation (IDF) [16]. This rate was surprisingly higher than those observed in licensing studies (Table 6). The IDF survey showed that 34% of patients experienced adverse reactions during the first administration of IVIG and who has had a recent bacterial infection. Reactions may develop 1 to 15% in the first 30 minutes of IVIG infusions. After second or third doses of the same IVIG product additionial infusion dependent reactions become less likely. Most IVIG reactions are mild, however anaphylaxis may occur occasionally. Adverse reactions are characterized by chills, headache, low grade fever, back or abdominal pain, nausea, vomiting, myalgias, rhinitis, asthma, flushing on face, vertigo, anxiety, conjunctival congestion, occasional rash and drop of arterial pressure. Varying rates of adverse events have been reported (Table 6) [53-56]. Thus, close monitoring of a patient during infusion is essential to identify and manage reactions [8,24,53]. Recently, manufacturing processes of immunoglobulins have been improved and new IVIG products have been developed. Several trials with these products demonstrated that the infusion related adverse reactions were reduced [24,53]. IVIG infusions have to be done at hospital or home by professionally educated staff if possible. Local anesthetic cream (EMLA Cream) could be applied on skin prior infusion to reduce pain in small children. Administration IVIG via indewelling venous catheter is not encouraged because of additional adverse events such as thrombotic and infectious complications.

Product	**Study Duration Months**	**Patients Treated**	**Dose**	**Acute Serious Bacterial Infect/subj/y**	**Other Bacterial Infect/subj/y**	**Related, Temporally Associated AEs (%of Infusions**	**Drug-Related SAEs**
CarimuneNF Liquid (12%)	6	42	200-800 mg/Kg/21–28 d	0	3.65	21.7% a	0
Flebogamma 5%	12	51	300–600 mg/Kg/21–28 d	0	061. NR	8.2% c	2
Flebogamma 5% DIF	12	46	300–600 mg/Kg/21–28 d	0.021	1. 96	11.8% c	0
Gammagard liquid 10%	12	61	300–600 mg/Kg/21–28 d	0	0.07	31.2% c	2 (1 patient)
Gamunex 10%	9	73	100–600 mg/Kg/21–28 d	0.07	0.18	5.7% a	0
Octagam 5%	12	46	300–600 mg/Kg/21–28d.	0.1	0	5.5% b	0
Privigen 10%	12	80	200–888 mg/Kg/21–28 d	0.08	3.55	18.5% b	5 (1 subject)
Vivaglobin 16%	15	51	34–352 mg/Kg/wk	0.04	4.4	Local, 49%; Systemic 5.4%	0

AE:Adverse event, infect/subj/y: infections per subject per year, NF:nanofiltration, SAE:serios adverse event a) 0-48 h postinfusion, b) 0-430 min postinfusion, c) 0-72 h postinfusion

Table 6. Clinical trials in patients with primary immunodeficiency disorders [22]

11. Late-onset side effects of IVIG

A variety of side effects due to IVIG therapy have been reported in different tissues [7-11,21-25,27,28,57]:

Central nervous system: rarely aseptic menengitis

Hematologic: hemolytic anemia, leukopenia, neutropenia, monocytopenia, disseminated intravascular coagulation and changes in blood rheology

Cardiovascular system: rarely heart attack, most commonly, drop in arterial blood pressure

Urogenital system: During the period between June 1985 and November 1998, 88 cases of kidney injuries had been reported to FDA. Acute renal failure occured with IVIG preparations stabilized with sucrose, where as those stabilized with D-sorbitol did not cause such an effect. Patients whose urinary output decreases, who suddenly gain weight with edeme on feet and ankles and those who experience dyspnea should be monitored very closely.

Liver Disease: The risk of Hepatitis C, Hepatitis B, HIV infection, prion disease disappeared after the initiation of viral inactivation (solvent-detergent or pasteurization) methods and PCR studies which took place after CDC's confirmation of 88 infections among 137 suspected hepatitis C cases (occuring after IVIG) in 1994. Therefore they are reliable preparations.

Skin: severe cutaneus vasculitis, dermatitis (egzema) and hair loss

Other: Life threatening parvovirus B19 has occured due to IVIG, hyperproteinemia, increased serum viscosity, pseudo-hyponatremia during infusions, transient serum sickness.

12. How to manage adverse reactions?

An expert monitoring is necessary for prompt diagnosis and treatment of adverse reactions. Most side effects resolve by themselves and are usually due to the speed of infusion. Infusion should temporarily be stopped 15 to 30 minutes if the symptoms appear or should be continued with slower rate once the symptoms disappear. Since the side effects are usually non-IgE dependent, the use of antihistamines is controversial, but diphenhydramine, acetaminophen or ibuprofen may be helpful. More severe reactions can be treated with 50 to 100 mg of hydrocortisone in adults and intravenous hydration is helpful.

Those who are reactive to IVIG should receive premedication. Thirty minutes prior to IVIG administration, oral nonsteroid anti-inflamatory agent (acetaminophen 15 mg/kg), antihistaminic agent (Benadryl 1mg/kg) or one hour prior to infusion intravenous hydrocortisone (6 mg/kg) should be administered [8,24].

13. Subcutaneos immunoglobulin

As an alternative to intravenous immunoglobulin treatment, immunoglobulins can be administered subcutaneously to patients with primary immunodeficiencies, Subcutaneous infusion of IgG was introduced more than 20 years ago but has gained ground in recent years [29,30,58-64]. Three ready-to-use liquid preparations of human IgG specifically formulated for subcutaneous infusions have been lisenced in US (Table 7). It can be stored at a temperature up to 25°C.

Product	Manufacturer	Dosage form	Sodium Content	Stabilizing agent /PH	Antimicrobial processes	IgA µg/mL	Osmolarity mOsm/kg
Gammagard S/D10%	Baxter Corporation	10% liquid <40 kg:20 mL/hr/site >40 kg:30 mL/hr/site	none	glycine PH 4.85	Cohn-Oncley fractionation, Ion exchange chromotography, 35 nmNanofiltration, Solvent-detergen, pH 4, elevated temperature incubation	37	240-300
Hizentra	BayerC CSL Behring CSL Behring	20% Liquid	Trace <10mmol/L	pH4.6-5.2	Cold alcohol fractionation, Octonic acid fractionation Anion exchange chromatography,Depth filtration Nanofiltration, pH4.0incubation TSE reduction steps include; Octonic acid fractionation, Depth filtration and virus filtration	<50	380
Vivaglobulin	CSL Behring	16% liquid	3mg/mL	none	Cold alcohol fractionation, Ethanol-fatty alcohol/pH precipitation, pasteurization, Diafiltered and ultrafiltered	<1700 µg/mL	445

Table 7. Commercial subcutaneous IG Products(Immune deficiency Foundation, October 2011)

The infusion can be applied through fine butterfly needles under the skin into the abdomen or thighs. Infusion pumps are used to administer the infusions and usually take 45 to 90 minutes. The amount of fluid given weekly to babies and children is 10 mls per site and 30 mls per site for older children. Subcutaneous infusion of 10-20% immunoglobulin, with the rate of 0.05-0.20 ml/kg/hour is advised. The recommended maintenance dose is 100 mg/kg/week. Immunoglobulin trough levels should be >5 g/L for patients with agammaglobulinaemia and 3 g/L greater than the initial IgG level for patients with CVID; however, the clinical response should be consider in choosing the dose and trough level [24]. Parents and patients can be educated on how to infuse the preparation at home. These infusions are better tolerated compared to IVIG and time sparing (home administration). Subcutaneous infusions are recommended to patients who are small children or reactive to IVIG or have poor veins.

Bioavailability and pharmacokinetics properties of subcutaneous IgG (SCIG) differs from intravenous IgG (IVIG). There are still debates about how the dose should be adjusted when switching from IVIG to SCIG. Berger M et al reported that the doses that will yield desired serum levels for IVIG and SCIG may be estimated with the help of pharmacokinetic studies [8]. Area under the curve (AUC) of serum IgG versus time and trough level ratios (TLRs) on SCIG/IVIG were evaluated as guides for adjusting the dose. The mean dose adjustments required for non-inferior AUCs with 2 different SCIG preparations were 137% (± 12%) and 153% (± 16%). However, there were wide variations between adjustments required by different subjects, and in the resulting TLRs. Recent studies allow estimation of the ratio of IgG levels with different dose adjustments, and of the steady state serum levels with different SCIG doses [8]. When switching a patient from IVIG to SCIG, practising immunologist can tailor the dosage based on measured serum IgG levels and the clinical response Skoda-Smith S et al recommended a sample calculation process for converting from IVIG to subcutaneous IG, thus weekly dose for subcutaneous Ig should calculate as 1.37 X IVIg dose [65].

Safety and therapeutic efficacy of subcutaneous immunoglobulin products has been demonstrated in children and pregnant women. Therapeutic efficacy of intravenous or subcutaneous immunoglobulin treatment in reducing infections was equal [5,28,57,65,66]. In an international study performed by Chapel et al. the efficacy of immunoglobulin replacement therapy given via intravenously or subcutaneously in patients with PAD was compared [60]. Forty patients received subcutaneous or intravenous immunoglobulin for the first year and switched to the alternative treatment in the second year, and the study showed that there was no difference in efficacy and adverse reactions between both routes. In another study, Fasth A et al. used a 16%, ready-to-use human normal immunoglobulin solution subcutaneously in children with PID previously receiving regular IVIG treatment, and the study showed that mild injection reactions were the adverse effects of the treatment, and the rate of bacterial infections was not different between both IVIG treatments. In the at home treatment there were fewer missed school days, low healthcare expenses [62].

The cost effectiveness of the use of subcutaneous IG compared to IVIG therapy had been investigated in several studies [67,68]. The mean cost of both immunoglobulins was evaluated in the study performed by Beaute J et al. and they showed that monthly doses were equal for both routes of administration. In addition SCIG and IVIG (hospital-based) costs were also similar, but the costs may differ from one country to another [52]. Although this theoretical model showed little difference between the costs, SCIG seems to be expensive compared to IVIG due to the doses of immunoglobulin, but further studies are needed. Overall costs may be higher in CVID, because these patients need higher doses of immunoglobulin [21,52].

The SCIG home therapy was reported to give better health and improved school/social functioning for the children, reduced emotional distress and limitations on personal time for the parents and fewer limitations on family activities [58-64]. Pharmacokinetic studies reveal a more physiologic profile, in peak and trough levels of serum IgG [62,66]. Local tissue reactions are more frequent but the systemic side effect profile is low. Local tissue reactions are often mild and tend to improve over time. Adults switching therapy reported improved vitality, mental health, and social functioning. Treatment satisfaction (TS) scores and health-related quality of life (HRQOL) was improved in adults and children with immunodeficiency [69].

According to ESID registry (http://www.esid.org), 4462 of 10,039 patients with PID receive IgG replacement (74% intravenous, 26% subcutaneous, <0.5% intramuscular). There is a wide variety of frequency of subcutaneous IgG replacement therapy in European countries. Sweden was the first country to deliver IgG via the SC route, therefore more than 80% of all patients with antibody deficiencies receive SCIg [3].

14. Conclusion

Replacement therapy with immunoglobulin either via intravenous or via subcutaneous is in patients with immunodeficiencies are associated with reduced infection frequency and organ damage and increased life expectancy. IVIG has been widely used in US and Europe for many years. Monthly IVIG treatment offered steady-state IgG level throughout the dosing cycle, dedicated viral inactivation steps improved safety concerns, pooled analyses confirmed the efficacy and safety, benefits of therapy and adverse events has been welll established.

Recent advances in the basic science of immunoglobulins and meta-analyses of patient data have provided new approaches in using polyclonal IgG to treat patients with primary immunodeficiencies. The old fashion subcutaneuos IG infusion reintroduced to treat patients with immunodeficiencies. The subcutaneous-IG therapy was reported to be effective, safe and well tolerated in children and adults. In addition, the SCIG home therapy high treatment satisfaction (TS) scores and health-related quality of life (HRQOL) was advantages of SCIG. Subcutaneous infusions are recommended to patients who are small children or reactive to IVIG or have problem with vascular access. Practicing immunologists can use new concepts in tailoring their approach to treat patients with primary immunodeficiencies.

Author details

Yıldız Camcıoğlu*
Istanbul University Cerrahpasa Medical School, Department of Pediatrics
Infectious Diseases, Clinical Immunology and Allergy Division, Cerrahpasa, Istanbul

15. References

[1] Stiehm ER, Vaerman JP, Fudenberg HH. Plasma infusions in immunologic deficiency states: metabolic and therapeutic studies. *Blood*, 1966. 28(6): p. 918-937.

* Corresponding Author

[2] Fischer A. Primary immune deficiencies of B-lymphocytes. *Rev Prat*, 1991. 41(9): p. 790-794.

[3] Gathmann B, Binder N, Ehl S, Kindle G. The European internet-based patient and research database for primary immunodeficiencies: update 2011. *Clin Exp Immunol.* 167(3): p. 479-491.

[4] Notarangelo LD. Primary immunodeficiencies. *J Allergy Clin Immunol.* 2010.125(2 Suppl 2): p. S182-194.

[5] van der Burg M, van Zelm MC, Driessen GJ, van Dongen JJ. New frontiers of primary antibody deficiencies. *Cell Mol Life Sci.* 2012. 69(1): p. 59-73.

[6] Driessen G, van der Burg M. Educational paper: primary antibody deficiencies. *Eur J Pediatr.* 2011.170(6): p. 693-702.

[7] Cunningham-Rundles C, Intravenous immune serum globulin in immunodeficiency. *Vox Sang*, 1985. 49 Suppl 1: p. 8-14.

[8] Berger M. Principles of and advances in immunoglobulin replacement therapy for primary immunodeficiency. *Immunol Allergy Clin North Am*, 2008. 28(2): p. 413-437.

[9] Thampakkul S. Replacement intravenous immune serum immunoglobulin therapy in patients with antibody immune deficiency. *Immunol Allergy Clin North America*, 2001. 21(1): p. 165-184.

[10] Wood P, Stanworth S, Burton J, Jones A, Peckham DG, Green T, Hyde C, Chapel H. Recognition, clinical diagnosis and management of patients with primary antibody deficiencies: a systematic review. *Clin Exp Immunol*, 2007. 149(3): p. 410-423.

[11] Lee ML, Gale RP, Yap PL. Use of intravenous immunoglobulin to prevent or treat infections in persons with immune deficiency. *Annu Rev Med*, 1997. 48: p. 93-102.

[12] Fontan G, Garcia MC, Pascual-Salcedo D, Lopez Trascasa M, Alvarez-Doforno R, Ferreira A. (New indications for gamma globulins). *An Esp Pediatr*, 1992. 36 Suppl 48: p. 135-138.

[13] Lemieux R, Bazin RNeron S. Therapeutic intravenous immunoglobulins. *Mol Immunol*, 2005. 42(7): p. 839-848.

[14] Imbach P, *Morell A.* Idiopathic thrombocytopenic purpura (ITP): immunomodulation by intravenous immunoglobulin (IVIg). *Int Rev Immunol.* 1989; 5(2):181-8.

[15] Abe TKawasugi K, Use of intravenous immunoglobulin in various medical conditions. A Japanese experience. *Cancer*, 1991. 68(6 Suppl): p. 1454-1459.

[16] Orange JS, Hossny EM, Weiler CR, Ballow M, Berger M, Bonilla FA, Buckley R, Chinen J, El-Gamal Y, Mazer BD, Nelson RP, Jr., Patel DD, Secord E, Sorensen RU. Wasserman RLCunningham-Rundles C, Use of intravenous immunoglobulin in human disease: a review of evidence by members of the Primary Immunodeficiency Committee of the American Academy of Allergy, Asthma and Immunology. *J Allergy Clin Immunol*, 2006. 117(4 Suppl): p. S525-553.

[17] Yong PL, Boyle J, Ballow M, Boyle M, Berger M, Bleesing J, Bonilla FA, Chinen J, Cunninghamm-Rundles C, Fuleihan R, Nelson L, Wasserman RL, Williams KC, Orange JS. Use of intravenous immunoglobulin and adjunctive therapies in the

treatment of primary immunodeficiencies: A working group report of and study by the Primary Immunodeficiency Committee of the American Academy of Allergy Asthma and Immunology. *Clin Immunol.*2010. 135(2): p. 255-263.

[18] Casanova JL. (Genetic predisposition to infectious diseases: identification of new genetic immunodeficiencies). *Bull Mem Acad R Med Belg,* 2004. 159(1-2): p. 132-136.

[19] Cohn EJ, Strong LE et al. Preparation and properties of serum and plasma proteins; a system for the separation into fractions of the protein and lipoprotein components of biological tissues and fluids. *J Am Chem Soc,* 1946. 68: p. 459-475.

[20] Bruton OC. Agammaglobulinemia. *Pediatrics,* 1952. 9(6): p. 722-728.

[21] Hooper JA. Intravenous immunoglobulins: evolution of commercial IVIG preparations. *Immunol Allergy Clin North Am,* 2008. 28(4): p. 765-778.

[22] Schwartz SA. Intravenous immunoglobulin treatment of immunodeficiency disorders. *Pediatr Clin North Am,* 2000. 47(6): p. 1355-1369.

[23] Maarschalk-Ellerbroek LJ, Hoepelman IM, Ellerbroek PM. Immunoglobulin treatment in primary antibody deficiency. *Int J Antimicrob Agents.* 2011. 37(5): p. 396-404.

[24] Hoernes M, Seger R, Reichenbach J. Modern management of primary B-cell immunodeficiencies. *Pediatr Allergy Immunol.*2011. 22(8): p. 758-769.

[25] Quinti I, Soresina A, Guerra A, Rondelli R, Spadaro G, Agostini C, Milito C, Trombetta AC, Visentini M, Martini H, Plebani A, Fiorilli M. Effectiveness of immunoglobulin replacement therapy on clinical outcome in patients with primary antibody deficiencies: results from a multicenter prospective cohort study. *J Clin Immunol.*2011. 31(3): p. 315-322.

[26] Kazatchkine MD, Kaveri SV. Immunomodulation of autoimmune and inflammatory diseases with intravenous immune globulin. *N Engl J Med,* 2001. 345(10): p. 747-755.

[27] Berkman SA, Lee ML, Gale RP, Clinical uses of intravenous immunoglobulins. *Ann Intern Med,* 1990. 112(4): p. 278-292.

[28] Cunningham-Rundles C, Bodian C. Common variable immunodeficiency: clinical and immunological features of 248 patients. *Clin Immunol,* 1999. 92(1): p. 34-48.

[29] Gardulf A, Hammarstrom L, Smith CI. Home treatment of hypogammaglobulinaemia with subcutaneous gammaglobulin by rapid infusion. *Lancet,* 1991. 338(8760): p. 162-166.

[30] Stiehm ER, Casillas AM, Finkelstein JZ, Gallagher KT, Groncy PM, Kobayashi RH, Oleske JM, Roberts RL, Sandberg ET, Wakim ME. Slow subcutaneous human intravenous immunoglobulin in the treatment of antibody immunodeficiency: use of an old method with a new product. *J Allergy Clin Immunol,* 1998. 101(6 Pt 1): p. 848-849.

[31] Teschner W, Butterweck HA, Auer W. Muchitsch EM, Weber A, Liu SL, Wah PS, Schwarz HP, A new liquid, intravenous immunoglobulin product (IGIV 10%) highly purified by a state-of-the-art process. *Vox Sang,* 2007. 92(1): p. 42-55.

[32] Roifman CM, Schroeder H, Berger M, Sorensen R, Ballow M, Buckley RH, Gewurz A, Korenblat P, Sussman G, Lemm G. Comparison of the efficacy of IGIV-C, 10% (caprylate/chromatography) and IGIV-SD, 10% as replacement therapy in primary

immune deficiency. A randomized double-blind trial. *Int Immunopharmacol*, 2003. 3(9): p. 1325-1333.
[33] Ochs HD, Pinciaro PJ. Octagam 5%, an intravenous IgG product, is efficacious and well tolerated in subjects with primary immunodeficiency diseases. *J Clin Immunol*, 2004. 24(3): p. 309-314.
[34] van der Meer JW, van Beem RT, Robak T, Deptala A, Strengers PF. Efficacy and safety of a nanofiltered liquid intravenous immunoglobulin product in patients with primary immunodeficiency and idiopathic thrombocytopenic purpura. *Vox Sang*. 2011. 101(2): p. 138-146.
[35] Durandy A, Kaveri SV, Kuijpers TW, Basta M, Miescher S, Ravetch JV, Rieben R. Intravenous immunoglobulins-understanding properties and mechanisms. *Clin Exp Immunol*, 2009. 158 Suppl 1: p. 2-13.
[36] Ibanez C, Sune P, Fierro A, Rodriguez S, Lopez M, Alvarez A, De Gracia J, Montoro JB. Modulating effects of intravenous immunoglobulins on serum cytokine levels in patients with primary hypogammaglobulinemia. *BioDrugs*, 2005. 19(1): p. 59-65.
[37] Aschermann S, Lux A, Baerenwaldt A, Biburger M, Nimmerjahn F. The other side of immunoglobulin G: suppressor of inflammation. *Clin Exp Immunol*. 2010. 160(2): p. 161-167.
[38] Bayry J, Lacroix-Desmazes S, Carbonneil C, Misra N, Donkova V, Pashov A, Chevailler A, Mouthon L, Weill B, Bruneval P, Kazatchkine MDKaveri SV, Inhibition of maturation and function of dendritic cells by intravenous immunoglobulin. *Blood*, 2003. 101(2): p. 758-765.
[39] Scott-Taylor TH, Green MR, Eren E, Webster AD. Monocyte derived dendritic cell responses in common variable immunodeficiency. *Clin Exp Immunol*, 2004. 138(3): p. 484-490.
[40] Geha RS, Notarangelo LD, Casanova JL, Chapel H, Conley ME, Fischer A. Hammarstrom L, Nonoyama S, Ochs HD, Puck JM, Roifman C, Seger R, Wedgwood J. Primary immunodeficiency diseases: an update from the International Union of Immunological Societies Primary Immunodeficiency Diseases Classification Committee. *J Allergy Clin Immunol*, 2007. 120(4): p. 776-794.
[41] Ballow M, Notarangelo L, Grimbacher B, Cunningham-Rundles C, Stein M, Helbert M, Gathmann B, Kindle G, Knight AK, Ochs HD, Sullivan KFranco JL, Immunodeficiencies. *Clin Exp Immunol*, 2009. 158 Suppl 1: p. 14-22.
[42] Chapel HCunningham-Rundles C. Update in understanding common variable immunodeficiency disorders (CVIDs) and the management of patients with these conditions. *Br J Haematol*, 2009. 145(6): p. 709-727.
[43] Bayrakci B, Ersoy F, Sanal O, Kilic S, Metin A, Tezcan I. The efficacy of immunoglobulin replacement therapy in the long-term follow-up of the B-cell deficiencies (XLA, HIM, CVID). *Turk J Pediatr*, 2005. 47(3): p. 239-246.

[44] Baris S, Ercan H, Cagan HH, Ozen A, Karakoc-Aydiner E, Ozdemir C, Bahceciler NN. Efficacy of intravenous immunoglobulin treatment in children with common variable immunodeficiency. *J Investig Allergol Clin Immunol*. 2011. 21(7): p. 514-521.

[45] Plebani A, Soresina A, Rondelli R, Amato GM, Azzari C, Cardinale F, Cazzola G, Consolini R, De Mattia D, Dell'Erba G, Duse M, Fiorini M, Martino S, Martire B, Masi M, Monafo V, Moschese V, Notarangelo LD, Orlandi P, Panei P, Pession A, Pietrogrande MC, Pignata C, Quinti I, Ragno V, Rossi P, Sciotto A, Stabile A. Clinical, immunological, and molecular analysis in a large cohort of patients with X-linked agammaglobulinemia: an Italian multicenter study. *Clin Immunol*, 2002. 104(3): p. 221-230.

[46] Quartier P, Debre M, De Blic J, de Sauverzac R, Sayegh N, Jabado N, Haddad E, Blanche S, Casanova JL, Smith CI, Le Deist F, de Saint Basile G, Fischer A. Early and prolonged intravenous immunoglobulin replacement therapy in childhood agammaglobulinemia: a retrospective survey of 31 patients. *J Pediatr*, 1999. 134(5): p. 589-596.

[47] Kaveri SV, Maddur MS, Hegde P, Lacroix-Desmazes S, Bayry J. Intravenous immunoglobulins in immunodeficiencies: more than mere replacement therapy. *Clin Exp Immunol*.2011. 164 Suppl 2: p. 2-5.

[48] Busse PJ, Razvi S, Cunningham-Rundles C. Efficacy of intravenous immunoglobulin in the prevention of pneumonia in patients with common variable immunodeficiency. *J Allergy Clin Immunol*, 2002. 109(6): p. 1001-1004.

[49] Misbah S, Kuijpers T, van der Heijden J, Grimbacher B, Guzman D, Orange J. Bringing immunoglobulin knowledge up to date: how should we treat today? *Clin Exp Immunol*. 2011. 166(1): p. 16-25.

[50] Bjorkander J, Hammarstrom L, Smith CI, Buckley RH, Cunningham-Rundles C, Hanson LA. Immunoglobulin prophylaxis in patients with antibody deficiency syndromes and anti-IgA antibodies. *J Clin Immunol*, 1987. 7(1): p. 8-15.

[51] Cunningham-Rundles C. Lung disease, antibodies and other unresolved issues in immune globulin therapy for antibody deficiency. *Clin Exp Immunol*, 2009. 157 Suppl 1: p. 12-16.

[52] Beaute J, Levy P, Millet V, Debre M, Dudoit Y, Le Mignot L, Tajahmady A, Thomas C, Suarez F, Pellier I, Hermine O, Aladjidi N, Mahlaoui N, Fischer A. Economic evaluation of immunoglobulin replacement in patients with primary antibody deficiencies. *Clin Exp Immunol*. 2011.160(2): p. 240-245.

[53] Ballow M. Safety of IGIV therapy and infusion-related adverse events. *Immunol Res*, 2007. 38(1-3): p. 122-132.

[54] Baxley A, Akhtari M. Hematologic toxicities associated with intravenous immunoglobulin therapy. *Int Immunopharmacol*. 2011. 11(11): p. 1663-1667.

[55] Pierce LR, Jain N. Risks associated with the use of intravenous immunoglobulin. *Transfus Med Rev*, 2003. 17(4): p. 241-251.

[56] Ochs HD, Fischer SH, Wedgwood RJ, Wara DW, Cowan MJ, Ammann AJ, Saxon A, Budinger MD, Allred RU, Rousell RH. Comparison of high-dose and low-dose

intravenous immunoglobulin therapy in patients with primary immunodeficiency diseases. *Am J Med,* 1984. 76(3A): p. 78-82.

[57] Pautard B, Hachulla E, Bagot d'Arc M, Chantreuil L. (Intravenous immunoglobulin (Endobulin) clinical tolerance: prospective therapeutic follow-up of 142 adults and children). *Rev Med Interne,* 2003. 24(8): p. 505-513.

[58] Bhole MV, Burton J, Chapel HM. Self-infusion programmes for immunoglobulin replacement at home: feasibility, safety and efficacy. *Immunol Allergy Clin North Am,* 2008. 28(4): p. 821-832.

[59] Jolles S, Sleasman JW. Subcutaneous immunoglobulin replacement therapy with Hizentra, the first 20% SCIG preparation: a practical approach. *Adv Ther.* 2011.28(7): p. 521-533.

[60] Chapel HM, Spickett GP, Ericson D, Engl W, Eibl MM, Bjorkander J. The comparison of the efficacy and safety of intravenous versus subcutaneous immunoglobulin replacement therapy. *J Clin Immunol,* 2000. 20(2): p. 94-100.

[61] Ochs HD, Gupta S, Kiessling P, Nicolay U, Berger M. Safety and efficacy of self-administered subcutaneous immunoglobulin in patients with primary immunodeficiency diseases. *J Clin Immunol,* 2006. 26(3): p. 265-273.

[62] Fasth A, Nystrom J. Safety and efficacy of subcutaneous human immunoglobulin in children with primary immunodeficiency. *Acta Paediatr,* 2007. 96(10): p. 1474-1478.

[63] Gustafson R, Gardulf A, Hansen S, Leibl H, Engl W, Linden M, Muller A, Hammarstrom L, Rapid subcutaneous immunoglobulin administration every second week results in high and stable serum immunoglobulin G levels in patients with primary antibody deficiencies. *Clin Exp Immunol,* 2008. 152(2): p. 274-279.

[64] Gardulf A, Nicolay U, Asensio O, Bernatowska E, Bock A, Carvalho BC, Granert C, Haag S, Hernandez D, Kiessling P, Kus J, Pons J, Niehues T, Schmidt S, Schulze I, Borte M. Rapid subcutaneous IgG replacement therapy is effective and safe in children and adults with primary immunodeficiencies--a prospective, multi-national study. *J Clin Immunol,* 2006. 26(2): p. 177-185.

[65] Skoda-Smith S, Torgerson TR, Ochs HD, Subcutaneous immunoglobulin replacement therapy in the treatment of patients with primary immunodeficiency disease. *Ther Clin Risk Manag.* 2010. 6: p. 1-10.

[66] Berger M, Rojavin M, Kiessling P, Zenker O. Pharmacokinetics of subcutaneous immunoglobulin and their use in dosing of replacement therapy in patients with primary immunodeficiencies. *Clin Immunol.*2011. 139(2): p. 133-141.

[67] Haddad E, Berger M, Wang EC, Jones CA, Bexon M, Baggish JS. Higher doses of subcutaneous IgG reduce resource utilization in patients with primary immunodeficiency. *J Clin Immunol.*2012. 32(2): p. 281-289.

[68] Membe SK, Ho C, Cimon K, Morrison A, Kanani A, Roifman CM. Economic assessment of different modalities of immunoglobulin replacement therapy. *Immunol Allergy Clin North Am,* 2008. 28(4): p. 861-874, x.

[69] Gardulf A, Borte M, Ochs HD, Nicolay U. Prognostic factors for health-related quality of life in adults and children with primary antibody deficiencies receiving SCIG home therapy. *Clin Immunol*, 2008. 126(1): p. 81-88.

Chapter 2

Stem Cell Transplantation for Primary Immunodeficiency

Mary A. Slatter and Andrew R. Gennery

Additional information is available at the end of the chapter

1. Introduction

In 1968, hematopoietic stem cell transplantation (HSCT) was first performed for patients with inherited cellular immunodeficiencies: a child with severe combined immune deficiency (SCID) and another with Wiskott–Aldrich syndrome (WAS) transplanted from matched siblings [1, 2]. Since then, HSCT techniques have advanced enormously due to refined HLA-tissue typing, the increased use of alternative donors, the availability of new stem cell sources including umbilical cord blood as well as less toxic chemotherapeutic conditioning [3], and graft-versus host disease (GVHD) prophylaxis. Supportive care has also improved, with molecular detection of viral infection enabling pre-emptive antiviral treatment before organ damage supervenes [4]. Greater awareness of primary immunodeficiency (PID) amongst general paediatricians, highlighted by campaigns promoting warning signs has lead to earlier diagnosis and referral to specialist centres[5]. Indications for HSCT increase as advances in molecular immunology better define PIDs while parallel studies of the natural history of PIDs reveal which will benefit most from early HSCT before organ damage is present[6]. There are now nearly 200 molecularly defined PIDs. HSCT aims to give stable donor stem cell engraftment after partial or full ablation of the recipient's marrow and immune system using a combination of chemotherapy, antibody therapy, and a graft-versus-marrow effect. [7] Nearly 1,500 children in Europe who have received allogeneic HSCT for PIDs[8] were reported recently, as well as over 1,000 children from Northern America in 2008.[9] Overall survival has increased to 90% for SCID babies with a genoidentical donor and nearly 70% for those given matched unrelated donor (URD) HSCT. For non-SCID PIDs, the survival for both genoidentical and URD HSCT is between 70% and 80%.[8] Together with improved survival advances have led, and continue to focus on, improved quality of life longterm.

2. Who, when, what to transplant

SCID is one of the most severe forms of PID. Early diagnosis and management are essential and HSCT is curative. For other forms of PID, management and in particular the indications for HSCT are evolving. New data is emerging on the natural history of patients with diseases such as CGD and CD40L deficiency and the outcome from HSCT has improved dramatically and so the risks of performing HSCT at a young age before organ damage from recurrent infection and inflammation need to be carefully assessed and discussed with families balanced against a potentially shortened life span with poor quality of life due to multiple hospital admissions.

Table 1 gives a current list of primary immunodeficiency diseases in which HSCT is indicated.

2.1. Importance of molecular diagnosis

Precise molecular diagnosis is very helpful as prognosis can then be accurately assessed. The outcome following HSCT for patients with B negative forms of SCID such as RAG deficiency is less good than for those with B positive forms. Furthermore those with artemis deficiency have a worse prognosis than those with RAG deficiency because of the associated cellular radiosensitivity. In the long term post HSCT human papilloma virus warts predominantly occur in patients with common gamma chain or JAK3 deficient SCID[10], but not other SCID genotypes.

Ill-defined combined immunodeficiencies (CID) are a challenge to treat, as the outcome with HSCT is variable, and often poor[8]. This is because, at least in part, decisions about when to transplant are not made until a disease-defining illness has occurred (Table 2), which may leave significant organ damage or a persisting viral burden, which alters the prognosis following transplantation. Identification of a specific gene defect in a patient cohort can alter management decisions. For example, clear molecular definition has changed the management of an autosomal recessive form of hyper IgE syndrome caused by mutations in the dedicator of the cytokinesis 8 (DOCK8) gene. Previously this disease was managed conservatively, as a form of hyper IgE syndrome. Accurate molecular definition enabled data to be gathered on a patient cohort leading to the realisation that there is a high risk of infection, skin malignancy and death. Reports of cases being successfully transplanted have lead to HSCT becoming the treatment of choice for this diagnosis.[11-15]

Reticular dysgenesis is an autosomal recessive form of SCID characterised by an early differentiation arrest in myeloid lineage and impaired lymphoid maturation. Affected individuals also have bilateral sensorineural deafness. Mutations in AK2 (adenylate kinase 2) published in 2008 demonstrated that AK2 is expressed in the stria vascularis region of the inner ear providing an explanation for the deafness in addition to it's role in specific haematopoietic lineages. Again this can lead to an earlier specific diagnosis and appropriate intervention.[16]

Severe combined immunodeficiency	Cytokine signalling	CγC JAK 3 IL7 Rα
	Nucleotide biosynthesis salvage pathway defects	ADA deficiency
	Defects affecting signalling through the T cell antigen receptor	CD45 CD3δ CD3ε CD3ζ
	VDJ recombination defects	RAG 1 & 2 Artemis Cernunnos DNA Ligase 4 DNA PK
	Other	AK2 deficiency (RD) ORAI1 STIM1
T cell immunodeficiency	CD4 lymphopenia Zap 70 kinase deficiency MHC class II deficiency PNP deficiency Omenn's syndrome CD40 ligand deficiency Wiskott Aldrich syndrome X-Linked lymphoproliferative disease MHC Class I deficiency Combined Immune Deficiency with skeletal dysplasia Cartilage hair hypoplasia Severe Di George syndrome (22q 11 del)* CHARGE association* Undefined	
Phagocytic cell disorders	Familial Hemophagocytic lymphohistiocytosis Griscelli disease Immunodeficiency with partial albinism Interferon-γ receptor deficiency Kostmann disease ** Shwachman-Diamond syndrome ** Leucocyte Adhesion Defect XL and AR Chronic Granulomatous Disease Chediak-Higashi syndrome Undefined	
Severe Immune dysregulation	Autoimmune lymphoproliferative syndrome (homozygotes) ** IPEX syndrome	

Abbreviations: CγC Common gamma chain, XL X linked, Jak 3 Janus associated kinase 3, AR Autosomal recessive, ADA Adenosine deaminase, RAG Recombinant activating gene, MHC Major histocompatibility, PNP Purine nucleoside phosphorylase, IPEX Immunodeficiency polyendocrinopathy enteropathy X linked, CHARGE coloboma, heart anomalies, choanal atresia, retardation of growth and development, and genital and ear anomalies due to CHD7 gene mutations.

*Thymic transplant recommended in preference to HSCT

**Not all require HSCT

Table 1. Indications for HSCT in immunodeficiencies

2.2. Severe combined immunodeficiency

Severe combined immunodeficiency is usually fatal by 1 year of age unless an infant receives a new immune system and should be considered a paediatric emergency which is immediately life threatening. In the most recent analysis of 699 SCID patients transplanted across Europe there was a survival of 90% for those transplanted with a genoidentical sibling donor and nearly 70% for those receiving a matched unrelated donor[8]. The outcome for those without pre-existing infection such as those diagnosed at birth is even better: in the UK series the survival for those transplanted having being diagnosed at or before birth was 91.5% compared to 61% for those transplanted having being diagnosed at a median age of 143 days and a significant number of these children died from infection before reaching transplant[5]. These data support neonatal screening programmes, which are being introduced in North America, and pick up patients with SCID in the newborn period, before infection supervenes[17]. Similar screening programmes are being considered in Europe. Recognition of the specific molecular defect may alter the approach to HSCT. Patients with adenosine deaminase-deficient SCID will develop adequate immunological reconstitution following an unconditioned infusion from HLA-identical sibling stem cells[18], whereas those with RAG-deficient SCID will require chemotherapy conditioning to achieve stem cell engraftment and immunological reconstitution.

2.3. Other primary immunodeficiencies

For other non-SCID PID, debate continues about the optimum age for transplantation. As registry data for specific diseases becomes available, the role of HSCT is increasingly clear, but the optimum age for transplantation remains to be determined. Earlier transplantation is favoured for T cell immunodeficiencies.

Filipovich et al published results of 170 transplants for Wiskott Aldrich syndrome and demonstrated that boys receiving an unrelated donor transplant before the age of 5 had as high a survival rate to matched sibling donor recipients of any age[19]. A recent international report of 194 patients with Wiskott Aldrich syndrome, transplanted in 12 centers, reported an overall survival of 84%, rising to 89% for those transplanted since the year 2000. Younger age and milder clinical phenotype was associated with better outcome[20]. Whilst survival has improved over the last decade, young age at transplant before complications of the underlying disease supervene, also improves outcome.[21]

The outcome of patients transplanted for CD40 ligand deficiency is also dependent on age at transplantation, with pre-existing lung disease being a significant factor in predicting survival[22, 23]. Thirty eight children were reported who were transplanted in Europe for CD40L between 1993 and 2002. Of the 34 engrafted, 26 survived (68%), and 20 no longer required immunoglobulin replacement therapy. This survival and cure rate was little better than the survival of non-transplanted patients at the age of 20 years. However, many patients in this series were over 10 years of age when transplanted and already had significant lung and/or liver damage. A total of 14 patients with CD40L deficiency have been transplanted in our centre: 2 received MSD and 10 URD; 4 died (overall survival 71%), but none since the year 2000, and 3 out of the 4 deaths were in children over 12 years of age who already had sclerosing cholangitis. All the survivors express CD40L and only one needs immunoglobulin. These data further emphasize the importance of early age at transplant before organ damage supervenes.

For non-T cell immunodeficiencies, timing of transplantation has been more controversial, although with registry data becoming available, the natural history of disease on conventional treatment is becoming more clear. Lifelong antibacterial and antifungal prophylaxis with cotrimoxazole and itraconazole has improved short- and medium-term survival for patients with chronic granulomatous disease. However, although steroids and aminosalicylates ameliorate colitis and other inflammatory complications they do not cure the underlying genetic defect and longterm immunosuppression is required to maintain symptom control. Quality of life is poor with frequent hospital admissions and poor growth. Even with the best prophylactic treatment, only 50% of patients are alive at 30 years[6] (Figure 1). HSCT can cure CGD with resolution of infection and colitis but was previously considered to be a high risk procedure. A European multicenter experience of replete marrow HSCT with mainly matched sibling donor stem cells following myeloablative conditioning gave good results; 23/27 patients survived, 22 were cured (81%), with deaths confined to high-risk patients with active fungal infection[24]. A more recent single centre study demonstrated similar outcomes with either matched sibling or matched unrelated donors, with a survival and cure of 90% and low incidence of significant GvHD. Mean weight and height for age Z scores on recovery from HSCT rose significantly. Transplant-associated complications were restricted to those with pre-existing infection or inflammation, supporting the argument for early HSCT for all CGD patients with a well matched donor[25]. As transplantation techniques improve, and survival increases, earlier transplantation becomes a more attractive option for other primary immunodeficiencies requiring long term antimicrobials and immunosuppression to control symptoms.

2.4. Donor choice and degree of HLA matching

Unlike patients with haematological malignancy in whom a graft versus leukaemia effect is desirable, GVHD confers no benefit to patients with PID. The best HLA matched donor is a sibling and so any siblings of the patient should be tissue typed. Many PID patients come from consanguineous families and so it may be possible to find a donor from the extended family. When tissue typing reveals more than one possible donor, other factors such as age, sex, parity, blood group and cytomegalovirus (CMV) status are taken into consideration. If no family donor is found a search of the National and International unrelated donor registries should be undertaken. There are currently 19 million adult and over 500,000 cord blood donors that can be accessed through the Bone Marrow Donors Worldwide registry (www.bmdw.org).

3. Stem cell source

Bone marrow has been the traditional source of stem cells and is harvested under general anaesthetic from the posterior iliac crests. Adult donors are increasingly being offered the option of donating peripheral blood stem cells (PBSC) rather than bone marrow. This may be especially useful for donors who may have a medical condition of their own that would increase the risks of general anaesthesia. PBSC collection is generally carried out as a day case procedure and some donors find this prospect less difficult than the short period of hospitalisation and general anaesthetic needed for bone marrow donation. However, PBSC will require the donor to receive a short course of injections of granulocyte-colony stimulating factor (G-CSF) prior to commencing the first collection. Typically G-CSF at 10 micrograms per kilogram is given daily for 5 days before 1-2 leukapheresis procedures are performed. This procedure is not licensed in children in most countries and so sibling donations from children continue to be bone marrow.

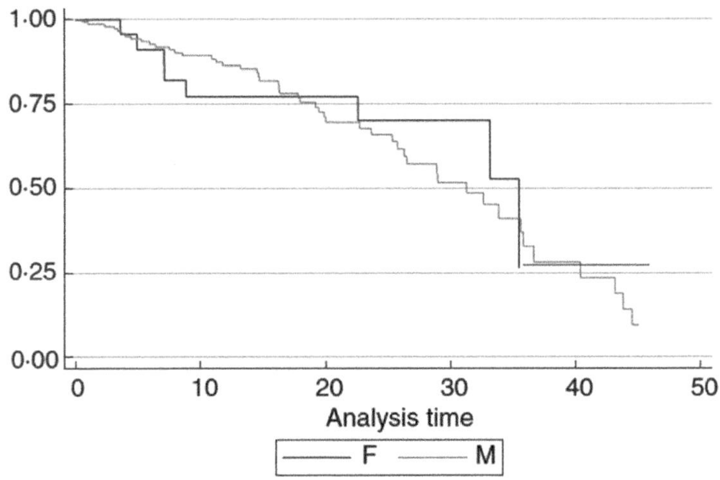

(Permission granted from Jones, *et al*[6]. Copyright by John Wiley and Sons, Ltd.)

Figure 1. Kaplan–Meier survival estimates, by sex for UK patients with chronic granulomatous disease.

Umbilical cord blood stem cell transplantation (UCSCT) offers a stem cell source when a matched sibling donor is unavailable.

Advantages of UCSCT include

i. quick access to the cord blood unit and ease of arranging date of transplant
ii. absence of risk to donor
iii. lower risk of latent viral transmission and graft versus host disease (GvHD)
iv. higher chance of matching rare HLA haplotypes.

Additionally, the HSC telomere length is longer in patients who have received UCSC than in those who have received PBSC from older donors. UCSCs may have greater self renewing capacity and longevity than those derived from an adult donor. As many transplanted PID patients are infants or young children, giving HSC with a greater proliferative life span is theoretically more attractive.

Disadvantages of UCSCT include

i. low stem cell dose, particularly for an older child,
ii. Lack of availability of the donor should any boost procedure be required
iii. Cord blood units are virologically naïve and have been reported to have slower engraftment which increases the risks from pre-existing infections.

However, the conditioning regimen employed may influence this, as omission of serotherapy enables viral clearance, albeit with an increased risk of GvHD[26].

For PID patients who often present before 1 year of age, UCSCT can offer a suitable stem cell source. In a recent European study mismatched-related donor HSCT was compared to unrelated donor cord HSCT in children with severe T cell deficiencies. There was no significant difference in survival, but cord blood recipients had a higher frequency of complete donor chimerism at day 100 and faster total lymphocyte recovery.[27]

4. Assessment of donor

A Physician or Paediatrician who is independent to that of the recipient should perform a pre-transplant assessment of any family donor. A medical history should be taken including:

- Vaccination history
- blood transfusion history
- allergy history
- history of travel to tropical countries
- number of pregnancies in women

A routine physical examination is performed and a chest radiograph and ECG if indicated.

For unrelated donors the examination is performed by the donor assessment centre. However the transplant centre will need to request blood for confirmatory tissue typing, DNA analysis for post transplant chimerism studies and the opportunity is usually taken to check the donor virology and serology status. The donor's fitness to donate must be ascertained before conditioning of the patient begins. The donor centre is responsible for the consent of the donor. The donor needs to be fully informed about the procedure for collecting the stem cells, the blood tests that will be performed including HIV status, the possibility of a second donation for the same patient and the emphasis on anonymity for the donor and patient. Anonymity may be relaxed in time and regulations may vary in different countries.

For related donors in the UK in addition to a physical examination, under the Human Tissue Act 2004, any potential donation of bone marrow or PBSC from adults who lack capacity to consent and children who lack competence to consent, must be assessed by an Accredited Assessor and a report submitted to the Human Tissue Authority for consideration.

Psychological aspects for the donor are important particularly when children are donating for siblings, for example if the recipient does not survive the donor may feel it is their fault. Therefore preparation and counselling for the donor is important

For cord blood donations at the time of cord collection tests for the following are performed on the mother:

The current minimum serology testing requirements for these products are summarised below:

Anti-HIV-1,2
HBsAg
Anti HBc (hepatitis B core antibody)
Anti-HCV-Ab (anti-hepatitis C antibody)
A validated testing algorithm to exclude the presence of syphilis/active infection
with Treponema pallidum (Anti-T. pallidum)
HTLV-I antibody testing for maternal donors living in, or originating from, high-incidence areas or with sexual partners originating from those areas, or where the donor's parents originate from those areas.

Furthermore, if the cord blood unit has been stored for more than 180 days the additional testing is required:

Nucleic acid testing for HIV (HIV-NAT)
Nucleic acid testing for hepatitis B (HBV-NAT)
Nucleic acid testing for hepatitis C (HCV-NAT)
Nucleic acid testing for HTLV-I (HTLV-I-NAT) of maternal donors living in, or originating from, high-incidence areas or with sexual partners originating from those areas, or where the donor's parents originate from those areas.

Confirmatory tests 3 to 6 months after delivery are also performed. The health of the baby is also assessed. Cord blood banks will supply the transplant centre with the required viral status of the mother and sometimes the cord blood itself. The cell doses contained within the cord donation and cell viability are also recorded. They will also perform extra tests for confirmatory tissue typing and virology and serology on small aliquots of the cord. Some centres may wish to perform their own confirmatory typing. A small sample is usually taken at the time of thawing for DNA analysis for post transplant chimerism studies.

5. Preparation of patient

The clinical condition of patients undergoing stem cell transplantation varies enormously depending on diagnosis, age, previous treatment, and organ damage. Once the decision to transplant has been made and a donor selected each organ system should be assessed so that any organ damage is known about prior to transplant and therefore potential harmful effects of chemotherapy, risks for GVHD and recurrence of infections can be anticipated. A full medical history should be taken and a physical examination performed. It is useful to perform the assessment at least 6 weeks before the transplant date in order that any necessary investigations can be arranged. A checklist is essential (Figure 2). It is helpful to perform microbiology screening for resistant bacteria e.g. methicillin resistant staphylococcus aureus (MRSA) and glycopeptide resistant enterococci (GRE/VRE). This will depend on unit policy.

Name of patient	MRN	D.O.B.
Description	**Date**	**Initials**
Full blood count		
Coagulation Screen		
Blood group		
Tissue typing		
DCT, Isohaemagglutinins		
U & E's, LFT's, Bone profile, Glucose		
Thyroid function tests		
Immunoglobulins (+Ig Subclasses)		
Specific antibodies (as appropriate)		
Lymphocyte subsets		
Proliferations		
Viral serology (CMV, EBV, Hep B & C, VZV, HSV, Measles, Toxoplasma, Treponema, HIV 1&2)		
Viral PCRs (CMV, HHV6, EBV, Adenovirus)		
DNA genetic markers		
Amino glycoside Study		
Other blood tests		
Referral for sperm donation (if applicable) **date:**		
Stool samples (C and S, Virology)		
Urine (C and S, +/- Virology)		
Nose /Throat Swab/NPA		
Chest X-ray		
Lung Function		
Ultrasound abdomen		
Echocardiogram		
Dental check		
Audiology		
Medical photography		
Height **Weight**		

With permission from Kath Grey. Liaison team nursing sister. Great North Children's Hospital, Newcastle upon Tyne

Figure 2. Checklist for patients requiring an immunology assessment for HSCT

A number of infectious agents, particularly viruses, can now be detected by sensitive molecular techniques such as polymerase chain reaction (PCR) at an early stage of the infectious process. This in turn means that pre-emptive therapy can be given before organ damage such as life threatening pneumonitis or hepatitis, occurs. Such early detection together with treatments such as cidofovir for Adenovirus has led to a dramatic improvement in outcome following viral infection.

Many children with PID fail to thrive and are malnourished and it is important to maximise nutritional status prior to transplant, which may mean high calorie enteral feeding via nasogastric tube or parenteral nutrition through a central venous catheter.

Some diseases such as IPEX syndrome require immunosuppression to control autoimmune enteropathy and it is important to suppress any active inflammation prior to transplant, but also to minimise immunosuppression in order to reduce risk of infection.

Familial haemophagocytic lymphohistiocytosis is a genetically determined disorder characterized by the early onset of fever, hepatosplenomegaly, central nervous system disease, thrombocytopenia, coagulation disorders, and haemophagocytosis. It is caused by genetic defects that impair T cell–mediated and natural cytotoxicity. Chemotherapy and/or immunotherapy-based treatments can achieve remission, but HSCT is the only curative option. Outcome of HSCT is much more favourable if active disease is controlled prior to transplantation[28].

Sometimes a combination of antimicrobials and immunosuppression may be the optimal treatment. For example, Leiding et al have described 9 cases of severe life threatening liver abscesses in patients with CGD that progressed despite appropriate antibacterial therapy and drainage but responded to moderately high doses of corticosteroids tapered over several months.[29]

It is essential to address family and psychosocial issues and so each patient should be referred to a social worker and psychologist. Each unit will have their own system for information giving including written information about the transplant procedure, a visit to the unit and a home visit. It may be appropriate for patients to meet the dietician and physiotherapist prior to transplant. Fertility issues need to be discussed. In particular sperm banking should be arranged if appropriate. It is vital that written consent is taken once the patient/family are fully aware of all the aspects of the transplant.

6. Conditioning

Conditioning aims to create space in the recipient marrow niche to enable donor stem cells to engraft more easily. A range of conditioning regimens are available from non conditioning, through immunosuppressive regimens to myeloablative combinations (Figure 3).

For many years, myeloablative chemotherapy with busulphan and cyclophosphamide was given prior to HSCT for PIDs. However, busulphan is associated with significant toxicity including veno-occlusive disease (VOD). A strong correlation between blood levels of cyclophosphamide metabolites and VOD has previously been shown due to depletion of glutathione from the liver[30]. Combinations of cyclophosphamide with reduced-dose busulphan may also lead to severe hepatic toxicity and VOD [31, 32]. The combination of fludarabine and full dose busulfan has gradually replaced the combination of busulfan and cyclophosphamide in most centres. Malar et al. have recently reported on the importance of therapeutic drug monitoring for intravenous busulphan therapy in 34 paediatric patients. Seven children all weighing less than 12 kg had VOD despite not exceeding the targeted area under the curve: six of them had AUCs below the target range, highlighting the difficulty in giving busulphan to this young group of children despite careful therapeutic monitoring.[33]

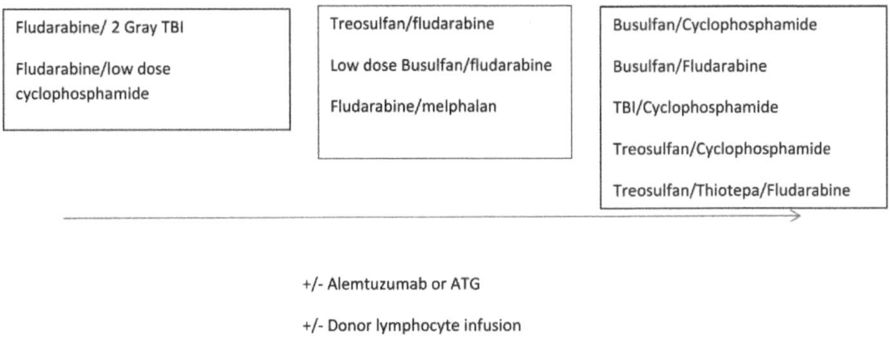

Figure 3. Chemotherapy regimens, increasing in intensity from left to right

Reduced-intensity conditioning regimens using drugs such as fludarabine and melphalan have diminished treatment-related toxicity in some PID patients,[3] but toxicity remains a problem for children under one year of age,[34] and cardiac toxicity is associated with melphalan[35]. Minimal-intensity conditioning with fludarabine and low dose cyclophosphamide can reduce toxicity even further, but may be associated with poor donor myeloid chimerism or an increased incidence of GVHD.[36] Consequently, new conditioning regimens for PIDs have been developed that give adequate myeloablation but less toxicity, particularly in patients under one year of age. Treosulfan (l-treitol-1, 4-bis-methanesulfonate) is the pro-drug of l-epoxybutane, a water-soluble bifunctional alkylating agent with myeloablative and immunosuppressive properties,[37] and is effective in HSCT conditioning with less toxicity, particularly in VOD, compared to busulphan. A recent study of 70 children in the UK, transplanted for various PIDs and given treosulfan with either fludarabine or cyclophosphamide, showed an overall survival of 81%. Of 46 children less than 12 months of age at HSCT, only eight died (overall survival 83%). Two children had VOD when treosulfan was given in combination with cyclophosphamide, but none when it was given with fludarabine. In the treosulfan cohort, there was no cardiactoxicity, such as seen with melphalan or pulmonary fibrosis as seen with busulphan[38-40]. T cell chimerism was significantly better when treosulfan was given in combination with fludarabine, and although numbers were small, there was a suggestion that chimerism was better when PBSCs were used as the stem source. Conversely, patients receiving cord blood stem cells in conjunction with serotherapy had a tendency to more mixed donor chimerism. While donor myeloid chimerism was sufficiently high to cure most patients with CGD and WAS with all donor types/stem cell sources, where 100% donor chimerism might be preferred in all cell lineages—for example, WAS[20] — then the use of PBSCs or full myeloablation with busulphan might be required. Early results using PBSCs with treosulfan and fludarabine look promising in terms of good chimerism without an increased incidence of greater than grade II GVHD. Prospective studies are needed comparing treosulfan/ fludarabine with busulphan and fludarabine,[41-43] where early reports also indicate reduced transplant-related toxicities and excellent survival. Long-term follow-up is needed to see if this "modified intensity" regimen results in less long-term toxicity and, in particular, infertility, as the gonadal toxicity of busulphan is already well documented[44]. Radioimmunotherapy, in which targeted irradiation of the bone marrow is achieved by using radiolabeled monoclonal antibodies, may be used as a potent myeloablative agent with low intrinsic organ toxicity. Schulz et al. recently reported on the use of radioimmunotherapy with 90Y-anti-CD66 for conditioning in 30 pediatric patients undergoing HSCT, including 16 with non-malignant disorders with high co-morbidities. Patients received radioimmunotherapy with fludarabine or melphalan alone or in combination, usually with ATG; one patient was given radioimmunotherapy alone. A highly favorable ratio of marrow dose to other organ dose was demonstrated, and stable engraftment was achieved with complete donor chimerism in 13 out of 16 (81%) patients. One patient with Griscelli syndrome and who had secondary graft failure after the first HLA haploidentical transplantation achieved stable complete donor chimerism with radioimmunotherapy alone[45].

Antibodies to eliminate host stem cells prior to transplantation could mean that toxic conditioning regimens would not be needed. Administration of ACK2 and an antibody that blocks c-Kit function led to transient removal of >98% of endogenous HSCs in immune-deficient mice[46]. Subsequent transplantation with donor HSCs led to chimerism levels up to 90% compared to only 3% in those without this preconditioning. The pharmacological agent AMD3100, which is a CXCR4 inhibitor, has been shown to induce egress of HSCs out of the marrow and improve levels of donor HSC engraftment relative to untreated recipients[47]. Plerixafor, a CXCR4 inhibitor, may also be a more effective mobilizer of stem cells for donors of PBSCs than granulocyte colony stimulating factor (G-CSF), allowing larger doses of stem cells to be administered, which may lead to more rapid engraftment.

7. Methods of T cell depletion

In 1981 the introduction of T lymphocyte depletion to remove of alloreactive lymphocytes from the bone marrow source enabled transplantation across HLA barriers. This meant that patients without an HLA-identical donor could receive T lymphocyte depleted marrow from an HLA-haploidentical parent.

Profound T-cell depletion is a fundamental prerequisite for haploidentical donor transplantation to avoid severe GVHD and B cell depletion lessens the risk of Epstein Barr Virus (EBV)-related lymphoproliferative disease. Various methods have been used to remove viable T lymphocytes from the graft, including E-rosette lectin depletion and in vitro anti CD52 (CAMPATH-1M anti-lymphocyte antibody which is no longer available). Since the late 1990s European centers performing T lymphocyte–depleted HSCT for patients with PID have used CD34+ stem cell selection rather than T-lymphocyte depletion. The most commonly used method, the Miltenyi Clini-MACS system, uses an organic iron bead attached to an anti-CD34 antibody to isolate purified CD34+ HSCs from the other cells by passing the HSC source through a magnetic column[48]. The purified CD34+ HSC fraction is infused into the patient. By using this method, 4 log depletions of T-lymphocyte numbers can be achieved. There are important differences between CD34+ stem cell–selected and T lymphocyte–depleted bone marrow. Although the residual T-lymphocyte count in anti-CD52–treated marrow can be relatively high, very few of the T lymphocytes remain viable because they are still coated with anti-CD52 when infused into the recipient and are then destroyed by complement-mediated lysis. In the anti-CD34 selected HSC product, although the number of T lymphocytes infused into the patient might be very low, those that are infused are viable and could cause GvHD. The anti-CD52– treated product contains component blood cell precursors and cells already in early differentiation from the stem cell, as well as other stromal factors that might aid engraftment of HSCs into the bone marrow space thus achieving better engraftment.

An alternative means of stem cell enrichment has been used with the aim of achieving an optimal balance between the competing risks of GVHD, poor engraftment and delayed immune reconstitution. By targeting T- and B- cells specifically CD3/CD19 depleted grafts not only retain CD34+ stem cells but also CD34 negative progenitors, natural killer, dendritic and graft-facilitating cells which enhance engraftment.

Further developments are now focusing on the depletion of TcRαβ+ T cells which can prevent GvHD after allogeneic stem cell transplantation from HLA non identical donors and may lead to more rapid immune reconstitution than CD3+ depletion of grafts. In contrast to depletion of CD3+ T cells valuable TcRγδ+ T cells are spared.[49]

8. Results

8.1. Severe combined immunodeficiency

A successful HSCT procedure in patients with primary immunodeficiency should result in a cure of the underlying defect with normal immuno-reconstitution leading to normal immune function and a normal life. The likelihood of a successful outcome depends on the underlying diagnosis, degree of HLA matching from the donor, and pre existing end organ damage. Overall the outcome for patients with SCID is better than that for patients with other PID and has improved over time[8]. The likelihood of cure following HSCT is up to 90% in those SCID patients with a genoidentical donor. Even for those with no HLA identical donor, survival following a T cell depleted haploidentical transplant is approaching 60%. Whilst infusion of the stem cell product without the use of chemotherapy eliminates the potentially fatal effects of conditioning including infection from aplasia and increased risk of pneumonitis and mucositis, the quality of engraftment is compromised. Thus for patients with common gamma chain or JAK3 SCID thymopoiesis may be achieved as T cell precursors engraft in the thymus[50], but B cell engraftment is unlikely and patients will remain on lifelong immunoglobulin replacement as recipient B cells are unable to produce IgM through the IL 21 mediated signalling path and do not undergo immunoglobulin class switching.[51] Patients thus remain at risk of bronchiectasis in the long term. However, for patients with VDJ recombination defects leading to T- B-NK+ SCID, stem cell infusion will lead to no B cell engraftment and only peripheral T cell engraftment with poor T cell numbers, no thymopoiesis and risk of immunosenescence in the medium term.[52]. So, although conditioning may increase the short term risks, immune function is better in the long term following chemotherapy. Full donor chimerism is not necessary as stable mixed donor chimerism may give adequate immune reconstitution. Best results are achieved in patients diagnosed early with no infection and no end organ damage. Newborn transplantation gives the best results of all[5, 53, 54], giving weight to the argument for newborn screening by detection of T cell receptor excision circles (TRECS) on the neonatal blood spot (Guthrie) card and thus detection of SCID before presentation with a SCID defining illness such as pneumocystis pneumonitis (Table 2).

Common Presentations	Rare Presentations
Persistent or recurrent viral gastroenteritis	**Bacterial septicaemia**
	Disseminated BCG infection
Persistent or recurrent viral lower respiratory tract infection	**Haemophagocytosis**
***Pneumocystis jiroveci* pneumonitis**	**Lymphoid malignancy**
Recurrent or recalcitrant candidiasis	**Autoimmune cytopenias**
Fungal abscess	**Maternofetal GvHD**
Recurrent bacterial lymphadenitis	
Persistant cutaneous human papillomavirus warts	
Persistant molluscum contagiosum	

Table 2. Disease defining illness in Primary Immunodeficiency

For those patients presenting late with infection, graft manipulation such as new methods of T cell depletion and add back of virus specific cytotoxic T cells has enabled more rapid immunoreconstitution and viral clearance[55]. For those patients requiring additional support through the transplant period, improvement in paediatric intensive care, close liaison between BMT and PICU teams, and earlier interventions are leading to improved outcomes of patients receiving HSCT but needing to go to PICU. Survival rates are now approaching up to 60%, better survival for those who receive only invasive ventilation and worse survival for those with multi organ failure[56].

8.2. Other primary immunodeficiencies

The results of transplant for other primary immunodeficiencies are historically not so good as those for patients with SCID but are improving over time[8]. This is likely due to a number of factors. Foremost is the adoption of stem cell transplant as a recognised therapy for the underlying condition. As transplant becomes an accepted treatment for a specific condition, patients with end organ disease undergo transplant, and some do not survive. Secondly, patients will need to undergo conditioning chemotherapy in order to prevent rejection of the graft and achieve donor chimerism and are therefore subject to the toxicities associated with conditioning. Thirdly, is the question of the optimum time to perform transplantation. Severe combined immunodeficiencies are usually fatal within the first 18 months of life, patients with other primary immunodeficiencies live longer and can survive into adulthood, albeit with a deteriorating quality of life as they accumulate end organ damage secondary to infection and inflammatory complications of the underlying disease. Registry data has provided good quality information about long term prognosis for some of these disorders, even when appropriate antimicrobial prophylaxis is available, enabling parents, patients and physicians to make informed choices about timing of transplantation[6, 11, 57]. Most non-SCID PIDs are life limiting in the medium to long term, rather than fatal in the first few months of life. As with SCID, results of transplant are better if patients are transplanted whilst younger, without end organ damage. For those with XLP, survival from transplant is significantly better for patients who do not experience haemophagocytic lymphohistiocytosis[58]. In a similar fashion, for patients with chronic granulomatous disease, outcome is better in those that have not had significant fungal infection or inflammatory sequalae[24]. Thus transplantation at an early age before onset of complications gives the best chance of survival and cure but some families may prefer not to put a healthy child through transplant, rather monitoring them closely for significant deterioration and transplant at the first sign of trouble. It is advisable that searches for an appropriate donor are made soon after diagnosis so that transplantation can proceed quickly once the decision to transplant has been made.

The amount of chimerism required to achieve cure depends on the underlying disease. Patients with CD40 ligand require only good T cell donor chimerism which will enable immunoglobulin class switching, whereas Wiskott Aldrich Syndrome patients with incomplete donor chimerism are much more likely to develop auto immune complications[20]. The cell lineage in which donor chimerism is required may not be obvious. A patient with IPEX syndrome was cured although T cells appeared to be recipient, because on detailed study, the only donor cells were found to be the FOXP3+ cells[59], required to cure the condition. On the other hand, donor B cells are required in CgC or JAK-3 deficient SCID to achieve independence from immunoglobulin substitution[51, 60], but recipient B cells are functional in SCID due to defects in IL7Ra.

9. Complications post HSCT

Complications following transplantation for primary immunodeficiency are similar to those for patients with malignancy. Infection through the transplant period is a risk, particularly when patients are aplastic (Figure 4). Any primary immunodeficiency patients may carry pre-existing infection (particularly viral infection) into transplant, as the underlying condition means that they are unable to clear infections effectively. Careful assessment of

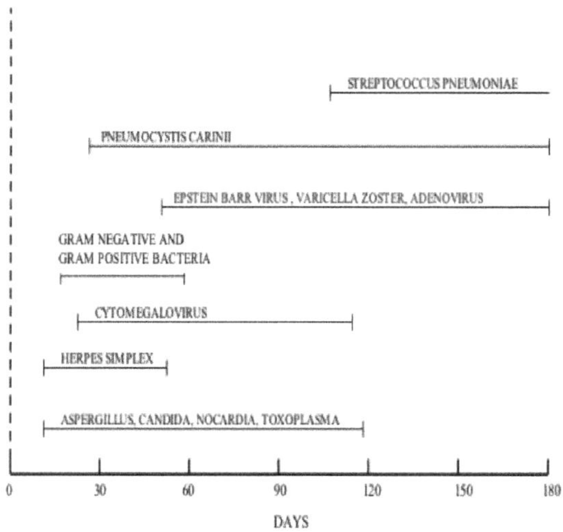

Figure 4.

pre-existing infection needs to be made pre-transplant so that treatment can be optimised as patients begin transplant to reduce the risk of infectious complications. Pneumonitis, particularly at engraftment is a risk, especially in those with pre-existing viral pneumonitis at time of transplantation[61]. Nebulised steroids may improve the outcome in these patients. Acute and chronic graft versus host disease may be significant complications in primary immunodeficiency patients post transplant. Unlike patients with malignancy, graft versus host disease is not encouraged as there is no graft versus leukaemia benefit to be gained. Therefore HLA matching, T cell depletion where appropriate and Graft versus host disease prophylaxis with a calcineurine inhibitor (with or without additional MMF/steroids/Methotrexate) should be utilised. Staging and treatment of established graft versus host disease (Table 3) is as for other transplant patients - methylprednisoline

(2mg/kg) is standard first line treatment. If the patient fails to respond to this, then a variety of other agents may be tried including monoclonal antibodies such as infliximab, alemtuzimab, antithymocyteglobulin, mesenchymal stem cells and extra corporeal phototherapy but none have yet proven to be consistently effective. Veno occlusive disease is a risk factor particularly in those with osteopetrosis, with pre-existing liver disease or under going conditioning with busulphan or cyclophosphamide. Prophylaxis with defibrotide is effective at preventing veno-occlusive disease and treating if necessary[62]. Haemorrhagic cystitis is a rare complication following HSCT, associated with adenovirus or BK virus infection, associated with T cell depletion or prolonged immunosuppression. Treatment is as for patients undergoing HSCT for other indications[63].

Stage	**Skin** **% body surface area**	**Liver** **Bilirubin µmol/l**	**Gut** **Diarrhoea vol. ml/kg/day** (or if >50kg body weight)
1	Maculopapular <25%	34-50	10-19.9 (or 500-1000ml/day)
2	25-50%	51-100	20-30 (or 1000-1500ml/day)
3	Generalised erythema	101-255	>30 (or>1500ml/day)
4	Exfoliation/vesicles	>256	Severe abdo pain +/- ileus

Grade	**Skin stage**	**Liver stage**	**Gut stage**	**Clinical performance**
I	1-2	0	0	normal
II	1-3	1	1	mild decrease
III	2-3	2-3	2-3	marked decrease
IV	2-4	2-4	2-4	incapacitated

Adapted from Jacobsohn DA[69]

Table 3. Staging of acute GVHD

10. Post transplantation immuno-reconstitution

Full immunoreconstitution can take up to 2 years post transplant. Most patients remain on immunoglobulin replacement for around 6 months post transplant or until evidence of immunoglobulin production (gauged by measuring IgM production). Ongoing immunosuppression or graft versus host disease will delay assessment of antibody production. Thymopoiesis can be measured by documenting an increase in recent thymic emigrants measured by TRECS or surrogate markers such as CD27 or CD31 on T cells. Thymopoiesis normally occurs around 120 days post transplant[64]. Graft versus host disease may impair or abrogate this process[65].

Once immunoglobulin production is established, immunoglobulin replacement should be discontinued. After a wash out period of 3 months, primary vaccinations with non-live antigens can begin, having assessed base line specific antibody levels. The response to vaccine antigens can be assessed once the primary vaccination schedule is complete. Vaccination with live vaccines such as MMR should only be considered once normal T cell proliferation has been demonstrated and an antibody response to the primary vaccination schedule has been confirmed. Prophylaxis against polysaccharide coated organisms should be continued for at least 2 years post transplant[66]. Patients should however have received the conjugated pneumococcal and meningococcal vaccines. Once the response to polysaccharide organisms has been demonstrated in those with normal splenic function, antibiotic prophylaxis can be discontinued. Patients should be monitored for evidence of endocrine dysfunction - particularly thyroid dysfunction[67]. Thyroid dysfunction occurs in up to 10% of post transplant patients. Usually this is hypothyroidism but more rarely hyperthyroidism has been described and each should be managed appropriately. In the long term there may be issues with fertility due to the conditioning regimens and patients should be counselled accordingly – referral to fertility clinics or endocrine specialists may be necessary. Growth is usually normal, and growth retardation due to the underlying illness may be reversed post transplant. Ongoing care of previous end organ damage such as bronchiectasis may require specialist input with regular monitoring of lung function and radiological changes. The quality of life post transplant has not been extensively assessed in primary immune deficiency patients. One study looking at the outcome of patients transplanted for severe primary immune deficiency demonstrated an increased risk of long term cognitive difficulties with associated emotional and behavioural difficulties. Specific genetic diagnosis and a severe clinical course were specifically associated with poor outcome[68]. Conversely a recent study looking at patients with CGD found significantly better quality of life skills in those who had undergone transplantation compared to those who were not transplanted, with the post transplant patients score similar to normal controls. As more patients survive the transplant procedure and a longer follow up is achieved further work will be needed in this area to determine quality of life.

11. Future prospects

Transplantation for primary immunodeficiency is a successful treatment leading to cure of disease and normal life quality for the majority of patients. Future work will need to address optimal timing of transplantation, which may be gauged as future registry data becomes available. Less damaging conditioning regimens, particularly for newborns identified with the newborn screening programmes will become important. Treosulfan, fludarabine containing regimens are less toxic than busulphan containing regimens but targeting conditioning using radiotherapy or monoclonal antibodies may play a great role in the future. Accelerating thymopoiesis and immuno-reconstitution will be important particularly when pre-existing viral infection is present. Agents including exogenous interleukin 7 or keratinous growth factor may have a role to play. Graft manipulation may improve outcomes for some patients - better use of T cell depleted donors when no matched donors are available and particularly improving immune reconstitution through TCR alpha beta depletion may be appropriate. Expansion of stem cells in cord blood transplantation, the use of multiple cords or the combined use of haplo-identical stem cells with an umbilical cord blood stem cell unit may also speed of immune reconstitution and lessen the risk from viral infection. Increased use of viral specific cytotoxic T cells will have a role to play. Finally better and more effective treatment of steroid resistant Graft versus host disease is needed and the use of extra corporeal phototherapy, the role of regulatory T cells and of mesenchymal stem cells needs to be explored.

Author details

Mary A. Slatter* and Andrew R. Gennery
The Institute for Cellular Medicine, Newcastle upon Tyne University, Newcastle upon Tyne, UK

12. References

[1] Gatti RA, Meuwissen HJ, Allen HD, Hong R, Good RA. Immunological reconstitution of sex-linked lymphopenic immunological deficiency. Lancet. 1968;2(7583):1366-9. Epub 1968/12/28.
[2] Bach FH, Albertini RJ, Joo P, Anderson JL, Bortin MM. Bone-marrow transplantation in a patient with the Wiskott-Aldrich syndrome. Lancet. 1968;2(7583):1364-6. Epub 1968/12/28.
[3] Rao K, Amrolia PJ, Jones A, Cale CM, Naik P, King D, et al. Improved survival after unrelated donor bone marrow transplantation in children with primary immunodeficiency using a reduced-intensity conditioning regimen. Blood. 2005;105(2):879-85. Epub 2004/09/16.
[4] Lion T, Baumgartinger R, Watzinger F, Matthes-Martin S, Suda M, Preuner S, et al. Molecular monitoring of adenovirus in peripheral blood after allogeneic bone marrow transplantation permits early diagnosis of disseminated disease. Blood. 2003;102(3):1114-20. Epub 2003/04/19.
[5] Brown L, Xu-Bayford J, Allwood Z, Slatter M, Cant A, Davies EG, et al. Neonatal diagnosis of severe combined immunodeficiency leads to significantly improved survival outcome: the case for newborn screening. Blood. 2011;117(11):3243-6. Epub 2011/01/29.
[6] Jones LB, McGrogan P, Flood TJ, Gennery AR, Morton L, Thrasher A, et al. Special article: chronic granulomatous disease in the United Kingdom and Ireland: a comprehensive national patient-based registry. Clinical and experimental immunology. 2008;152(2):211-8. Epub 2008/04/16.
[7] Wynn RF, Boelens JJ. Bone-marrow transplantation in non-malignant disease. Lancet. 2009;374(9693):856-8. Epub 2009/09/05.
[8] Gennery AR, Slatter MA, Grandin L, Taupin P, Cant AJ, Veys P, et al. Transplantation of hematopoietic stem cells and long-term survival for primary immunodeficiencies in Europe: entering a new century, do we do better? The Journal of allergy and clinical immunology. 2010;126(3):602-10 e1-11. Epub 2010/08/03.

* Corresponding Author

[9] Griffith LM, Cowan MJ, Kohn DB, Notarangelo LD, Puck JM, Schultz KR, et al. Allogeneic hematopoietic cell transplantation for primary immune deficiency diseases: current status and critical needs. The Journal of allergy and clinical immunology. 2008;122(6):1087-96. Epub 2008/11/11.

[10] Laffort C, Le Deist F, Favre M, Caillat-Zucman S, Radford-Weiss I, Debre M, et al. Severe cutaneous papillomavirus disease after haemopoietic stem-cell transplantation in patients with severe combined immune deficiency caused by common gammac cytokine receptor subunit or JAK-3 deficiency. Lancet. 2004;363(9426):2051-4. Epub 2004/06/23.

[11] Zhang Q, Davis JC, Lamborn IT, Freeman AF, Jing H, Favreau AJ, et al. Combined immunodeficiency associated with DOCK8 mutations. The New England journal of medicine. 2009;361(21):2046-55. Epub 2009/09/25.

[12] McDonald DR, Massaad MJ, Johnston A, Keles S, Chatila T, Geha RS, et al. Successful engraftment of donor marrow after allogeneic hematopoietic cell transplantation in autosomal-recessive hyper-IgE syndrome caused by dedicator of cytokinesis 8 deficiency. The Journal of allergy and clinical immunology. 2010;126(6):1304-5 e3. Epub 2010/09/03.

[13] Barlogis V, Galambrun C, Chambost H, Lamoureux-Toth S, Petit P, Stephan JL, et al. Successful allogeneic hematopoietic stem cell transplantation for DOCK8 deficiency. The Journal of allergy and clinical immunology. 2011;128(2):420-22 e2. Epub 2011/05/07.

[14] Gatz SA, Benninghoff U, Schutz C, Schulz A, Honig M, Pannicke U, et al. Curative treatment of autosomal-recessive hyper-IgE syndrome by hematopoietic cell transplantation. Bone marrow transplantation. 2011;46(4):552-6. Epub 2010/07/14.

[15] Bittner TC, Pannicke U, Renner ED, Notheis G, Hoffmann F, Belohradsky BH, et al. Successful long-term correction of autosomal recessive hyper-IgE syndrome due to DOCK8 deficiency by hematopoietic stem cell transplantation. Klinische Padiatrie. 2010;222(6):351-5. Epub 2010/11/09.

[16] Lagresle-Peyrou C, Six EM, Picard C, Rieux-Laucat F, Michel V, Ditadi A, et al. Human adenylate kinase 2 deficiency causes a profound hematopoietic defect associated with sensorineural deafness. Nature genetics. 2009;41(1):106-11. Epub 2008/12/02.

[17] Verbsky J, Thakar M, Routes J. The Wisconsin approach to newborn screening for severe combined immunodeficiency. The Journal of allergy and clinical immunology. 2012;129(3):622-7. Epub 2012/01/17.

[18] Hassan A, Booth C, Brightwell A, Veys P, Rao K, Gennery A, Slatter M, Bredius R, Finocchi A, Aiuti A, Porta F, Ridella M, Steward C, Filipovich A, Bordon V, Almuhsen S, Al-Mousa H, Speckmann C, Fischer A, Mahlaoui N, Nichols K, Grunebaum E, Honig M, Friedrich W, Boelens J, Davies EG, Roifman C, Cavazzana-Calvo M, Notarangelo L, Gaspar HB. Outcome of Haematopoietic Stem Cell Transplantation for Adenosine Deaminase Deficient Severe Combined Immunodeficiency. Blood 2012 (in press).

[19] Filipovich AH, Stone JV, Tomany SC, Ireland M, Kollman C, Pelz CJ, et al. Impact of donor type on outcome of bone marrow transplantation for Wiskott-Aldrich syndrome: collaborative study of the International Bone Marrow Transplant Registry and the National Marrow Donor Program. Blood. 2001;97(6):1598-603. Epub 2001/03/10.

[20] Moratto D, Giliani S, Bonfim C, Mazzolari E, Fischer A, Ochs HD, et al. Long-term outcome and lineage-specific chimerism in 194 patients with Wiskott-Aldrich syndrome

treated by hematopoietic cell transplantation in the period 1980-2009: an international collaborative study. Blood. 2011;118(6):1675-84. Epub 2011/06/11.
[21] Shin CR, Kim MO, Li D, Bleesing JJ, Harris R, Mehta P, et al. Outcomes following hematopoietic cell transplantation for Wiskott-Aldrich syndrome. Bone marrow transplantation. 2012. Epub 2012/03/20.
[22] Khawaja K, Gennery AR, Flood TJ, Abinun M, Cant AJ. Bone marrow transplantation for CD40 ligand deficiency: a single centre experience. Archives of disease in childhood. 2001;84(6):508-11. Epub 2001/05/23.
[23] Gennery AR, Khawaja K, Veys P, Bredius RG, Notarangelo LD, Mazzolari E, et al. Treatment of CD40 ligand deficiency by hematopoietic stem cell transplantation: a survey of the European experience, 1993-2002. Blood. 2004;103(3):1152-7. Epub 2003/10/04.
[24] Seger RA, Gungor T, Belohradsky BH, Blanche S, Bordigoni P, Di Bartolomeo P, et al. Treatment of chronic granulomatous disease with myeloablative conditioning and an unmodified hemopoietic allograft: a survey of the European experience, 1985-2000. Blood. 2002;100(13):4344-50. Epub 2002/10/24.
[25] Soncini E, Slatter MA, Jones LB, Hughes S, Hodges S, Flood TJ, et al. Unrelated donor and HLA-identical sibling haematopoietic stem cell transplantation cure chronic granulomatous disease with good long-term outcome and growth. British journal of haematology. 2009;145(1):73-83. Epub 2009/02/19.
[26] Chiesa R, Gilmour K, Qasim W, Adams S, Worth AJ, Zhan H, et al. Omission of in vivo T-cell depletion promotes rapid expansion of naive CD4+ cord blood lymphocytes and restores adaptive immunity within 2 months after unrelated cord blood transplant. British journal of haematology. 2012;156(5):656-66. Epub 2012/01/10.
[27] Fernandes JF, Rocha V, Labopin M, Neven B, Moshous D, Gennery AR, et al. Transplantation in patients with SCID: mismatched related stem cells or unrelated cord blood? Blood. 2012;119(12):2949-55. Epub 2012/02/07.
[28] Ouachee-Chardin M, Elie C, de Saint Basile G, Le Deist F, Mahlaoui N, Picard C, et al. Hematopoietic stem cell transplantation in hemophagocytic lymphohistiocytosis: a single-center report of 48 patients. Pediatrics. 2006;117(4):e743-50. Epub 2006/03/22.
[29] Leiding JW, Freeman AF, Marciano BE, Anderson VL, Uzel G, Malech HL, et al. Corticosteroid therapy for liver abscess in chronic granulomatous disease. Clinical infectious diseases : an official publication of the Infectious Diseases Society of America. 2012;54(5):694-700. Epub 2011/12/14.
[30] McDonald GB, Slattery JT, Bouvier ME, Ren S, Batchelder AL, Kalhorn TF, et al. Cyclophosphamide metabolism, liver toxicity, and mortality following hematopoietic stem cell transplantation. Blood. 2003;101(5):2043-8. Epub 2002/10/31.
[31] Kroger N, Schetelig J, Zabelina T, Kruger W, Renges H, Stute N, et al. A fludarabine-based dose-reduced conditioning regimen followed by allogeneic stem cell transplantation from related or unrelated donors in patients with myelodysplastic syndrome. Bone marrow transplantation. 2001;28(7):643-7. Epub 2001/11/13.
[32] Slavin S, Nagler A, Naparstek E, Kapelushnik Y, Aker M, Cividalli G, et al. Nonmyeloablative stem cell transplantation and cell therapy as an alternative to conventional bone marrow transplantation with lethal cytoreduction for the treatment

of malignant and nonmalignant hematologic diseases. Blood. 1998;91(3):756-63. Epub 1998/02/03.

[33] Malar R, Sjoo F, Rentsch K, Hassan M, Gungor T. Therapeutic drug monitoring is essential for intravenous busulfan therapy in pediatric hematopoietic stem cell recipients. Pediatric transplantation. 2011;15(6):580-8. Epub 2011/07/09.

[34] Straathof KC, Rao K, Eyrich M, Hale G, Bird P, Berrie E, et al. Haemopoietic stem-cell transplantation with antibody-based minimal-intensity conditioning: a phase 1/2 study. Lancet. 2009;374(9693):912-20. Epub 2009/09/05.

[35] Ritchie DS, Seymour JF, Roberts AW, Szer J, Grigg AP. Acute left ventricular failure following melphalan and fludarabine conditioning. Bone marrow transplantation. 2001;28(1):101-3. Epub 2001/08/11.

[36] Burroughs LM, Storb R, Leisenring WM, Pulsipher MA, Loken MR, Torgerson TR, et al. Intensive postgrafting immune suppression combined with nonmyeloablative conditioning for transplantation of HLA-identical hematopoietic cell grafts: results of a pilot study for treatment of primary immunodeficiency disorders. Bone marrow transplantation. 2007;40(7):633-42. Epub 2007/07/31.

[37] Sjoo F, Hassan Z, Abedi-Valugerdi M, Griskevicius L, Nilsson C, Remberger M, et al. Myeloablative and immunosuppressive properties of treosulfan in mice. Experimental hematology. 2006;34(1):115-21. Epub 2006/01/18.

[38] Bacher U, Klyuchnikov E, Wiedemann B, Kroeger N, Zander AR. Safety of conditioning agents for allogeneic haematopoietic transplantation. Expert opinion on drug safety. 2009;8(3):305-15. Epub 2009/06/10.

[39] Akasheh MS, Freytes CO, Vesole DH. Melphalan-associated pulmonary toxicity following high-dose therapy with autologous hematopoietic stem cell transplantation. Bone marrow transplantation. 2000;26(10):1107-9. Epub 2000/12/07.

[40] Bruno B, Souillet G, Bertrand Y, Werck-Gallois MC, So Satta A, Bellon G. Effects of allogeneic bone marrow transplantation on pulmonary function in 80 children in a single paediatric centre. Bone marrow transplantation. 2004;34(2):143-7. Epub 2004/06/01.

[41] Horn B, Baxter-Lowe LA, Englert L, McMillan A, Quinn M, Desantes K, et al. Reduced intensity conditioning using intravenous busulfan, fludarabine and rabbit ATG for children with nonmalignant disorders and CML. Bone marrow transplantation. 2006;37(3):263-9. Epub 2005/12/06.

[42] Jacobsohn DA, Duerst R, Tse W, Kletzel M. Reduced intensity haemopoietic stem-cell transplantation for treatment of non-malignant diseases in children. Lancet. 2004;364(9429):156-62. Epub 2004/07/13.

[43] Seger RA. Modern management of chronic granulomatous disease. British journal of haematology. 2008;140(3):255-66. Epub 2008/01/26.

[44] Slatter MA, Rao K, Amrolia P, Flood T, Abinun M, Hambleton S, et al. Treosulfan-based conditioning regimens for hematopoietic stem cell transplantation in children with primary immunodeficiency: United Kingdom experience. Blood. 2011;117(16):4367-75. Epub 2011/02/18.

[45] Schulz AS, Glatting G, Hoenig M, Schuetz C, Gatz SA, Grewendorf S, et al. Radioimmunotherapy-based conditioning for hematopoietic cell transplantation in

children with malignant and nonmalignant diseases. Blood. 2011;117(17):4642-50. Epub 2011/02/18.

[46] Czechowicz A, Kraft D, Weissman IL, Bhattacharya D. Efficient transplantation via antibody-based clearance of hematopoietic stem cell niches. Science. 2007;318(5854):1296-9. Epub 2007/11/24.

[47] Chen J, Larochelle A, Fricker S, Bridger G, Dunbar CE, Abkowitz JL. Mobilization as a preparative regimen for hematopoietic stem cell transplantation. Blood. 2006;107(9):3764-71. Epub 2006/01/28.

[48] Laurenti L, Sora F, Piccirillo N, Chiusolo P, Cicconi S, Rutella S, et al. Immune reconstitution after autologous selected peripheral blood progenitor cell transplantation: comparison of two CD34+ cell-selection systems. Transfusion. 2001;41(6):783-9. Epub 2001/06/16.

[49] Schumm M, Depletion of TcRab+ and CD19-positive cells from leukapheresis products with the CliniMACS device. Bone Marrow Transplant. 2011;46: 339 Suppl 1:P1093.

[50] Neven B, Leroy S, Decaluwe H, Le Deist F, Picard C, Moshous D, et al. Long-term outcome after hematopoietic stem cell transplantation of a single-center cohort of 90 patients with severe combined immunodeficiency. Blood. 2009;113(17):4114-24. Epub 2009/01/27.

[51] Recher M, Berglund LJ, Avery DT, Cowan MJ, Gennery AR, Smart J, et al. IL-21 is the primary common gamma chain-binding cytokine required for human B-cell differentiation in vivo. Blood. 2011;118(26):6824-35. Epub 2011/11/01.

[52] Borghans JA, Bredius RG, Hazenberg MD, Roelofs H, Jol-van der Zijde EC, Heidt J, et al. Early determinants of long-term T-cell reconstitution after hematopoietic stem cell transplantation for severe combined immunodeficiency. Blood. 2006;108(2):763-9. Epub 2006/07/11.

[53] Kane L, Gennery AR, Crooks BN, Flood TJ, Abinun M, Cant AJ. Neonatal bone marrow transplantation for severe combined immunodeficiency. Archives of disease in childhood Fetal and neonatal edition. 2001;85(2):F110-3. Epub 2001/08/23.

[54] Myers LA, Patel DD, Puck JM, Buckley RH. Hematopoietic stem cell transplantation for severe combined immunodeficiency in the neonatal period leads to superior thymic output and improved survival. Blood. 2002;99(3):872-8. Epub 2002/01/25.

[55] Qasim W, Derniame S, Gilmour K, Chiesa R, Weber M, Adams S, et al. Third-party virus-specific T cells eradicate adenoviraemia but trigger bystander graft-versus-host disease. British journal of haematology. 2011;154(1):150-3. Epub 2011/04/20.

[56] Cole TS, Johnstone IC, Pearce MS, Fulton B, Cant AJ, Gennery AR, et al. Outcome of children requiring intensive care following haematopoietic SCT for primary immunodeficiency and other non-malignant disorders. Bone marrow transplantation. 2012;47(1):40-5. Epub 2011/03/02.

[57] Engelhardt KR, McGhee S, Winkler S, Sassi A, Woellner C, Lopez-Herrera G, et al. Large deletions and point mutations involving the dedicator of cytokinesis 8 (DOCK8) in the autosomal-recessive form of hyper-IgE syndrome. The Journal of allergy and clinical immunology. 2009;124(6):1289-302 e4. Epub 2009/12/17.

[58] Booth C, Gilmour KC, Veys P, Gennery AR, Slatter MA, Chapel H, et al. X-linked lymphoproliferative disease due to SAP/SH2D1A deficiency: a multicenter study on the

manifestations, management and outcome of the disease. Blood. 2011;117(1):53-62. Epub 2010/10/12.
[59] Seidel MG, Fritsch G, Lion T, Jurgens B, Heitger A, Bacchetta R, et al. Selective engraftment of donor CD4+25high FOXP3-positive T cells in IPEX syndrome after nonmyeloablative hematopoietic stem cell transplantation. Blood. 2009;113(22):5689-91. Epub 2009/05/30.
[60] White H, Thrasher A, Veys P, Kinnon C, Gaspar HB. Intrinsic defects of B cell function in X-linked severe combined immunodeficiency. European journal of immunology. 2000;30(3):732-7. Epub 2000/03/31.
[61] Crooks BN, Taylor CE, Turner AJ, Osman HK, Abinun M, Flood TJ, et al. Respiratory viral infections in primary immune deficiencies: significance and relevance to clinical outcome in a single BMT unit. Bone marrow transplantation. 2000;26(10):1097-102. Epub 2000/12/07.
[62] Corbacioglu S, Cesaro S, Faraci M, Valteau-Couanet D, Gruhn B, Rovelli A, et al. Defibrotide for prophylaxis of hepatic veno-occlusive disease in paediatric haemopoietic stem-cell transplantation: an open-label, phase 3, randomised controlled trial. Lancet. 2012;379(9823):1301-9. Epub 2012/03/01.
[63] Harkensee C, Vasdev N, Gennery AR, Willetts IE, Taylor C. Prevention and management of BK-virus associated haemorrhagic cystitis in children following haematopoietic stem cell transplantation--a systematic review and evidence-based guidance for clinical management. British journal of haematology. 2008;142(5):717-31. Epub 2008/06/11.
[64] Muller SM, Kohn T, Schulz AS, Debatin KM, Friedrich W. Similar pattern of thymic-dependent T-cell reconstitution in infants with severe combined immunodeficiency after human leukocyte antigen (HLA)-identical and HLA-nonidentical stem cell transplantation. Blood. 2000;96(13):4344-9. Epub 2000/12/09.
[65] Fallen PR, McGreavey L, Madrigal JA, Potter M, Ethell M, Prentice HG, et al. Factors affecting reconstitution of the T cell compartment in allogeneic haematopoietic cell transplant recipients. Bone marrow transplantation. 2003;32(10):1001-14. Epub 2003/11/05.
[66] Slatter MA, Bhattacharya A, Flood TJ, Spickett GP, Cant AJ, Abinun M, et al. Polysaccharide antibody responses are impaired post bone marrow transplantation for severe combined immunodeficiency, but not other primary immunodeficiencies. Bone marrow transplantation. 2003;32(2):225-9. Epub 2003/07/03.
[67] Slatter MA, Gennery AR, Cheetham TD, Bhattacharya A, Crooks BN, Flood TJ, et al. Thyroid dysfunction after bone marrow transplantation for primary immunodeficiency without the use of total body irradiation in conditioning. Bone marrow transplantation. 2004;33(9):949-53. Epub 2004/03/09.
[68] Titman P, Pink E, Skucek E, O'Hanlon K, Cole TJ, Gaspar J, et al. Cognitive and behavioral abnormalities in children after hematopoietic stem cell transplantation for severe congenital immunodeficiencies. Blood. 2008;112(9):3907-13. Epub 2008/07/23.
[69] Jacobsohn DA. Acute GVHD in children. Bone Marrow Transplant 2008;41:215-221

Chapter 3

"Wrapped Up" Vaccines in the Context of HIV-1 Immunotherapy

Winni De Haes, Charlotte Pollard, Guido Vanham and Joanna Rejman

Additional information is available at the end of the chapter

1. Introduction

The Human Immunodeficiency Virus-1 (HIV-1), the causative agent of the acquired immunodeficiency syndrome (AIDS), was described for the first time in 1983 [1, 2]. In the meantime, various classes of anti-retroviral drugs have been developed and combination therapy has improved the quality of life for millions of people affected. At the end of 2010 more than 34 million people were living with HIV infection worldwide [3]. Despite the increased access to antiretroviral therapy, an extensive treatment gap persists between the low-/middle-income countries and well-developed ones. This resulted in 1.8 million HIV related deaths and 2.6 million newly infected persons in 2009 [3]. Even for those who have access to treatment, there is no cure, as current therapy regimens cannot eradicate the virus. Therefore, the control and ultimate eradication of this pathogen remains one of the most important challenges in today's biomedical research.

HIV belongs to the family of *Retroviridae* and the genus *Lentivirus* (*lenti*, Latin for "slow"), which is characterized by a long incubation period causing long-lasting illnesses [4]. An HIV particle has a spherical shape and a size of about 100 nm. It consists of an outer coat, called the viral envelope, and an inner capsid enclosing two copies of positive single stranded ribonucleic acid (RNA). The RNA genome is 9.5 kB large and is composed of nine genes encoding structural (Gag, Pol and Env), regulatory (Tat and Rev) and accessory (Nef, Vif, Vpr and Vpu) proteins [5]. HIV-1 mainly infects $CD4^+$ cells such as $CD4^+$ T cells, macrophages and dendritic cells (DCs). Infection is initiated by the binding of the viral envelope glycoprotein 120 (gp120) to the CD4 receptor of the host cell, resulting in a conformational change that allows gp120 to interact with one of the co-receptors, CCR5 or CXCR4.

Binding of gp120 to the co-receptor induces further conformational changes that lead to the exposure of the fusion domain on glycoprotein 41 (gp41). Fusion of this domain with the lipid cell membrane allows entry of the viral core into the host cell cytoplasm. This is followed by reverse transcription of the single-stranded RNA into double-stranded DNA, which becomes integrated into the host genome [6]. After DNA integration, HIV remains present as a latent DNA provirus which becomes active upon cell activation [7]. Transcription of the viral proteins eventually leads to the formation of mature and infectious virions [8].

HIV-1 can be transmitted "horizontally" through hetero- or homosexual contact or blood-blood contact (e.g. blood transfusion or intravenous drug use) as well as "vertically" from mother-to-child [9]. The transmission of HIV strongly depends on the concentration of virus in the body fluids (genital secretions, plasma or breast milk), viral "fitness" properties and the host susceptibility at both the immunological and the cellular level [10].

Clinically, an HIV-1 infection course can be divided in three stages: the primary or acute infection phase, the chronic phase (first asymptomatic and later non-AIDS defining symptoms) and the terminal AIDS defining illness. The first days after infection, the virus spreads from the portal of entry via regional lymph nodes throughout the body. It readily infects $CD4^+$ T cells, producing new virions, which results in a high plasma viral load (VL). The virus finds its way to all lymphoid organs, but with a particularly massive viral production by the gastro-intestinal associated lymphoid tissue (GALT) is often observed. Remarkably, only a proportion of the newly infected patients experiences a clinical "acute phase syndrome", characterized by mononucleosis- or flu-like symptoms, including fever, fatigue, sore throat, skin rash, enlarged lymph nodes, diarrhea, nausea and general malaise. In the first three to six weeks a rapid decline of $CD4^+$ T cells is observed in the peripheral blood and even more pronounced in the GALT, which nonetheless remains an important HIV reservoir [11]. The appearance of HIV-1 specific cellular immune responses and the subsequent production of HIV-1 specific antibodies results in a sharp drop of viral load reaching a steady state viraemia, called the viral setpoint (usually within six months after infection). A dynamic equilibrium is then established between viral replication (fitness) and viral suppression by the immune system. Nevertheless, because of the limited regeneration capacity of the immune system (including thymic atrophy in adults) the number of $CD4^+$ T cells will continue to gradually decrease during the chronic phase. This stage can last up to ten years and is characterized by lack of clinical symptoms of illness or relatively mild symptoms that often do not raise suspicion of HIV infection. Eventually the immune system becomes exhausted due to chronic immune activation and T-cell depletion as a result of direct cytopathic effects of infected cells, but even more by induction of apoptosis of uninfected bystander cell ($CD4^+$ and $CD8^+$ T cells) and degeneration of lymphoid organs. Opportunistic diseases, including serious infections or malignant tumors that are no longer controlled due to a loss of immune surveillance are the cause of AIDS-related deaths [10, 12, 13].

The majority (> 90 %) of infected individuals progresses to AIDS within about ten years after primary infection (normal progressors). Some individuals (around 5 %) remain asymptomatic for more than ten years with stable numbers of $CD4^+$ T cells and low to intermediate viral loads (long term survivors and long term non progressors) [14]. Less than

1 % of infected individuals have viral loads below 50 copies per ml for at least 1-2 years while untreated (elite controllers or HIV controllers) [15]. Some individuals remain uninfected, despite being highly exposed to HIV-1 (exposed seronegatives) [16].

The first effective antiretroviral drugs (all nucleoside analogues) became available at the end of the nineties. They were used in single and later in dual combinations, but could suppress the viral load (VL) only temporarily. This was due to the appearance of drug resistance [17]. Triple drug combinations called "highly active antiretroviral therapy" (HAART), are able to suppress VL in a more sustained way and hence can prevent the emergence of drug resistance. For a number of years viral suppression was only possible at the cost of a high medication burden and many side effects. During the last decade, however, HAART has become less complicated and better tolerated, which has converted HIV-1 infection into a chronic but treatable disease [18].

It should be kept in mind, however, that HAART is not a treatment devoid of shortcomings. Firstly, a life-long commitment to the therapy remains mandatory to keep the virus under control and delay disease progression. Secondly, the treatment may cause toxic drug-related adverse effects such as cardiovascular complications [19], renal and hepatic diseases [20], lipodystrophy and diabetes mellitus, collectively called "metabolic syndrome" [21]. Thirdly, even though HAART restores the number of circulating $CD4^+$ T cells to near normal levels, responses against HIV itself remain deficient [11, 22]. Finally, this costly treatment is not available for all infected persons, especially not in low- and middle-income countries in Africa, Asia and Latin America, where the numbers of patients are the highest and still increasing [3].

Therefore, there is a clear need for cheaper and more widely available therapies that can suppress and/or eliminate the viral reservoir even if the treatment is stopped or interrupted. Improving HIV-specific cell-mediated immunity by therapeutic vaccination is a generally accepted approach to tackle the problem.

During the last decade immunotherapeutic vaccination strategies have been sought after to boost the immune system in order to control virus replication and to eliminate infected cells. These vaccines are largely based on ex vivo loading of dendritic cells with antigens and immune-stimulating molecules. This personalized process is time-consuming, labor intensive, and requires strict quality control. It should be stressed that high costs of the procedure together with the need to use sophisticated equipment, restrains its application in less developed countries.

Recently, particulate antigen vehicles have been introduced in the field of vaccine design with the purpose to improve antigen delivery and to induce antigen specific immune responses. A variety of nano- and micro-carriers has been developed to deliver protein, peptides and/or nucleic acids to cells of the immune system. The intracellular fate of these particles depends on their physicochemical characteristics such as size, stability and charge. These in turn determine the efficiency with which the specific cargo is delivered to antigen-presenting cells (APC) and the extent of antigen-specific immune responses induced.

2. HIV and the immune system

2.1. Immune activation

Chronic HIV-related immune activation is characterized by the inappropriate production of pro-inflammatory cytokines and overexpression of cellular activation and exhaustion markers. Most of these inflammatory responses induced by HIV are not directed toward HIV. They rather enhance susceptibility of target cells to HIV infection and enhance virus replication in already infected cells, which accelerates disease progression. This chronic, non-specific T cell activation leads to T cell exhaustion and apoptosis of $CD4^+$ and $CD8^+$ T cells [23]. Increased expressions of HLA-DR and CD38 molecules on $CD8^+$ T cells correlate with a higher level of immune activation and constitute markers for bad prognosis, which are partly independent from actual CD4 T count and VL [24].

It remains unclear whether there is a single key mechanism behind this HIV-associated immune activation. A so-called "leaky gut syndrome" hypothesis proposes that massive loss of $CD4^+$ T cells in the GALT may affect the protective barrier of the intestinal mucosa, allowing bacterial toxins such as lipopolysaccharide (LPS) to enter the bloodstream [25]. This "microbial translocation" could in consequence induce a pathological over-activation of both the innate and adaptive immune system. Another hypothesis puts more emphasis on intrinsic regulation of type I interferon (IFN) [26]. It has been shown indeed that patterns of type I IFNs produced by plasmacytoid DCs (pDCs) are different in non-pathogenic SIV infections of natural hosts (like sooty mangabeys, African green monkeys and mandrills) and pathogenic SIV infections of rhesus macaques. High and robust type I IFN responses are observed in natural hosts during acute infection. Expression of type I IFNs is, however, down-regulated during the chronic infection phase. By contrast, the type I IFNs are persistently produced in SIV infected rhesus macaques [27]. Sooty mangabeys, the natural hosts of SIV, show no immune activation and rarely progress to AIDS, despite high levels of virus replication and severe $CD4^+$ T cell depletion in the GALT. In contrast, rhesus macaques, infected with the same or closely related SIV, progress to AIDS [28].

Another enigma remains the role of CD25 and forkhead box (FOX) P3 expressing regulatory $CD4^+$ T (Treg) cells. On the one hand, they may suppress chronic immune activation. On the other hand, they could undermine the effective T cell responses [29]. It has been shown that the number of Treg cells increases in the GALT, but not in the peripheral blood, during HIV infection in untreated individuals [30]. Whether this accumulation of Treg cells delays disease progression by inhibition of immune activation or increases the susceptibility of the gastrointestinal tract to opportunistic infections remains a matter of debate [29].

2.2. HIV-specific humoral immune response

The humoral immune response is mediated by antibody producing B cells (**figure 1**). In general, by preventing infections of the host cells, virus-specific antibodies play an important role in the control of many viral infections [31]. This arm of the adaptive immune system is activated after uptake of viral proteins by antigen presenting cells (DCs, macrophages and B cells) that digest the proteins into small peptides and present them on MHC II molecules to CD4+ T helper (Th) cells. Specifically activated Th2 cells that produce B cell stimulating cytokines (including IL-4, IL-5, IL-6, IL-10, TGF–β) will activate naive B cells. The latter are recognized by specific epitopes or intact virus through their surface IgM and promote B cell differentiation into plasma cells producing large amounts of IgG, IgA, IgE antibodies and memory B cells. During HIV-1 infection antibodies against gp120, gp41, the nucleocapsid (p24) and the matrix (p17) arise few weeks to several months after infection. This process is commonly referred to as seroconversion.

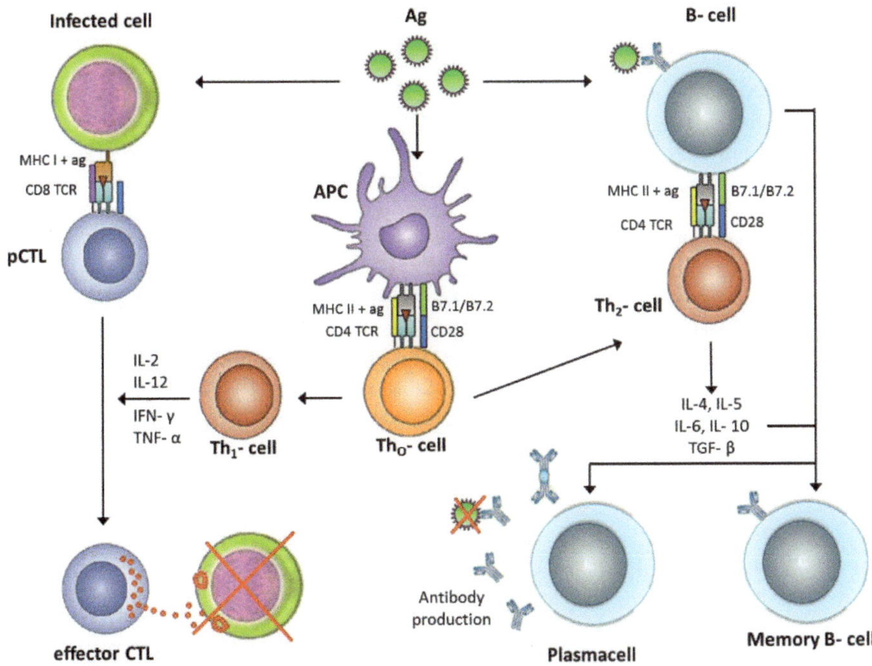

Figure 1. Overview of the adaptive immune responses after virus recognition by antigen presenting cells. Virus antigens are presented by dendritic cells and B cells to T cells. Infected cells present peptides together with MHC I molecules on the plasma membrane. The peptide-MHC I complex is recognized by precursor cytotoxic CD8+ T lymphocytes (CTLs). Th1 cells, induced by antigen presenting cells, produce IL-2, IFN-γ, and TNF-α. This results in activation and differentiation of the precursor CTLs into memory or effector CTLs. Effector CTLs can directly kill infected cells by the production of perforines and granzymes. Activated Th2 cells, also induced by antigen presenting cells, produce B cell stimulating cytokines (including IL-4, IL-5, IL-6, IL-10, TGF–β) that activate naive B cells. This facilitates/induces B cell differentiation into memory B cells and plasma cells that produce large amounts of IgG, IgA, IgE antibodies that prevent further virus infection. Ab: antibody, Ag: antigen, APC: Antigen Presenting Cell, DC: Dendritic Cell, IL: Interleukin, TCR: T Cell Receptor, Th: CD4+ T helper cell.

The virus neutralization is characterized by the interaction of specific antibodies with the viral envelope spikes. This interferes with virus attachment or viral entry in target cells and results in the inhibition of infection. Only a minority of anti-HIV Env antibodies, at any time, exerts immune pressure by autologous neutralization. However, the virus easily mutates and readily escapes from these potentially protective immune responses [32]. During the chronic course of infection only 20% of the infected individuals will generate broadly neutralizing antibodies (bNAbs) having the ability to neutralize heterologous viruses [33]. In addition to classical neutralization, antibodies can attach to HIV infected cells and kill them via antibody dependent cellular cytotoxicity (ADCC) mediated through their Fc moiety and natural killers cells (NK) [34, 35].

2.3. HIV-specific cellular immune response

The cellular immune response is the other arm of the adaptive immune system (**figure 1**) and it is crucial to combat viral infections. $CD8^+$ cytotoxic T lymphocytes (CTLs), which eliminate infected cells, play a key role in this process. The initial step involves processing of intracellular antigens by the proteasome. The resulting peptides are then presented together with MHC I molecules on the membrane of infected somatic cells. The peptide-MHC I complex is recognized by precursor cytotoxic $CD8^+$ T lymphocytes (CTLs). Also in that case a $CD4^+$ T cell help, induced by antigen presenting cells, is crucial. In this case so-called Th1 cells, producing IL-2, IFN-γ, and TNF-α, activate and differentiate the CTLs into memory or effector CTLs. Effector CTLs can directly kill infected cells by the production of perforines and granzymes (**figure 2**) [36]. Alternatively, CTLs can induce apoptosis of the infected cells after interaction of Fas ligand on CTLs with Fas receptor on infected T cells [37]. $CD8^+$ T cells also display a non-cytotoxic antiviral activity involving several cytokines, chemokines and a yet unidentified soluble $CD8^+$ cell antiviral factor (CAF) [38].

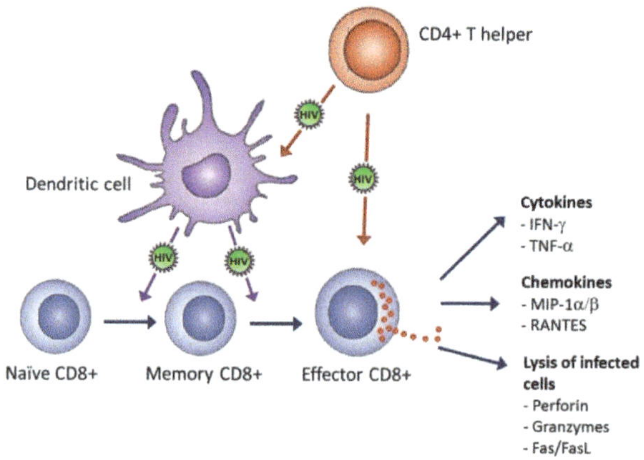

Figure 2. HIV-induced T cell responses. HIV specific $CD8^+$ effector cells produce chemokines and cytokines in order to eliminate infected cells. $CD4^+$ T helper cells help to stimulate both dendritic cells and $CD8^+$ T-cells to maintain a $CD8^+$ T-cell memory response. HIV interferes with this supportive function of $CD4^+$ T-cells.

The first T cell responses during HIV infection arise when the viraemia peak is approached and reach maximum 1-2 weeks later. In non-controllers, the virus evades the $CD8^+$ mediated T cell response by introducing mutations in CTL epitopes [39], by Nef-mediated down-regulation of MHC I and by influencing cytokine production and T-cell signaling [40]. Since an optimal $CD8^+$ T cell response, similar to the B cell response, depends on help of $CD4^+$ T lymphocytes, the deterioration of CD8 mediated viral control is also related to the weakening of $CD4^+$ T cell function [41, 42].

There are many indications that HIV-specific $CD8^+$ T cell responses are responsible for at least partial VL control. In the macaque model, depletion of $CD8^+$ T cells during SIV-infection resulted in an increased viral load [43, 44]. In HIV-infected human subjects, who initially control the virus, escape mutations in specific $CD8^+$ T cell epitopes were responsible for the loss of control and increase in VL [45, 46].

3. Correlates of protection

To date no definite biological markers have been unambiguously shown to correlate with patients' ability to control HIV infection by suppressing virus production and eliminating infected cells. Defining these factors would be crucial for the development of preventive and therapeutic vaccination strategies. For that reason, research groups focusing on preventive vaccines carefully study individuals that can avoid infection (exposed seronegatives) or partly control the virus load without the need of HAART.

3.1. Natural resistance and genetic factors of the host

Individuals that have the homozygote deletion Δ32 in co-receptor CCR5 are largely resistant to HIV-1 infection [47]. It has been recently reported that an HIV patient, who received *CCR5* Δ32/Δ32 stem cells for transplantation, remained without viral rebound for several years [48, 49].

Certain intracellular molecules, expressed by the host, can at least partly protect against cellular infection or virus release. The most important factors identified so far are APOBEC3G, APOBEC3F, TRIM5α and tetherin. APOBEC3G is a cytosine deaminase that incorporates adenosine instead of guanosine during synthesis of the viral DNA, which results in defective proviral DNA [50]. In addition APOBEC3G promotes natural killer cell-mediated lysis [51]. Individuals expressing large amounts of APOBEC3G have lower viral loads during acute infection phase [52]. TRIM5a binds to the viral capsid, blocking replication early in the viral life cycle [53]. Tetherin interferes with the virion release by attaching the mature virions to each other and to the host membrane [54].

Certain polymorphisms in the human leukocyte antigen (HLA type) and T or NK cell receptor can affect the cellular HIV-specific immune responses. It has been shown that human leukocyte antigens B*27, B*57 and B*58 are associated with better control of HIV-1 and slower disease progression [55-57]. Interestingly HLA B*57 also plays a role in the innate protective immune responses, acting as a natural ligand for inhibitory killer immunoglobulin-like receptors (KIRs). KIR3DL1 and KIR3DS1 are also associated with delay in disease progression [58, 59].

3.2. Suggested immune correlates

High and broadly neutralizing antibody titers at the port of the virus entry are likely essential to prevent (new) infections of host cells. Indeed high levels of HIV-neutralizing IgA were detected at mucosal surfaces of some exposed seronegative individuals [60-62]. Moreover, in several models of transmission, passive immunization with neutralizing monoclonal antibodies could protect macaques from infection. In contrast, once infection has been established, neutralizing antibodies seem to be unable to control the virus spread [63]. In order to eliminate infected cells, strong $CD8^+$ T cell responses seem to be of importance. As already discussed, most infected individuals show strong $CD8^+$ T cell responses in reaction to the first viraemia peak, resulting in a decline of the viral load in early infection. Unfortunately, in most cases (except for elite controllers) these responses are not able to maintain full control, mainly due to iterative immune escape [39] and chronic immune activation [23], ultimately resulting in T cell exhaustion [64]. In contrast, HIV-specific $CD8^+$ T cells preserve their function and new effective $CD8^+$ T cell responses can arise against viral escape variants in elite controllers [55]. Additionally, a strong avidity of the T cell receptor for the epitope-MHC-I-complex has been shown to promote polyfunctional $CD8^+$ T cells [65] and to initiate more rapid lysis of the target cell [66, 67]. Furthermore, the presence of polyfunctional $CD8^+$ T cells, that have the capacity to exert different effector functions by producing IFN-γ, TNF-α, IL-2, MIP-1β, perforines and/or granzymes and to proliferate upon antigen stimulation, has been associated with the "controller" status [68, 69]. Another important observation came from the study of Geldmacher and colleagues who reported that responses directed against Gag epitopes are dominant and potentially protective in long term non progressors and elite controllers [70]. One of the reasons for this observation could be escape mutations, in particular HLA-restricted epitopes of Gag, that come at a cost of great loss in viral fitness [71-73].

As already explained, maturation and differentiation of $CD8^+$ T cells into functional memory and effector subsets are also dependent on functional $CD4^+$ T helper cells. The remaining $CD4^+$ T cells, after massive depletion during acute infection, need to be polyfunctional by producing at least both IFN-γ an IL-2 in order to proliferate upon antigen stimulation [41] and provide help to CTL. This Th1 function is impaired in HIV non-controllers [74].

Unfortunately, none of these factors can truly predict protection against HIV infection [75]. Therefore, at present it seems wise to conclude that all potential correlates (**table 1**) should be taken into account while designing HIV therapies. This includes the preservation of functional Th1 HIV-specific $CD4^+$ T cells and the availability of central memory and memory effector HIV-specific CD8 T cells, with strong avidity for particular difficult-to-mutate epitopes. In addition also a broad functional activity, including production of several effector cytokines and lytic factors are important to result in high and broad HIV-suppressive immune responses [75].

Level of protection	Suggested correlates of protection
Viral factors	Deletion in Nef [76]
Host genetic factors	CCR5 D32/D32 [48, 49]
Host restriction factors	High levels of antiviral fator APOBEC3G [51, 52]
	High production of TRIM5α [53]
	Up-regulation of tetherin [54]
	HLA types B*27, B*57, B*58 [55, 56]
	KIR3DL1, KIR3DS1 [58, 59]
Humoral immunity	Neutralizing Abs: IgA antibodies at the mucosal surfaces [60-63]
Cellular immunity	Polyfunctional T cells [66, 69]
	Proliferative $CD4^+$ and $CD8^+$ T cells [68, 70]
	Avidity of HIV specific T cell responses [65, 66, 74]

Table 1. Suggested correlates of protection.

4. Vaccination strategies against HIV-1

Many infection-related hurdles complicate the development of an HIV vaccine. These include the high genetic variability, the potential of cell-to-cell transmission and other evasion strategies such as down-regulating MHC I in infected cells and latency of the virus [77]. In addition, correlates conferring protection against HIV remain to be established. A number of potential markers have been suggested to prevent or control HIV infection. These comprise: production of high titers of neutralizing antibodies with broad specificities, concomitant HIV-specific activation of $CD4^+$ and $CD8^+$ T cells, polyfunctional T cell responses (production of several immune mediators by the same T cell) and induction of long- term memory cells [78].

4.1. Prophylactic vaccines

Prophylactic vaccines rely on the production of antibodies that bind to free virus particles thereby preventing viral entry into host cells (defined as neutralization) and thus block infection. Vaccines are designed to mimic natural infections, by using live-attenuated virus (measles, mumps), chemically inactivated virus (polio) or recombinant subunits of the virus (Hepatitis B). There is circumstantial evidence that neutralizing antibodies could play a role in the protection against HIV. HIV-neutralizing IgA antibodies have been isolated in frequently exposed individuals, who remained uninfected [62, 79]. In addition, passive immunization with several HIV neutralizing IgG monoclonal antibodies protects macaques against infectious SHIV (simian immune deficiency virus with an HIV envelope) [80, 81]. Although attenuated SIV vaccines provided some level of protection against super-infection in macaques, attenuated HIV is considered too risky to be ever tried in humans [82]. Therefore, much effort has been invested in the development of subunit vaccines that could elicit production of neutralizing antibodies. It should be taken into account that broadly neutralizing antibodies (bNAbs) that inhibit also heterologous viruses *in vitro,* can be detected in 20% of naturally infected individuals. This implies that the production of these antibodies is not sufficient to provide full protection against established HIV, but could still be efficient in prevention of cell-free transmission. The most important reason why it is difficult to induce bNAbs is the extreme variability of HIV Env antigenic epitopes. Moreover, the virus is shielded by non-immunogenic glycans, which hinder binding of antibodies to the envelope proteins [83, 84]. Due to these problems, prophylactic vaccine trials in humans have failed to elicit protection. The only exception till now is the recent Thai vaccine trial (RV144).

Nevertheless neutralizing antibodies with activity against easy-to-neutralize so-called "Tier 1" viruses have been induced in a number of animal trials, but these antibodies failed to broaden and faded rapidly, even upon repeated heterologous boosts [85]. The failure to induce high titers of NAbs moved the field towards strategies aiming at stimulating polyfunctional and sustained $CD4^+$ T help responses [69] to support high quality cytotoxic T cells (both central memory and effector memory). These cells would be necessary to rapidly eliminate infected cells, if antibodies fail to prevent cellular infection [86, 87]. This "second line prevention" hypothesis was further supported by the observations that HIV-specific $CD4^+$ and/or $CD8^+$ T cells as well as particular human leukocyte antigen (HLA) class I markers, and not antibodies, correlate with resistance to HIV in some highly exposed seronegative children (potential vertical transmission) [88] or women (potential heterosexual transmission) [89-91].

In this connection, current HIV vaccines are also aiming at the induction (prophylactic field) or enhancing (therapeutic field) of HIV specific T cell responses. Such vaccines would elicit or boost HIV specific cytotoxic T cells (CTLs) to eliminate infected cells and $CD4^+$ T cells, which can help to induce and maintain B cell and $CD8^+$ T cells responses [92]. Several strategies are currently under investigation to establish effective T cell responses in either a preventive or therapeutic setting either based on protein [93, 94] or peptide [95] vaccinations, virus like particles (VPLs) [96], DNA vaccination using viral vectors [97, 98], prime-boost vaccinations [99, 100] or DC-based vaccines [101-109].

4.2. Viral vaccine delivery

Whereas the use of live attenuated HIV is considered to be unsafe for the use in humans, the development of vaccines based on HIV-inactivated with formalin is compromised by the fact that the antigenicity of the envelope gets lost. Milder formalin treatment of the virus, followed by heat-inactivation has been shown to circumvent this hurdle and induce modest neutralizing antibodies titer in non-human primates [110].

During the last decade, a variety of vaccines was designed using (plasmid) DNA/RNA vaccine candidates for priming followed by live vectored recombinant vaccines for boosting, some of which have already been tested in advanced stages of clinical trials [111, 112]. We will highlight here some of the specific characteristics of viral vectors, which have been used in preclinical and early clinical preventive vaccinations against SIV and HIV, respectively.

Adenoviruses, poxviruses and lentiviruses are the most frequently used viral vector systems. The major advantages of these vectors are the high transduction efficiency resulting in high level expression of the encoded protein and the possibility to target specific cells achieved by altering the viral tropism (e.g. by pseudotyping with envelope or counter receptors of another virus) [113, 114]. Major drawbacks are the high risk of insertional mutagenesis, high production cost of large amounts high-titered viral stocks and a limited size of nucleic acids that can be packed [113, 114]. The first trial of a preventive HIV vaccine that was designed to elicit a strong cellular immune response was the STEP trial done by Merck. It involved immunization of almost 3000 healthy uninfected volunteers with three recombinant adenovirus serotype-5 (rAD5) vectors, Ad5-*gag*, Ad5-*pol* and Ad5-*nef*. Unfortunately, it failed to induce protection against infection [115, 116]. Moreover, the vaccine increased the rate of HIV infection in individuals with pre-existing immunity to adenoviruses [117]. The exact mechanism that underlies this phenomenon remains to be elucidated, but it has been suggested that the activation of pre-existing vector specific T cells may have increased numbers of HIV target cells. This might be avoided by the use of less prevalent adenovirus serotypes (e.g. Ad11, Ad24 or Ad35) instead of the Ad5 vector in designing future HIV vaccines [118, 119].

Alternatively, poxvirus-based vectors should be taken into account since they do not pose any problems with pre-existing immunity. In addition, they are used as highly attenuated vaccinia virus strains. Three of the best characterized highly attenuated pox vectors are the recombinant viral canary pox vectors such as the highly attenuated vaccinia virus strain ALVAC [120], the recombinant modified vaccinia Ankara (MVA) vectors [121-123] and canarypox-derived NYVAC [120, 124, 125]. Recombinant pox vectors, encoding HIV antigens, have been shown to be safe in humans and to induce HIV specific immune responses. No protection against HIV infection has been achieved with the exception of the preventive RV144 phase III clinical trial. In this clinical trial, involving 16 000 uninfected individuals, a canary pox vector coding HIV Gag and Env was used as prime immunization followed by a recombinant Env gp120 protein boost (RV144). A 31% efficacy of protection against HIV infection was demonstrated after three years [126]. Very recently, Barouch *et al.* reported that rhesus monkeys, receiving heterologous vector regimes (adeno with MVA), were protected with an efficacy of 80% after SIV challenges [127].

Another type of vectors that could avoid the pre-existing immunity issue is based on lentiviruses. These vectors have been explored extensively in the field of gene therapy since they efficiently transduce non-dividing cells, such as DCs [128, 129], and promote long term antigen expression [130]. Lentiviral vector vaccines have been shown to induce both high short term and long-term anti-HIV immune responses in mice [131, 132]. Even in the absence of circulating $CD4^+$ T cells, induction of specific CTLs was obtained [133]. Despite reassuring safety and tolerability results in a phase I clinical trial [134], the major concern remains the risk of insertional mutagenesis [135]. Attempts to overcome this risk, have led to the design of self-inactivating vectors, vectors with targeted integration and non-integrating vectors [135].

Replicating and persistent recombinant cytomegalovirus (CMV) vectors have recently been shown to be a promising system in rhesus macaques [136]. Prophylactically vaccinated animals maintained CD4+ and CD8+ T effector memory (T_{EM}) cell responses, regardless to pre-existing CMV immunity, and were more resistant to challenge than the control group even in the absence of neutralizing antibodies [137]. The authors suggest that T_{EM} responses are crucial in the protection against HIV infection after sexual exposure. This is obviously also the scope of HIV immunotherapy where sustained effector and memory T cells can eliminate infected cells.

Virus-like-particles (VLPs) have recently emerged as novel delivery systems. They contain envelope and core proteins from SIV/HIV in their native structure. These pseudo-virions are produced in baculovirus or vaccinia virus expression systems where Gag and Env proteins from HIV or SIV are co-expressed and spontaneously assembled. The immunogenicity of these vaccines was only modest in non-human primates [96], however, efficiency was greatly improved when combined with a HIV DNA vaccine prime [138].

Safety concerns and difficulties related to repeated administrations of viral vectors that may evoke dangerous immune reactions are the most important bottlenecks in regard to clinical application in humans. To improve the general safety profile and circumventing the drawbacks inherited to viral delivery, well-defined particulate vaccines have emerged as promising candidates in the field of vaccine development.

5. HIV Immunotherapy with DC-based vaccines

5.1. Therapeutic vaccines

Since the introduction of HAART, HIV-1 infection has evolved into a chronic but treatable disease. Although HAART suppresses viral replication and partially reconstitutes both CD4+ T cell numbers [139] and T cell immune responses to opportunistic infections, it cannot restore effective HIV specific T cell responses [140], resulting in a rapid rebound of HIV-1 replication upon treatment interruption [141]. This implies that infected individuals are bound to lifelong treatment, imposing a high burden in terms of adherence, costs and the risk of drug related metabolic disorders [142]. Therefore, therapeutic vaccination has emerged as an option to boost and improve the cellular immune responses in infected individuals [143]. This concept is supported by increasing evidence that strong HIV-1 specific CD4+ helper T cells and CD8+ CTLs are responsible for viral control both in macaques [144] and humans [145]. During acute infection CD8+ T cell responses contribute to control of the initial viraemia peak. However, in most infected subjects, this CD8+ T cell response loses its efficacy during chronic infection. This is due to a high mutation rate of the virus, the absence of proliferative and highly functional CD4+ T cells [145, 146] and the appearance of impaired or apoptotic HIV-specific CD8 T cells [147]. Clearly, the major challenge for therapeutic vaccination is to elicit strong CD4+ and CD8+ responses that would allow stopping of HAART. *In vitro* modulation of DCs to efficiently present target antigens to elicit cellular immune responses has been shown to be a promising strategy in cancer immunotherapy [148], which constituted a model for development of similar HIV immunotherapies.

5.2. Dendritic cells

DCs are the sentinels of the immune system, bridging innate and adaptive immunity, in response to pathogens crossing the mucosal or dermal barrier. Immature DCs (iDCs) continuously sample their environment and take up autologous and foreign antigens [149]. They undergo maturation in response to signals that originate from pathogen-associated molecular patterns (PAMPs). These PAMPs activate a set of pattern recognition receptors (PRRs) such as Toll like receptors (TLRs), nucleotide-binding oligomerization domain (NOD)-like receptors (NLRs), C-lectin receptors (CLRs) and retinoic acid-inducible gene protein (RIG)- like receptors (RLRs). Triggering of PPR results in an increased expression of major histocompatibility complex I and II (MHC I and MHC II), co-stimulatory molecules (CD80 and CD86) as well as secretion of T cell stimulatory cytokines (e.g. IL-12). During this maturation process DCs lose their ability to take up antigens and chemokine receptors (e.g. CCR7) are up-regulated in order to promote their migration to lymph nodes. Mature DCs process endogenous antigens via proteasome into 8-9 amino-acid peptides which are then loaded on MHC I and presented to $CD8^+$ T cells. Exogenous antigens are processed via the endolysosome into longer peptides to be load onto MHC II for presentation to $CD4^+$ T cells. The capacity of DCs to present exogenous antigens also via MHC I pathway (i.e. cross presentation), distinguishes them from other APCs, such as macrophages and B cells. To stimulate effective T cell responses, peptide-MHC complex on DCs should interact with T cell receptors (TCR). This is accompanied by binding of co-stimulatory molecules on DCs with CD28 present on T cells (**figure 3**). Finally, produced cytokines determine the differentiation of the effector cells into Th1, Th2 or CTL [150]. The latter is achieved after DCs' licensing by the interaction of CD40 on the mature DCs with CD40L expressed on $CD4^+$ T cells. IL-4 secretion promotes $CD4^+$ Th2 cells, stimulating the production of antibody producing B cells. IL-12 promotes $CD4^+$ Th1 cells, providing help to CTL to kill infected cells. Secretion of IL-10 has a negative impact on Th1 or Th2 cells and induces immune tolerance. Licensed DCs also induce differentiation of $CD8^+$ T cells into CTL via peptide-MHC I complex and promote survival of $CD8^+$ T cells via co-stimulation through CD137L (4-1BBL) [151].

Roughly five DC subsets can be distinguished [152]. Classical or tissue resident DCs are located in lymphoid organs such as spleen and lymph nodes. Migratory DCs, found in non-lymphoid organs such as skin, intestines and lungs, sample their environment and migrate to lymph nodes to present tissue derived antigen to T cells. Langerhans cells reside in the multi-layerd epithelium of the skin, oral and genital surfaces. Plasmacytoid DCs (pDCs) and myeloid or monocyte-derived DCs may be present in various tissues, yet they mainly circulate in the blood. pDCs are known as major producers of type I interferons (IFNs) in response to virus-associated molecules such as single-stranded (ss) RNA and unmethylated cytosine-phosphate-guanine (CpG)-rich DNA that trigger TLR7 and TLR9, respectively [153]. Myeloid DCs represent the major fraction of APCs in the blood that responds to TLR ligation by producing IL-12 [154]. Noteworthy, the APC function of DCs is impaired by

HIV, which could contribute to the dysfunction of HIV specific T cell responses since maturation of DCs and IL-12 secretion are diminished, thereby suppressing T cell responses [155]. HIV-infected DCs preferably secrete IL-10 thus limiting T cell proliferation and activation and rather induce tolerance [156]. HIV-1 infected DCs also act as a Trojan horse to infect new T cells by promoting tolerance of T cells to HIV-1 [157].

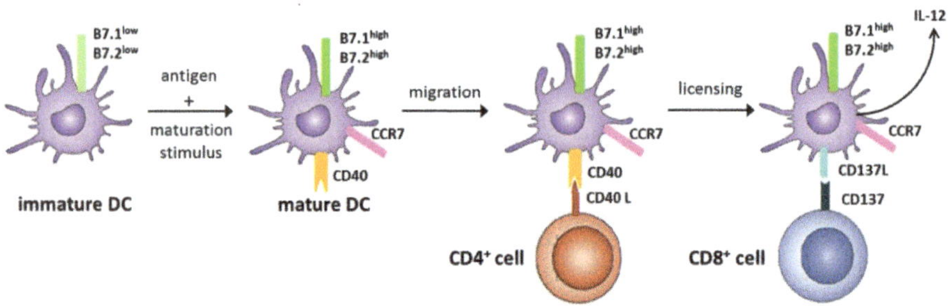

Figure 3. Differentiation process of dendritic cells. Immature DCs take up antigens. Activation of PPRs results in the differentiation towards mature DCs. The co-stimulatory molecules (B7-1, and B7-2) are overexpressed and the expression of the lymph node homing receptor CCR7 is induced. Mature DCs migrate to the draining lymph node, where they present antigens to cognate CD4+ T cells. Cross-linking CD40 on the DCs by CD40L expressed on the antigen-activated CD4+ T cell, induces the mature DCs to differentiate further, a process known as licensing. Licensed DCs up-regulate additional cell surface proteins, such as CD137L. The licensed DCs now present antigens to cognate CD8+ T cells. CD137L–mediated co-stimulation through CD137 on the antigen-activated CD8+ T cells enhances the survival and proliferative capacity of the activated CD8+ T cells.

5.3. HIV-1 antigen loaded dendritic cells tested in clinical trails

To obtain a large population of DCs to be used in immunotherapy, DCs are derived from blood monocytes that are cultured in the presence of granulocyte and macrophage colony stimulation factor (GM-CSF) and IL-4 [158, 159]. Various approaches for loading DCs with antigens have been applied. They include the use of inactivated virus [104, 160], recombinant viral proteins [107, 161-163], peptides [101, 164], DNA [165-167] and mRNA [168-172]. After loading, DCs are matured using various maturation cocktails composed of cytokines (such as type 1 (α,β) or type 2 (γ) interferons, TNF-α, IL-6) prostaglandines (PG), TLR ligands, T cell derived products (CD40L) or small interfering RNA (siRNA) against suppressors of cytokine signaling (SOCS)-1 [98, 151].

To this date at least ten DC-based immunotherapeutic vaccine trials (**table 2**) have been tested in infected individuals (recently reviewed by García and Routy [173]. Kundu *et al.* were the first to perform a human clinical trial, in which treatment-naïve HIV infected individuals were vaccinated with protein or peptides pulsed autologous DCs [107]. The vaccine was well tolerated and resulted in an increase of HIV specific CD8+ T cell response in 3 out of 6 individuals, but no effect on viral load was observed. Three other clinical trials tested peptides pulsed DCs [101, 105, 106]. In two of these trials an increase in HIV-specific

T cell responses in the absence of virological responses was shown [101, 105], whereas in the third study a transient decrease in viral load was found in 50% of vaccinated individuals [106]. Lu *et al.* were the first to demonstrate *in vivo* that a vaccine made of autologous monocyte-derived DCs, pulsed with autologous, aldithriol-2-inactivated HIV-1 was capable of inducing HIV-1-specific T cell responses. Moreover, there was an 80% decrease in plasma viral load levels over the first 112 days after vaccination. A prolonged suppression of viral load (of more than 90%) was seen for at least 1 year after vaccination in 8 out of 19 vaccinated patients. This suppression of viral load correlated with HIV-1-specific IL-2 and IFN-γ expressing $CD4^+$ T cells and with HIV-1 Gag-specific perforin-expressing $CD8^+$ effector cells [108]. Unfortunately, the lack of a control group does not allow a proper evaluation of the results obtained. The group of García *et al.* performed two clinical trials with autologous DCs pulsed with heat-inactivated virus [103, 104]. In a double blind placebo controlled study with a similar setup as Lu *et al.*, García *et al.* observed a small but significant decrease in viral loads for at least 48 weeks, concomitant with a weak increase in HIV-1 specific T cell responses in therapy naïve HIV infected individuals [103]. Another study performed by the same group in HAART treated patients showed a lengthening of the rebound after therapy interruption and a moderate increase in HIV specific T cell responses [104].

Form of antigen	Vaccine strategy	Subjects	Clinical trial outcome
Inactivated virus	DCs pulsed with autologous AT2 inactivated virus (10^9)	Untreated patients (n= 18)	Suppression of viral load was correlated with HIV specific IL-2 or IFN-γ producing CD4+ T cells and perforin producing CD8+ effector T cells. [108]
	DCs pulsed with autologous heat inactivated virus (10^6)	HAART treated patients followed by therapy interruption (n=18)	Lengthening of viral rebound correlated with numbers of HIV-specific proliferative $CD4^+$ and $CD8^+$ T cells. [104]
	DCs pulsed with autologous heat inactivated virus (10^9)	Untreated patients (n= 18)	Inverse correlation between decrease in viral load and HIV-specific T cell responses. [103]
Peptides	DCs pulsed with Gag, Pol and Env peptides	Untreated patients (n= 6)	In 3/6 cases Env-specific and proliferative immune responses were observed. [107]
	DCs pulsed with HLA A*0201 binding epitopes in Gag, Nef and Env	HAART treated patients followed by therapy interruption (n=4)	In 2/4 patients moderate $CD8^+$ T cell responses were observed. No lower viral setpoints after therapy interruption. [105]

Form of antigen	Vaccine strategy	Subjects	Clinical trial outcome
	DCs pulsed with HLA A*0201 binding epitopes in Gag, Pol and Env	HAART treated patients (n=18)	Increase in CTL responses against vaccine epitopes. [101]
	DCs pulsed with HLA A*0201 binding epitopes in Gag, Pol, Env, Vpu and Vif and Th epitopes in Gag and Env	Untreated patients (n= 12)	Generation of new T cell responses despite high viral loads. [106]
DNA	ALVAC pulsed DCs vs AlVAC alone	HAART treated patients followed by therapy interruption (n=29)	No differences in T cell responses against HIV antigens. Did not lower VL setpoint after therapy interruption. [102]
	ALVAC-Remune	HAART treated patients followed by therapy interruption (n=48)	No lowering of viral setpoint after vaccination, but VL rebound was delayed. [177]
mRNA	*Ex vivo* electroporated DCs with mRNA encoding CD40L and autologous HIV proteins (Gag, Ref, Nef, Vpr)	HAART treated patients (n=10)	HIV specific proliferative immune responses preferentially targeted to $CD8^+$ T cells. Correlation with viral control during therapy interruption. [109]
	Ex vivo electroporated DCs with mRNA and autologous HIV proteins (Gag, Tat, Rev, Nef)	HAART treated patients (n=6)	Breadth of IFN-γ response and T-cell proliferation were correlated with $CD4^+$ and $CD8^+$ polyfunctional T-cell responses. Autologous $CD8^+$ T cells inhibited HIV superinfection in *vitro*. [176]
	Ex vivo electroporated DCs with mRNA and autologous HIV proteins (Tat, Rev, Nef)	HAART treated patients followed by therapy interruption (n=17)	Induced or enhanced $CD4^+$ and $CD8^+$ T cell responses specific for the vaccine antigens. [175]

Table 2. Overview of therapeutic DC-based clinical trials.

Nucleic acids are also used as a source of antigens in DC-based immunotherapies. Phase I and II clinical trials were conducted to evaluate the potential of a canarypox HIV-vaccine (ALVAC), containing DNA encoding Env, Gag as well as parts of Nef and Pol to either directly vaccinate HAART-treated patient or *ex vivo* load autologous DCs. The results obtained did not demonstrate clear differences in the immunological or virological outcome and a control group was lacking [102]. In a very recent study, DNA encoding HIV proteins was complexed with polymers and topically administrated with a patch method named DermaPrep [174]. The results showed that vaccination induced new HIV-specific immune responses in HAART treated patients. Moreover, a better control of viral replication during treatment interruption was observed [167]. DCs loaded with mRNA have also been tested in clinical trials. Routy *et al.* reported the results of a trial in which HAART-treated patients received autologous DCs *ex vivo* electroporated with mRNA encoding autologous HIV sequences and CD40L [173]. This pilot study showed $CD8^+$ T cells specific for the presented HIV antigen were preferentially targeted. Two other clinical trials employing autologous DCs electroporated *ex vivo* with mRNA encoding Tat, Rev, Nef and Gag were recently concluded [175, 176]. Both studies showed that vaccine-specific $CD4^+$ and $CD8^+$ T cell responses were enhanced. In one study vaccinated individuals interrupted treatment. Six out of 17 individuals remained off therapy 96 weeks after cessation [175].

One should keep in mind, however, that *ex vivo* manipulation of DCs is a complex personalized vaccination procedure, which prevents its accessibility to large numbers of patients. Therefore, there is a constant need for new approaches that could target DCs directly *in vivo*. In the following paragraphs we will discuss various non-viral delivery approaches which promote antigen uptake by DCs and induce potent immune responses.

6. The way forward: Antigen delivery by non-viral carriers

Even though viral vectors are generally considered more efficient, non-viral delivery vehicles receive increasing attention since they are safer, more versatile, easier to prepare and hence more accessible for up-scaling [178]. In addition, they allow delivery of larger quantities of antigens. Importantly, encapsulation protects antigens from their environment and therefore permits a prolonged release of antigens in tissues or particular cells [179]. The usual size of particulate vaccines, ranging from a few hundred nanometers to a few microns, is ideal for uptake by DCs [180]. Moreover, the nature of non-viral carriers allows their functionalization with moieties permitting specific targeting to DCs. Additionally they allow co-delivery of immunostimulatory molecules which can direct the immune system toward the humoral or cellular arm [181]. The simultaneous delivery of antigens and immune-stimulators to the same DC is a feature which has been reported to significantly augment the strength of the induced adaptive immune responses [182-184]. In the following paragraphs we will discuss different lipid- and polymer-based carrier systems employed to deliver proteins and nucleic acids relevant for HIV-specific immunotherapy (**table 3**).

6.1. Choice of antigen

Peptides, proteins or nucleic acids (DNA or RNA) have been used as a source of antigen in the majority of therapeutic vaccination strategies. Each of them comes with specific characteristics in terms of safety, stability, potential to cover antigenic variability, requirements for delivery and nature of the immune response induced [185]. Recombinant proteins or peptides utilized as subunit vaccines are safe and simple forms of antigens. However, their production at clinical grade quality is very expensive. As a consequence, only one or a few antigenic variants can be produced at an affordable price. Moreover, they are susceptible to pre-mature proteolytic degradation. Since DCs recognize them as exogenous antigens, they are preferentially presented in a MHC class II context [143] and to a lesser extent onto MHC I molecules via cross-presentation [180]. Therefore, they will not induce strong and broad CD8$^+$ T cell responses, which are considered as a prerequisite for a therapeutic vaccine. These limitations can partially be resolved by their encapsulation. Encapsulation protects proteins and peptides from being prematurely degraded by proteolytic enzymes. Additionally, particulate antigen delivery favors cross-presentation thereby enhancing CD8$^+$ T cell responses [186, 187]. In the context of HIV immunotherapy, however, the use of proteins as antigens is not ideal since HIV generates escape variants during the course of infection which remain present as a latent reservoir in cells [188]. With the technology available, it is not feasible to produce hundreds of variants of the same protein and include them in a therapeutic vaccine.

Delivery vehicle	**Form of antigen**	**Advantages**	**Disadvantages**
PLA-PLGA particles	Proteins	FDA approved, induction of specific antibodies and Th1 cellular responses	Harsh preparation process, expensive to upscale.
Polyelctrolyte capsules	Proteins, peptides	Induction of both Th1 and Th2 responses. Easy to tailor with immunostimulators. Stability and release kinetics correlate with a number of bilayers.	Not (yet) FDA-approved
Polyplexes	Nucleic acids	Protect nucleic acids, facilitate escape from the endosomal compartment.	Strong electrostatic interactions may hamper release of nucleic acids from the carrier
Liposomes	Proteins, peptides, nucleic acids	Good protection of antigens, facilitate intracellular uptake. Induction of both Th1 and Th2 responses.	Poorly immunogenic
Lipoplexes	Nucleic acids	Protect nucleic acids, facilitate escape from the endosomal compartment.	Might aggregation in the presence of serum

Table 3. Advantages and disadvantages of different non-viral delivery systems.

Nucleic acids, such a plasmid DNA (pDNA) or messenger RNA (mRNA), encoding viral proteins, can more easily cover the wide range of viral quasi species [189, 190]. As compared to pDNA, mRNA-based delivery may hold several advantages. First of all, mRNA is easier to engineer; there is no need for specific promoters and terminators to be present in the construct. Secondly, the synthesis of proteins encoded by mRNA is transient, which ensures a controlled antigen exposure [191]. Thirdly, in contrast to pDNA, mRNA does not need to cross the nuclear membrane to be effective and therefore offers the possibility to produce proteins in slow or non-dividing cells [192]. Furthermore, the use of mRNA excludes the risk of integration into the cell genome, eliminating possible insertional mutagenesis [189, 193]. For years, the application of mRNA has been hampered by a general believe that it is too labile to guarantee sufficient protein expression. Nowadays, however, mRNA vaccination strategies are being thoroughly investigated in the field of allergy [194, 195], cancer [193, 196-198] and HIV [109, 170, 171] immunotherapy. These studies mostly rely on the *ex vivo* electroporation of dendritic cells. We and others focus on complexing mRNA with cationic lipids and polymers (**figure 4**), which could protect mRNA. Moreover, we believe that complexing mRNA with cationic carriers might hold potential for their application *in vivo*. This approach could serve as an alternative for laborious *ex vivo* loading of DCs.

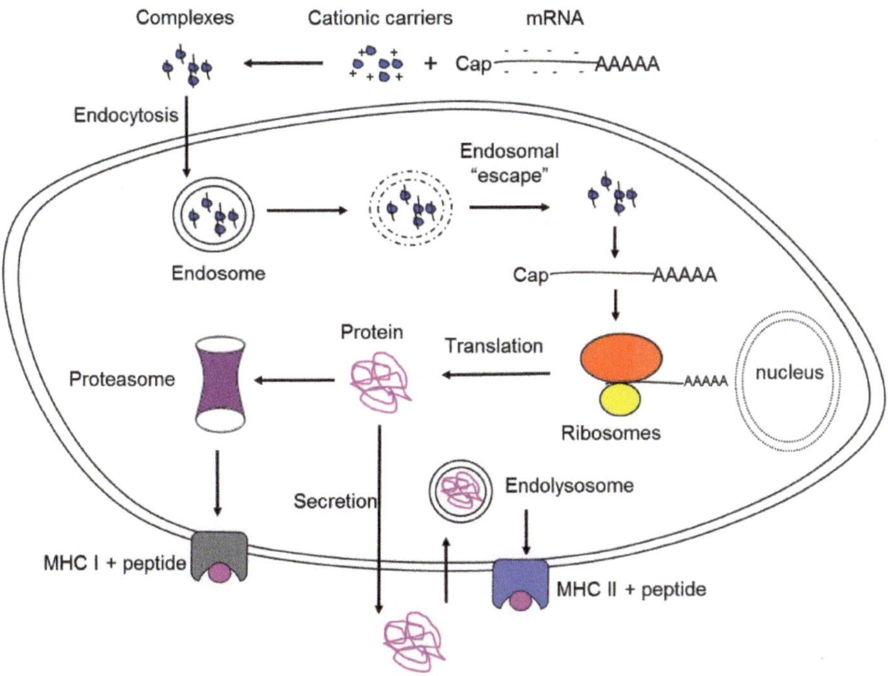

Figure 4. Internalisation and intracellular trafficking of mRNA/cationic carrier complexes. Negatively charged mRNA is complexed with cationic carriers (lipid or polymer based). After endocytosis, complexes end up in endosomes, from where they should release their cargo mRNA into the cytoplasm to enable translation by ribosomes .Translated protein is either secreted or can directly be processed via proteaseome to be presented with MHC class I. Secreted protein can be taken up and promote presentation in a MHC class II way after cleavage in the endolysosomes.

6.2. Polymer-based antigen delivery systems

Various polymers have been used to prepare nano- and micro- particles for antigen delivery. Here, we will focus on polymers that have shown to be promising in terms of immunotherapeutic vaccination.

6.2.1. Polymers based on lactic acid (PLA) and glycolic acid (PLGA)

The most studied polymers for antigen delivery in the context of vaccination are the biodegradable poly(D,L-lactide) (PLA) and poly(D,L-lactic-*co*-glycolic acid) (PLGA), which have been FDA approved for human use. These particles have mainly been evaluated for their potential to deliver proteins and peptides to DCs or macrophages with the aim to induce $CD8^+$ cytotoxic T cell immune responses in the context of prophylactic vaccination. It has been demonstrated that PLGA particles are phagocytosed by APCs [199] and ensure prolonged antigen presentation by DCs [200]. Whereas empty PLGA particles do not influence the maturation status of DCs [201, 202], DC activation can be induced, if the PLGA polymer is employed to encapsulate TLR ligands (poly I:C, MPLA) or surface loaded with anti-CD40 antibodies clear activation of DCs was observed [203-205]. PLA particles carrying p24 protein have been shown to induce both mucosal antibody production as well as CTL responses [206, 207].

The main drawback of these polymers is that some antigens tend to aggregate during the encapsulation process. Moreover, the exposure of proteins to organic solvents, required to dissolve the polymer, makes them highly susceptible to denaturation leading to the loss of antigenic epitope recognition [208]. This can partially be overcome by adsorption of proteins on the particle surface [209, 210]. Additionally, a rather expensive up-scaling process and clean-up procedure to ensure sterile production constitute difficult obstacles [211]. Due to the harsh preparation process and the hydrophobic nature of PLGA and PLA, these carriers are not suitable for nucleic acids delivery [212-214].

6.2.2. Polyelectrolyte microcapsules

Polyelectrolyte microcapsules (PeMCs) fabricated using a so-called layer-by-layer (LbL) technology are a relatively novel class of particles [215]. The process of their preparation is less harsh as compared to that of PLGA/PLA particles. A template containing an antigen and colloid nanoparticles is used as a sacrificial core. This core is coated with several bilayers of polymers of opposite charges. At the end of the procedure the template core is dissolved (**figure 5**). Since the encapsulation process is performed in a purely aqueous environment, minimal stress for a protein antigen is ensured. With appropriate choice of polymers, these particles can be fully biodegradable. De Koker *et al.* used ovalbumin as a model antigen and showed the benefit of antigen encapsulation in PeMCs to stimulate antigen presentation to T cells by murine bone marrow-derived DCs [186, 216].

PeMCs containing p24 and poly I:C (TLR-3 ligand) have been shown to be promising as an HIV-1 immunotherapeutic vaccine. Both antigen and maturation stimulus could be delivered in the same particle to DCs inducing maturation and stimulation of HIV-specific responses both *in vitro* and *in vivo* [184]. PeMCs were also used for the delivery of Gag-peptides to APCs. These APCs could activate SIV-specific T cells in an *ex vivo* non-human primate model [217]. Immune responses could be further improved by sensitizing the PeMCs to enzymatic or reductive degradation upon cellular uptake, thereby assuring release of its cargo [218, 219].

PeMCs have been also employed to deliver pDNA [213, 220]. When considering their use for the delivery of mRNA, however, one should make sure that the preparation process is rigorously RNase-free, which might present a challenge.

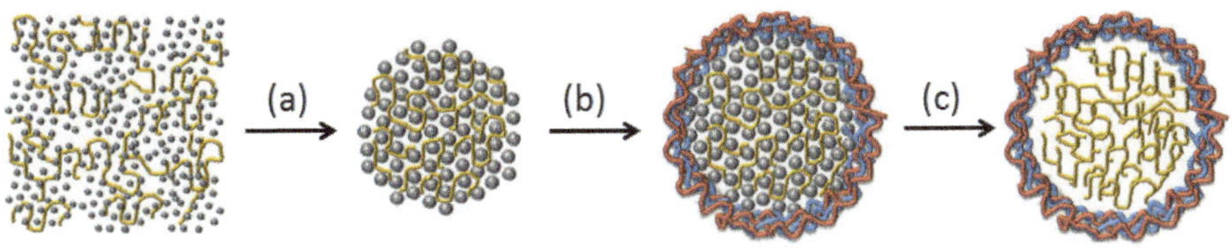

Figure 5. Preparation of polyelectrolyte microcapsule [186]. (a) In the first step an antigen (yellow) of interest is mixed with colloid nanoparticles (grey) to form a core template. (b) In the next step a layer of negatively charged polymer is deposited (blue). The non-adsorbed polymer is removed by washing. This is followed by applying a positively charged polymer (red) and another washing step. (c) When the desired number of polyelectrolyte layers is obtained, the core is dissolved.

6.2.3. Polyethyleneimine-based polyplexes

Polyethyleneimine (PEI) has been extensively used to deliver pDNA and siRNA to cells [221-223]. PEI consists of repeating units that contain two carbon atoms and a protonatable nitrogen atom. It exists in a linear or branched conformation (**figure 6**), both appearing in a broad range of molecular weights. PEI can efficiently bind pDNA to form so-called polyplexes. The linear form has been shown to release complexed pDNA more easily than the more stable branched form and thus results in higher transfection efficiencies [224]. The net positive charge of the polyplexes promotes their adhesion to the overall negative charge of the cellular membrane and facilitates their uptake. The protonatable units of PEI have a buffering capacity resulting in an influx of hydrogen ions into the endosomes upon polyplex uptake. Due to osmotic pressure thus building up, the endosomes are disrupted resulting in complex release into the cytosol [222, 225]. This mechanism of escape from the endosomes is called the proton sponge mechanism [226].

The group of Lisziewicz developed a therapeutic HIV vaccine, DermaVir, consisting of PEI-mannose complexed with pDNA encoding several HIV-1 antigens [227]. The vaccine was administered using a patch (DermaVir Patch) and was meant to target Langerhans cells (LCs) [174]. The vaccine induced specific and long lasting immune responses resulting in reduced viral load in SIV-infected macaques [228]. The safety of the vaccine formulation and of the delivery method was demonstrated in a phase I clinical trial in humans. A phase II clinical trial started in 2009 and aims at evaluating immunogenicity and efficacy of the vaccine in treatment-naïve and HAART-treated patients [229, 230].

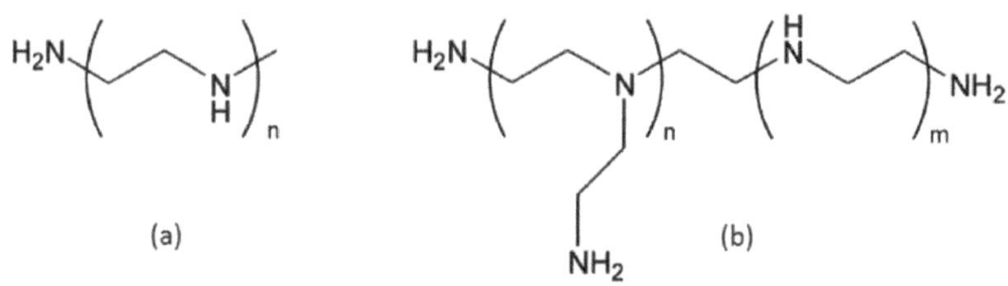

Figure 6. Structures of polyethyleneimine: (a) Linear backbone. (b) Branched backbone.

The main drawback of using PEI is its toxicity and non-specific interactions with cellular compartments. Another challenge is the aggregation of polyplexes in the presence of serum.

Rejman *et al.* reported that complexes made of mRNA and cationic lipids are much more efficient in transfecting different cell lines than PEI polyplexes. The authors suggest that this was likely due to the strong affinity of the polymer to mRNA impeding the release of the nucleic acid from the complexes. [191]. Bettinger *et al.* tested the potency of different protein derivatives for the delivery of mRNA. They demonstrated that complexing mRNA with short peptides results in better transfection efficiencies, likely due to a weaker electrostatic interaction with the nucleic acid. It should be noted, however, that the expression levels obtained were in general very low [192].

6.3. Lipid-based antigen delivery systems

6.3.1. Liposomes

Liposomes are spherical entities consisting of a phospholipid bilayer and an aqueous inner compartment. They have been used for drug delivery to treat cancer and infectious diseases. Until now, few liposomal formulations reached the pharmaceutical market of the U.S.A. Liposomes have been also employed to deliver antigens [231]. Given the liposome structure, the antigen can be encapsulated in its core (hydrophilic molecules) or accommodated within the lipid bilayer (hydrophobic molecules) [232]. It has been demonstrated that the lipid composition determines the immunogenicity of liposomes. For example, the incorporation of cationic lipids has been shown to elicit elevated CTL responses compared to neutral or anionic lipids [233]. Liposomal particles can be modified with specific ligands or antibodies to improve the uptake or to enhance/skew the immune response. Virosomes or virus like particles that consist of functional viral envelope proteins, anchored in a lipid membrane, have proven to be promising vaccine candidates [234]. Importantly, antigenic proteins encapsulated in liposomes can elicit both MHC I and II mediated immune responses as demonstrated by Zheng *et al.* [235]. These authors showed that HIV-1 Gag, Pol and Env proteins delivered to DCs by cationic liposomes induced stimulation of HIV-1 specific $CD8^+$ T cell responses. This was not observed when DCs were pulsed with the soluble proteins. It has been reported recently that mice immunized with Gag protein encapsulated in liposomes functionalized with lipid A induced both humoral and cellular immunity [236]. Another strategy to increase immunogenic potential of liposomal formulations involves the use of so-called lipopeptides. These structures consist of lipids linked to peptides that contain potential $CD4^+$ and $CD8^+$ T cell epitopes. These vaccines aim at the induction of strong T cell responses in HIV-1 infected patients [237-239]. Currently, a lipopeptide-pulsed DC vaccine is under evaluation in a phase I/II clinical trial in HAART-treated patients chronically infected with HIV-1 [240].

6.3.2 Cationic lipid based lipoplexes

The combination of positively charged lipids and negatively charged nucleic acids results in spontaneous formation of complexes called lipoplexes (**figure 7c**). These systems typically consist of two lipid species: a cationic lipid (such as DOTAP - 1,2-dioleoyl-3-trimethylammonium-propane) and a helper lipid with long unsaturated fatty acid chains (such as DOPE - dioleoylphosphatidylethanolamine) (**figure 7**). New cationic lipids are being synthesized almost daily aiming at introducing additional positive charges and reducing toxicity. Helper lipids are introduced to facilitate endosomal escape of these complexes [241].

The positive charge of lipoplexes promotes their cellular uptake, which was found to occur via clathrin-dependent and independent endocytosis [243-245]. The route of lipoplex uptake is determined by their size, chemical nature of the lipids and the cell line. After being internalised, the lipoplexes are located in endosomes. Escape from these compartments probably occurs via a mechanism proposed by Xu and Szoka [246]. It implies formation of neutral molecular pairs of lipoplex-derived cationic lipids and negatively charged phospholipids present in the endosomal membrane, eventually leading to release of the nucleic acid into the cytoplasm.

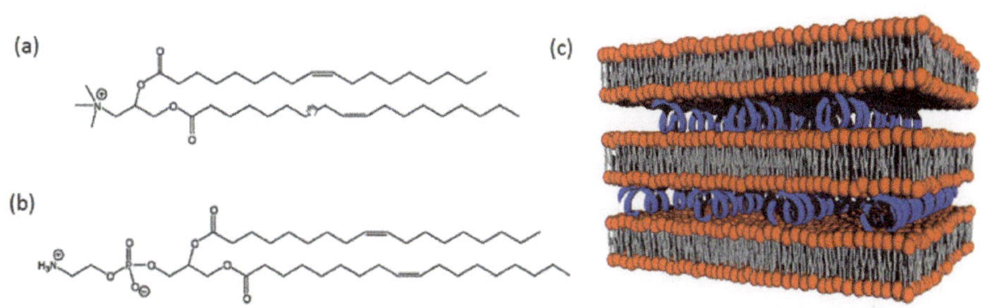

Figure 7. Chemical structures of DOTAP, cationic lipid, and DOPE, neutral helper lipid, used to form lipoplexes [213, 242]. DOTAP (a) and DOPE (b) contain a hydrophilic head group, a glycerol linker and two hydrophobic fatty acid chains. (c) Schematic representation of a lipoplex containing nucleic acids (blue) stabilized by bilayer of lipids: hydrophilic groups (red), hydrophobic fatty acid chain (grey).

Lipoplexes are mainly used to transfect primary cells or cell lines *in vitro*. However, since the rise of DNA vaccines, cationic lipids are considered as a versatile method to replace the hazardous viral vectors. In mice DNA lipoplexes have been shown to induce antitumor activity [247] and both antibody and Th1 cellular responses against hepatitis C virus [248, 249]. In the late eighties the first transfection with mRNA-lipoplexes was performed [250]. Generally it is established that mRNA transfection using non-viral cationic carriers is more efficient with cationic lipids than with cationic polymers [191, 192, 251, 252]. For both types of mRNA complexes the onset of protein expression was faster, but also lasted shorter than that produced by pDNA-complexes [191, 252]. The potential of mRNA-lipoplexes as an anti-cancer or influenza vaccine dates back to the nineties [253, 254]. Since then most anti-cancer and anti-virus immunotherapies have been focused on the *ex vivo* loading of DCs mainly by means of electroporation [109, 196, 198, 255, 256].

One of the most serious challenges of the use of lipoplexes is the extrapolation from the *in vitro* to the *in vivo* situation. Optimal transfection conditions are maintained *in vitro*, while *in vivo* lipoplexes encounter serum proteins causing their aggregation [257]. Depending on the target cells or tissue, this aggregation can either negatively or positively affect the uptake of the lipoplexes [258, 259]. Additional coating of the lipoplexes with polyethyleneglycol (PEG) can prevent the formation of aggregates [260], yet brings along other problems. Concerns have been raised that PEGylation of lipoplexes may be unfavorable in the context of vaccination as this could inhibit uptake of nanoparticles by APCs and negatively interfere with the release of complexes from the endosomal compartment [213]. However, a study performed by Singh and colleagues demonstrated that subcutaneous immunization of rabbits with PEGylated lipoplexes carrying a synthetic gp41 epitope of HIV-1 induced two times higher immune responses and prolonged persistence of antibodies than liposomes carrying epitopes without PEG moieties [261].

6.4. Targeting of DCs

Conceptually, particulate vaccines mimic the particulate nature of pathogens, including the size (nano- to micro-meter range), which facilitates their uptake by APCs. The actual size of the particles influences the uptake mechanism by APCs and the way of antigen presentation. Generally, larger particles are predominantly internalised via phagocytosis or macropinocytosis, while smaller particles are taken up by other endocytic mechanisms [262-264]. Internalisation through phagocytosis is known to lead to antigen cross-presentation in DCs [265, 266]. This emphasizes the enhanced potential of particulate antigen delivery to induce cellular immune responses as compared to soluble antigens, which are poorly cross-presented and preferentially presented via the MHC class II pathway.

Most nano- or microparticles can be functionalized with ligands or antibodies directed against cell surface receptors to target specific tissues or cells [267]. DCs express lectin-like receptors such as mannose receptor, DEC-205 and DC-SIGN which are believed to be involved in the phagocytosis of pathogens [268]. One way of increasing or promoting particle uptake by DCs is the attachment of mannose groups recognized by the mannose receptors present on DCs and macrophages. This has been shown to increase transfection efficiency of DNA-based vaccines [269, 270], antigen presentation following protein delivery [271] and the induction of cellular T cell responses in cancer and HIV immunotherapeutic strategies using lipoplexes and polyplexes [228, 270]. Another way of targeting is the use of ligands or antibodies directed against DEC-205 or DC-SIGN, which have shown potential to improve antigen uptake by immature and mature DCs [272-275]. It should be kept in mind, however, that attaching the desired ligand or protein is not always a straightforward process. The engraftment of chelator lipids on the surface of liposomes or lipoplexes, such as histidine tags, is crucial to ensure the functionality of the coupled target molecule [276-278]. In this context, the use of nanobodies directed against DCs could be of particular interest as they are mostly generated with a histidine tag for purification purposes. Alternatively, ligands could also be linked to liposomes via palmitoylation of the ligand [279].

In summary, targeting of particles may not only enhance efficacy but also the specificity of interaction with the surface receptors on DCs [179]. Moreover, coupling of specific adjuvants (e.g. TLR ligands), with the aim to promote the desired immune response, can also positively influence the uptake by DCs [280].

6.5. Co-delivery of antigens and adjuvants to improve immunogenicity of DCs

Although particulate antigen delivery improves antigen uptake and presentation by DCs, most particles are not immunogenic by themselves. This offers a possibility to use a specific adjuvant that can skew towards the desired type of immune responses [187]. Despite some positive results in animal models, one should be aware of the toxicity of potential immunomodulators in humans, that jeopardizes their clinical use [281]. Aluminum salts (referred to as alum) are the oldest and most widely used adjuvants for human vaccines. It has been shown that antigens can be precipitated with alum to form colloid particles, creating a depot effect after vaccination, that elicits strong humoral immune responses [282]. These results, together with further observations clearly showed that the physical linkage of antigen and immunomodulator is crucial to induce strong immune responses [182, 183, 283].

Immunostimulating complexes (ISCOMs) are another interesting delievery system. It is a sort of liposomal delivery vehicle with a built-in adjuvant. They are composed of a protein antigen, phosopholipids and the saponin Quil A adjuvant, derived from the bark of the *Quillaja saponaria*, a South American tree. It has been demonstrated that the use of ISCOMs improves CTL responses of influenza virus based vaccines [284, 285]. ISCOM-based vaccines have been tested in animal models and in clinical trials against cancer [286] and viral infections [287-289] [290, 291]. In all studies satisfactory safety and tolerance were shown and both humoral and cellular responses were induced.

Several studies have reported the use of ISCOMs as a system to deliver HIV or SIV antigens. In non-human primate models, incorporation of HIV or SIV peptides into ISCOMs has been shown to induce protective immunity [288, 292, 293]. Moreover, studies in mice demonstrated that ISCOMs can be used to elicit immune responses against HIV-1 antigens [287]. To generate mucosal immunity, Koopman and colleagues immunized rhesus maquaqes intranasally or via lymph nodes with HIV-1 peptides formulated into PR8-Flu ISCOMs [294]. Intranodal injection of these ISCOMs induced strong systemic and mucosal immune responses. In contrast, intranasal application resulted in very weak responses. Currently, ISCOM-based vaccines have been approved for veterinary use and are undergoing clinical trials for human use [295].

As described before, for an optimal immune response it is crucial that DCs, besides actively taking up the antigen, undergo activation and maturation to stimulate effective T cell responses. Ligands mimicking PAMPs that can target PPRs are therefore of potential interest. Extracellular and intracellular PPRs are divided into four groups: TLRs, NLRs, CLRs and RLRs [181]. Depending on the receptor that is triggered, DCs produce and secrete various sets of cytokines, determining the type of immune response [296]. Moreover, the incorporation of TLR ligands promotes phagocytosis of APCs [280]. TLRs represent the majority of PPRs studied in the development of effective adjuvants [281]. TLRs can be divided into two groups: the surface bound receptors (TLR 1, 2, 4, 5, 6) and the intracellular receptors present in the endosomes (TLR 3, 7, 8, 9) (**table 4**).

TLR	TLR ligand	DC subset	Effect of activation
1:2	Triacyl lipoproteins	Mo-DCs, myeloid DCs	Upregulation of CCR7, IL-6, IL-10, IL-12p70,TNF-α
2	Lipoproteins	Mo-DCs, myeloid DCs	Upregulation of CCR7, IL-6, IL-10, IL-12p70,TNF-α
3	Double stranded RNA	Mo-DCs, myeloid DCs	IFN-α/β activation and up-regulation IL-12p70
4	Lipopolysaccharide	Mo-DCs, myeloid DCs	Upregulation of CD80, CD86, CD83, CCR7. Secretion of IL-6, IL-8, IL-10, IL-12p70, IFN-β
5	Flagellin	Mo-DCs, myeloid DCs	Upregulation of CD80, CD86, CD83, CCR7. Secretion IFN-α/β , IL-1 , TNF-α, IL-8, IL-12p40
6:2	Triacyl lipoproteins	Mo-DCs, myeloid DCs	Upregulation of CCR7, IL-6, IL-10, IL-12p70,TNF-α
7	Single stranded mRNA	pDC, myeloid DCs	Upregulation of CCR7,CD40, CD80 and CD86. Secretion of IL-12p70 (myeloid DCs). Secretion of IFN-α (pDCs).
8	Single stranded mRNA	Mo-DCs	Increased TNF , IL-8, IL-12p40, MCP-1, CCL2, CCL3, CCL4, CCL5
9	Double stranded DNA	pDC	Upregulation of CD40, CD80, CD86, CD83, HLA-DR, CCR7. Upregulation of IFN-α (very high), IFN-β (lower), IL-6, TNF-α (low), IL-8

Table 4. Overview of Toll like receptors (TLRs) with their ligands and effect of activation [297].

The extracellular TLRs mainly recognize bacterial invaders, but also fungi and some enveloped viruses. Bacterial lipoproteins are recognized by the heterodimers TLR1:2 (triacyl lipoproteins) and TLR2:6 (diacyl lipoproteins). Liposomes engrafted with palmitoyl chain lipopeptides have been shown to up-regulate DC maturation markers *in vitro* [298]. Lipopolysaccharide (LPS), a gram negative bacterial carbohydrate, is recognized by TLR4. Recently, a phase I clinical trial has started evaluating the potential of autologous dendritic cells, *ex vivo* loaded with lipopeptides and activated with LPS, as an immunotherapy in HIV infected patients (NCT00796770). Lipopolysaccharide (LPS), a gram negative bacterial carbohydrate, is recognized by TLR4. Since the *in vivo* use of LPS for human purposes is not possible due to the risk of septic shocks, a derivative, monophosphoryl lipid A from *Salmonella Minnesota* referred to as MPLA, was proposed as a substitute. It has been shown to be less toxic than LPS and thus preferable for human vaccine applications. MPLA has been incorporated in PLGA particles and liposomes [299, 300]. Furthermore, MPLA is already used in combination with alum (AS04) as an adjuvant in Cervarix®, a human papilloma virus vaccine from GlaxoSmithKline. Another bacterial component, flagellin, is recognized by TLR5 and is also used as a potential adjuvant. Flagellin-related peptides containing a His-tag and incorporated in liposomes containing a tumor antigen, induced antitumor responses resulting in complete tumor regression in mice [278]. The advantage of flagellin is that it can be co-integrated as a protein into particulate vehicles or integrated as His-tagged peptides into liposomes.

The intracellular TLRs specifically recognize nucleic acids and are of major importance to the recognition of double stranded DNA (dsDNA) from viral or bacterial intruders. TLR-9, only expressed in pDCs, recognizes unmethylated cytosine-phosphate-guanine (CpG) oligodeoxynucleotides (ODNs). CpG motifs were demonstrated to induce cell-mediated responses *in vivo* when incorporated into PLGA particles [301, 302], liposomes [303] and other microparticles [304]. All these studies reported enhanced Th1 biased immune responses. Viral single stranded RNA (ssRNA) is recognized by TLR7 (expressed by all DC subsets and B-cells) and TLR8 (expressed by macrophages, monocytes and myeloid DCs) [181]. Agonists used to trigger these receptors are the synthetic imidazoquinoline drug compounds imiquimod and resiquimod (R848) or polyuridylic acid (polyU). Only few studies so far have used TLR7/8 ligands for particulate antigen delivery. Johnston *et al.* demonstrated that the combination of TLR 7 ligand with liposomes increased the cellular immune responses against OVA protein in a mice model [305]. Another study reported that co-encapsulation of OVA antigen and polyU in PLA-DOTAP microparticles increased the antibody titers and numbers of IFN-γ secreting T cells [306]. Finally, the endosomal TLR3 recognizes dsRNA, which can be mimicked by the synthetic polyinosinic:polycytidylic acid (poly I:C). This dsRNA analog is widely evaluated as a potential adjuvant since it strongly promotes the maturation of DCs [184, 204]. Furthermore, the combination of poly I:C with protein antigens encapsulated in either polymeric [183, 184, 307] or liposomal [308] particles favors enhanced Th1 immune responses. With regard to mRNA vaccination, the use of endosomal TLR ligands is problematic, since upon recognition by their receptor, high levels of type I interferon are produced leading to the activation of RNases [309, 310]. However, mRNA by itself can also trigger endosomal TLRs, implying the crucial importance of stabilizing the antigen encoding mRNA (reviewed by Tavernier *et al.*) [189].

Another possibility to improve immunogenicity is the addition of co-stimulatory molecules. The addition of CD40L to DCs loaded with liposome-complexed HIV-1 proteins could prime HIV-1 specific $CD8^{+}$ T cells *in vitro* [162]. Within the scope of mRNA transfection, mRNA encoding co-stimulatory molecules can be co-transfected with mRNA encoding an antigen, which has been shown to strongly enhance the capacity of electroporated DCs to stimulate HIV-specific T cell responses [311].

7. Concluding remarks

Ex vivo loading of DCs shows promising results as an immunotherapy for HIV and cancer. However, the currently applied strategy is not applicable on a large scale, especially in Africa where the largest incidence of HIV infections is observed. The use of particulate vehicles able to directly deliver the antigen of interest, be it proteins, peptides or nucleic acids, into DCs *in vivo* is a very attractive concept. Different antigen formulations can be further tailored with targeting antibodies or immunomodulatory ligands to promote uptake by DCs and to trigger the desired type of immune response. In the context of HIV immunotherapy a large number of epitopes needs to cover a broad panel of quasi species. Therefore, mRNA-based vaccination strategies present an attractive option. In contrast to pDNA, mRNA needs to be delivered only into the cytoplasm and induces transient antigen expression without the risk of genomic insertion. Further research will be required for designing an optimal carrier system preferably comprising an adjuvant, necessary to achieve strong HIV-specific CTL responses with the ultimate goal to control viral replication in the absence of additional HAART therapy.

Author details

Winni De Haes

Institute of Tropical Medicine of Antwerp, Department of Biomedical Sciences, Virology Unit, Antwerp, Belgium

Charlotte Pollard

Institute of Tropical Medicine of Antwerp, Department of Biomedical Sciences, Virology Unit, Antwerp, Belgium
Laboratory of Molecular Immunology, Ghent University, Belgium

Guido Vanham

Institute of Tropical Medicine of Antwerp, Department of Biomedical Sciences, Virology Unit, Antwerp, Belgium
Faculty of Pharmaceutical, Veterinary and Biomedical Sciences, University of Antwerp, Belgium
Faculty of Medicine and Pharmacology, Vrije Universiteit Brussel, Belgium

Joanna Rejman

Laboratory of General Biochemistry and Physical Pharmacy, Ghent University, Belgium

Acknowledgement

This work was supported by grants from IUAP (Inter-University Attraction Poles, P6/41 of the Belgian government), FWO (Fund for Scientific Research Flanders, project number G.0226.10) and SOFI-B (Secondary Research Funding ITM). W. De Haes is a doctoral fellow of the Institute for Science and Technology (IWT), Flanders. There is no conflict of interest.

8. References

[1] Barre-Sinoussi F, Chermann JC, Rey F, Nugeyre MT, Chamaret S, Gruest J, et al. Isolation of a T-lymphotropic retrovirus from a patient at risk for acquired immune deficiency syndrome (AIDS). Science. 1983;220(4599):868-71.

[2] Gallo RC, Sarin PS, Gelmann EP, Robert-Guroff M, Richardson E, Kalyanaraman VS, et al. Isolation of human T-cell leukemia virus in acquired immune deficiency syndrome (AIDS). Science. 1983;220(4599):865-7.

[3] UNAIDS. UNAIDS Global report 2010. wwwunaidsorg. 2010.

[4] Coffin J, Haase A, Levy JA, Montagnier L, Oroszlan S, Teich N, et al. Human immunodeficiency viruses. Science. 1986;232(4751):697.

[5] Haseltine WA. Molecular biology of the human immunodeficiency virus type 1. FASEB J. 1991;5(10):2349-60.

[6] Gotte M, Li X, Wainberg MA. HIV-1 reverse transcription: a brief overview focused on structure-function relationships among molecules involved in initiation of the reaction. Arch Biochem Biophys. 1999;365(2):199-210.

[7] Farnet CM, Haseltine WA. Determination of viral proteins present in the human immunodeficiency virus type 1 preintegration complex. J Virol. 1991;65(4):1910-5.

[8] Sierra S, Kupfer B, Kaiser R. Basics of the virology of HIV-1 and its replication. J Clin Virol. 2005;34(4):233-44.

[9] Jaffe HW, Bregman DJ, Selik RM. Acquired immune deficiency syndrome in the United States: the first 1,000 cases. J Infect Dis. 1983;148(2):339-45.

[10] Levy JA. HIV pathogenesis: 25 years of progress and persistent challenges. AIDS. 2009;23(2):147-60.

[11] Guadalupe M, Reay E, Sankaran S, Prindiville T, Flamm J, McNeil A, et al. Severe CD4+ T-cell depletion in gut lymphoid tissue during primary human immunodeficiency virus type 1 infection and substantial delay in restoration following highly active antiretroviral therapy. J Virol. 2003;77(21):11708-17.

[12] Cowley S. The biology of HIV infection. Lepr Rev. 2001;72(2):212-20.

[13] Pantaleo G, Fauci AS. Immunopathogenesis of HIV infection. Annu Rev Microbiol. 1996;50:825-54.

[14] Buchbinder S, Vittinghoff E. HIV-infected long-term nonprogressors: epidemiology, mechanisms of delayed progression, and clinical and research implications. Microbes Infect. 1999;1(13):1113-20.

[15] Saez-Cirion A, Pancino G, Sinet M, Venet A, Lambotte O. HIV controllers: how do they tame the virus? Trends Immunol. 2007;28(12):532-40.

[16] Shearer G, Clerici M. Historical perspective on HIV-exposed seronegative individuals: has nature done the experiment for us? J Infect Dis. 2010;202 (Suppl 3):329-32.

[17] Palella FJ, Delaney K, Moorman A, Loveless M, Fuhrer J, Satten G, et al. Declining morbidity and mortality among patients with advanced human immunodeficiency virus infection. HIV Outpatient Study Investigators. N Engl J Med. 1998;338(13):853-60.

[18] Pomerantz RJ, Horn DL. Twenty years of therapy for HIV-1 infection. Nat Med. 2003 Jul;9(7):867-73.

[19] Friis-Moller N, Reiss P, Sabin CA, Weber R, Monforte AdA, El-Sadr W, et al. Class of antiretroviral drugs and the risk of myocardial infarction. N Engl J Med. 2007;356(17):1723-35.

[20] Hawkins T. Understanding and managing the adverse effects of antiretroviral therapy. Antiviral Res. 2010 Jan;85(1):201-9.

[21] Carr A, Samaras K, Thorisdottir A, Kaufmann GR, Chisholm DJ, Cooper DA. Diagnosis, prediction, and natural course of HIV-1 protease-inhibitor-associated lipodystrophy, hyperlipidaemia, and diabetes mellitus: a cohort study. Lancet. 1999;353(9170):2093-9.

[22] Autran B, Carcelaint G, Li TS, Gorochov G, Blanc C, Renaud M, et al. Restoration of the immune system with anti-retroviral therapy. Immunol Lett. 1999;66(1-3):207-11.

[23] Day CL, Kaufmann DE, Kiepiela P, Brown JA, Moodley ES, Reddy S, et al. PD-1 expression on HIV-specific T cells is associated with T-cell exhaustion and disease progression. Nature. 2006;443(7109):350-4.

[24] Liu Z, Cumberland WG, Hultin LE, Prince HE, Detels R, Giorgi JV. Elevated CD38 antigen expression on CD8+ T cells is a stronger marker for the risk of chronic HIV disease progression to AIDS and death in the Multicenter AIDS Cohort Study than CD4+ cell count, soluble immune activation markers, or combinations of HLA-DR and CD38 expression. J Acquir Immune Defic Syndr Hum Retrovirol. 1997;16(2):83-92.

[25] Brenchley JM, Price DA, Schacker TW, Asher TE, Silvestri G, Rao S, et al. Microbial translocation is a cause of systemic immune activation in chronic HIV infection. Nat Med. 2006;12(12):1365-71.

[26] Mandl JN, Barry AP, Vanderford TH, Kozyr N, Chavan R, Klucking S, et al. Divergent TLR7 and TLR9 signaling and type I interferon production distinguish pathogenic and nonpathogenic AIDS virus infections. Nat Med. 2008;14(10):1077-87.

[27] Harris LD, Tabb B, Sodora DL, Paiardini M, Klatt NR, Douek DC, et al. Downregulation of robust acute type I interferon responses distinguishes nonpathogenic simian immunodeficiency virus (SIV) infection of natural hosts from pathogenic SIV infection of rhesus macaques. J Virol. 2010;84(15):7886-91.

[28] Silvestri G, Sodora DL, Koup RA, Paiardini M, O'Neil SP, McClure HM, et al. Nonpathogenic SIV infection of sooty mangabeys is characterized by limited bystander immunopathology despite chronic high-level viremia. Immunity. 2003;18(3):441-52.

[29] Sempere JM, Soriano V, Benito JM. T regulatory cells and HIV infection. AIDS Rev. 2007;9(1):54-60.
[30] Epple H-J, Loddenkemper C, Kunkel D, Troger H, Maul J, Moos V, et al. Mucosal but not peripheral FOXP3+ regulatory T cells are highly increased in untreated HIV infection and normalize after suppressive HAART. Blood. 2006;108(9):3072-8.
[31] Burton DR. Antibodies, viruses and vaccines. Nat Rev Immunol. 2002;2(9):706-13.
[32] Wei X, Decker JM, Wang S, Hui H, Kappes JC, Wu X, et al. Antibody neutralization and escape by HIV-1. Nature. 2003;422(6929):307-12.
[33] Stamatatos L, Morris L, Burton DR, Mascola JR. Neutralizing antibodies generated during natural HIV-1 infection: good news for an HIV-1 vaccine? Nat Med. 2009;15(8):866-70.
[34] Aasa-Chapman MMI, Holuigue S, Aubin K, Wong M, Jones NA, Cornforth D, et al. Detection of antibody-dependent complement-mediated inactivation of both autologous and heterologous virus in primary human immunodeficiency virus type 1 infection. J Virol. 2005;79(5):2823-30.
[35] Hessell AJ, Hangartner L, Hunter M, Havenith CEG, Beurskens FJ, Bakker JM, et al. Fc receptor but not complement binding is important in antibody protection against HIV. Nature. 2007;449(7158):101-4.
[36] McMichael AJ, Rowland-Jones SL. Cellular immune responses to HIV. Nature. 2001;410(6831):980-7.
[37] Gehri R, Hahn S, Rothen M, Steuerwald M, Nuesch R, Erb P. The Fas receptor in HIV infection: expression on peripheral blood lymphocytes and role in the depletion of T cells. AIDS. 1996;10(1):9-16.
[38] Saksena NK, Wu JQ, Potter SJ, Wilkinson J, Wang B. Human immunodeficiency virus interactions with CD8+ T lymphocytes. Curr HIV Res. 2008;6(1):1-9.
[39] Bernardin F, Kong D, Peddada L, Baxter-Lowe LA, Delwart E. Human immunodeficiency virus mutations during the first month of infection are preferentially found in known cytotoxic T-lymphocyte epitopes. J Virol. 2005;79(17):11523-8.
[40] Collins KL, Chen BK, Kalams SA, Walker BD, Baltimore D. HIV-1 Nef protein protects infected primary cells against killing by cytotoxic T lymphocytes. Nature. 1998;391(6665):397-401.
[41] Rosenberg ES, Billingsley JM, Caliendo AM, Boswell SL, Sax PE, Kalams SA, et al. Vigorous HIV-1-specific CD4+ T cell responses associated with control of viremia. Science. 1997;278(5342):1447-50.
[42] Lichterfeld M, Kaufmann DE, Yu XG, Mui SK, Addo MM, Johnston MN, et al. Loss of HIV-1-specific CD8+ T cell proliferation after acute HIV-1 infection and restoration by vaccine-induced HIV-1-specific CD4+ T cells. J Exp Med. 2004;200(6):701-12.
[43] Jin X, Bauer DE, Tuttleton SE, Lewin S, Gettie A, Blanchard J, et al. Dramatic rise in plasma viremia after CD8(+) T cell depletion in simian immunodeficiency virus-infected macaques. J Exp Med. 1999;189(6):991-8.

[44] Schmitz JE, Kuroda MJ, Santra S, Sasseville VG, Simon MA, Lifton MA, et al. Control of viremia in simian immunodeficiency virus infection by CD8+ lymphocytes. Science. 1999;283(5403):857-60.

[45] Feeney ME, Tang Y, Roosevelt K, Leslie A, McIntosh K, Karthas N, et al. Immune escape precedes breakthrough human immunodeficiency virus type 1 viremia and broadening of the cytotoxic T-lymphocyte response in an HLA-B27-positive long-term-nonprogressing child. J Virol. 2004;78(16):8927-30.

[46] Kemal KS, Beattie T, Dong T, Weiser B, Kaul R, Kuiken C, et al. Transition from long-term nonprogression to HIV-1 disease associated with escape from cellular immune control. J Acquir Immune Defic Syndr. 2008;48(2):119-26.

[47] Samson M, Libert F, Doranz BJ, Rucker J, Liesnard C, Farber CM, et al. Resistance to HIV-1 infection in caucasian individuals bearing mutant alleles of the CCR-5 chemokine receptor gene. Nature. 1996;382(6593):722-5.

[48] Hutter G, Ganepola S. Eradication of HIV by transplantation of CCR5-deficient hematopoietic stem cells. ScientificWorldJournal. 2011;11:1068-76.

[49] Hutter G, Nowak D, Mossner M, Ganepola S, Mussig A, Allers K, et al. Long-term control of HIV by CCR5 Delta32/Delta32 stem-cell transplantation. N Engl J Med. 2009;360(7):692-8.

[50] Chiu Y-L, Greene WC. Multifaceted antiviral actions of APOBEC3 cytidine deaminases. Trends Immunol. 2006;27(6):291-7.

[51] Croxford JL, Gasser S. Damage control: how HIV survives the editor APOBEC3G. Nat Immunol. 2011;12(10):925-7.

[52] Ulenga NK, Sarr AD, Thakore-Meloni S, Sankale J-L, Eisen G, Kanki PJ. Relationship between human immunodeficiency type 1 infection and expression of human APOBEC3G and APOBEC3F. J Infect Dis. 2008;198(4):486-92.

[53] Johnson WE, Sawyer SL. Molecular evolution of the antiretroviral TRIM5 gene. Immunogenetics. 2009;61(3):163-76.

[54] Neil SJD, Zang T, Bieniasz PD. Tetherin inhibits retrovirus release and is antagonized by HIV-1 Vpu. Nature. 2008;451(7177):425-30.

[55] Bailey JR, Williams TM, Siliciano RF, Blankson JN. Maintenance of viral suppression in HIV-1-infected HLA-B*57+ elite suppressors despite CTL escape mutations. J Exp Med. 2006;203(5):1357-69.

[56] Kiepiela P, Leslie AJ, Honeyborne I, Ramduth D, Thobakgale C, Chetty S, et al. Dominant influence of HLA-B in mediating the potential co-evolution of HIV and HLA. Nature. 2004;432(7018):769-75.

[57] Migueles SA, Sabbaghian MS, Shupert WL, Bettinotti MP, Marincola FM, Martino L, et al. HLA B*5701 is highly associated with restriction of virus replication in a subgroup of HIV-infected long term nonprogressors. Proc Natl Acad Sci U S A. 2000;97(6):2709-14.

[58] Martin MP, Qi Y, Gao X, Yamada E, Martin JN, Pereyra F, et al. Innate partnership of HLA-B and KIR3DL1 subtypes against HIV-1. Nat Genet. 2007;39(6):733-40.

[59] Qi Y, Martin MP, Gao X, Jacobson L, Goedert JJ, Buchbinder S, et al. KIR/HLA pleiotropism: protection against both HIV and opportunistic infections. PLoS Pathog. 2006;2(8):79.

[60] Devito C, Broliden K, Kaul R, Svensson L, Johansen K, Kiama P, et al. Mucosal and plasma IgA from HIV-1-exposed uninfected individuals inhibit HIV-1 transcytosis across human epithelial cells. J Immunol. 2000;165(9):5170-6.

[61] Kaul R, Trabattoni D, Bwayo JJ, Arienti D, Zagliani A, Mwangi FM, et al. HIV-1-specific mucosal IgA in a cohort of HIV-1-resistant Kenyan sex workers. AIDS. 1999;13(1):23-9.

[62] Mazzoli S, Trabattoni D, Lo Caputo S, Piconi S, Ble C, Meacci F, et al. HIV-specific mucosal and cellular immunity in HIV-seronegative partners of HIV-seropositive individuals. Nat Med. 1997;3(11):1250-7.

[63] Gupta P, Balachandran R, Ho M, Enrico A, Rinaldo C. Cell-to-cell transmission of human immunodeficiency virus type 1 in the presence of azidothymidine and neutralizing antibody. J Virol. 1989;63(5):2361-5.

[64] El-Far M, Halwani R, Said E, Trautmann L, Doroudchi M, Janbazian L, et al. T-cell exhaustion in HIV infection. Curr HIV/AIDS Rep. 2008;5(1):13-9.

[65] Almeida JR, Sauce D, Price DA, Papagno L, Shin SY, Moris A, et al. Antigen sensitivity is a major determinant of CD8+ T-cell polyfunctionality and HIV-suppressive activity. Blood. 2009;113(25):6351-60.

[66] Almeida JR, Price DA, Papagno L, Arkoub ZA, Sauce D, Bornstein E, et al. Superior control of HIV-1 replication by CD8+ T cells is reflected by their avidity, polyfunctionality, and clonal turnover. J Exp Med. 2007;204(10):2473-85.

[67] Derby M, Alexander-Miller M, Tse R, Berzofsky J. High-avidity CTL exploit two complementary mechanisms to provide better protection against viral infection than low-avidity CTL. J Immunol. 2001;166(3):1690-7.

[68] Zimmerli SC, Harari A, Cellerai C, Vallelian F, Bart P-A, Pantaleo G. HIV-1-specific IFN-gamma/IL-2-secreting CD8 T cells support CD4-independent proliferation of HIV-1-specific CD8 T cells. PNAS. 2005;102(20):7239-44.

[69] Betts MR, Nason MC, West SM, De Rosa SC, Migueles SA, Abraham J, et al. HIV nonprogressors preferentially maintain highly functional HIV-specific CD8+ T cells. Blood. 2006 Jun 15;107(12):4781-9.

[70] Geldmacher C, Currier JR, Herrmann E, Haule A, Kuta E, McCutchan F, et al. CD8 T-cell recognition of multiple epitopes within specific Gag regions is associated with maintenance of a low steady-state viremia in human immunodeficiency virus type 1-seropositive patients. J Virol. 2007;81(5):2440-8.

[71] Martinez-Picado J, Prado JG, Fry EE, Pfafferott K, Leslie A, Chetty S, et al. Fitness cost of escape mutations in p24 Gag in association with control of human immunodeficiency virus type 1. J Virol. 2006;80(7):3617-23.

[72] Sanchez-Merino V, Farrow MA, Brewster F, Somasundaran M, Luzuriaga K. Identification and characterization of HIV-1 CD8+ T cell escape variants with impaired fitness. J Infect Dis. 2008;197(2):300-8.

[73] Schneidewind A, Brockman MA, Yang R, Adam RI, Li B, Le Gall S, et al. Escape from the dominant HLA-B27-restricted cytotoxic T-lymphocyte response in Gag is associated with a dramatic reduction in human immunodeficiency virus type 1 replication. J Virol. 2007;81(22):12382-93.

[74] Harari A, Petitpierre S, Vallelian F, Pantaleo G. Skewed representation of functionally distinct populations of virus-specific CD4 T cells in HIV-1-infected subjects with progressive disease: changes after antiretroviral therapy. Blood. 2004;103(3):966-72.

[75] Makedonas G, Betts MR. Living in a house of cards: re-evaluating CD8 T-cell immune correlates against HIV. Immunol Rev. 2011;239(1):109-24.

[76] Deacon NJ, Tsykin A, Solomon A, Smith K, Ludford-Menting M, Hooker DJ, et al. Genomic structure of an attenuated quasi species of HIV-1 from a blood transfusion donor and recipients. Science. 1995;270(5238):988-91.

[77] Walker BD, Burton DR. Toward an AIDS vaccine. Science. 2008;320:760-4.

[78] Wijesundara DK, Jackson RJ, Ramshaw IA, Ranasinghe C. Human immunodeficiency virus-1 vaccine design: where do we go now? Immunol Cell Biol. 2011;89:367-74.

[79] Hirbod T, Broliden K. Mucosal immune responses in the genital tract of HIV-1-exposed uninfected women. J Intern Med. 2007;262:44-58.

[80] Hessell AJ, Rakasz EG, Poignard P, Hangartner L, Landucci G, Forthal DN, et al. Broadly neutralizing human anti-HIV antibody 2G12 is effective in protection against mucosal SHIV challenge even at low serum neutralizing titers. PLoS Pathog. 2009;5(5):e1000433.

[81] Ruprecht RM, Hofmann-Lehmann R, Smith-Franklin BA, Rasmussen RA, Liska V, Vlasak J, et al. Protection of neonatal macaques against experimental SHIV infection by human neutralizing monoclonal antibodies. Transfus Clin Biol. 2001;8:350-8.

[82] Reynolds MR, Weiler AM, Weisgrau KL, Piaskowski SM, Furlott JR, Weinfurter JT, et al. Macaques vaccinated with live-attenuated SIV control replication of heterologous virus. J Exp Med. 2008;205:2537-50.

[83] Burton DR, Desrosiers RC, Doms RW, Koff WC, Kwong PD, Moore JP, et al. HIV vaccine design and the neutralizing antibody problem. Nat Immunol. 2004;5:233-6.

[84] Roux KH, Taylor KA. AIDS virus envelope spike structure. Curr Opin Struct Biol. 2007;17:244-52.

[85] Derby NR, Kraft Z, Kan E, Crooks E, Barnett S, Srivastava I, et al. Antibody responses elicited in macaques immunized with human immunodeficiency virus type 1 (HIV-1) SF162-derived gp140 envelope immunogens: comparison with those elicited during homologous simian/human immunodeficiency virus SHIVSF162P4 and heterologous HIV-1 infection. J Virol. 2006;80(17):8745-62.

[86] Wilson NA, Reed J, Napoe G, Piaskowski S, Szymanski A, Furlott J, et al. Vaccine-induced cellular immune responses reduce plasma viral concentrations after repeated low-dose challenge with pathogenic simian immunodeficiency virus SIVmac239. J Virol. 2006;80(12):5875-85.

[87] Genescà M. Characterization of an effective CTL response against HIV and SIV infections. J Biomed Biotechnol. 2011;2011:103924.
[88] Cheynier R, Langlade-Demoyen P, Marescot MR, Blanche S, Blondin G, Wain-Hobson S, et al. Cytotoxic T lymphocyte responses in the peripheral blood of children born to human immunodeficiency virus-1-infected mothers. Eur J Immunol. 1992;22:2211-7.
[89] Schenal M, Lo Caputo S, Fasano F, Vichi F, Saresella M, Pierotti P, et al. Distinct patterns of HIV-specific memory T lymphocytes in HIV-exposed uninfected individuals and in HIV-infected patients. AIDS. 2005;19:653-61.
[90] Jennes W, Vuylsteke B, Borget M-Y, Traore-Ettiegne V, Maurice C, Nolan M, et al. HIV-specific T helper responses and frequency of exposure among HIV-exposed seronegative female sex workers in Abidjan, Cote d'Ivoire. J Infect Dis. 2004;189:602-10.
[91] Kaul R, Dong T, Plummer FA, Kimani J, Rostron T, Kiama P, et al. CD8(+) lymphocytes respond to different HIV epitopes in seronegative and infected subjects. J Clin Invest. 2001;107:1303-10.
[92] McElrath MJ, Haynes BF. Induction of immunity to human immunodeficiency virus type-1 by vaccination. Immunity. 2010;33:542-54.
[93] Goepfert PA, Tomaras GD, Horton H, Montefiori D, Ferrari G, Deers M, et al. Durable HIV-1 antibody and T-cell responses elicited by an adjuvanted multi-protein recombinant vaccine in uninfected human volunteers. Vaccine. 2007;25:510-18.
[94] Jones NG, DeCamp A, Gilbert P, Peterson ML, Gurwith M, Cao H. AIDSVAX immunization induces HIV-specific CD8+ T-cell responses in high-risk, HIV-negative volunteers who subsequently acquire HIV infection. Vaccine. 2009;27:1136-40.
[95] Taneichi M, Tanaka Y, Kakiuchi T, Uchida T. Liposome-coupled peptides induce long-lived memory CD8 T cells without CD4 T cells. PLoS One. 2010;5(11):e15091.
[96] Doan LX, Li M, Chen C, Yao Q. Virus-like particles as HIV-1 vaccines. Rev Med Virol. 2005;15:75-88.
[97] Papagno L, Alter G, Assoumou L, Murphy RL, Garcia F, Clotet B, et al. Comprehensive analysis of virus-specific T-cells provides clues for the failure of therapeutic immunization with ALVAC-HIV vaccine. Aids. 2011 Jan 2;25(1):27-36.
[98] Sandstrom E, Nilsson C, Hejdeman B, Brave A, Bratt G, Robb M, et al. Broad immunogenicity of a multigene, multiclade HIV-1 DNA vaccine boosted with heterologous HIV-1 recombinant modified vaccinia virus Ankara. J Infect Dis. 2008;198:1482-90.
[99] Peters BS, Jaoko W, Vardas E, Panayotakopoulos G, Fast P, Schmidt C, et al. Studies of a prophylactic HIV-1 vaccine candidate based on modified vaccinia virus Ankara (MVA) with and without DNA priming: effects of dosage and route on safety and immunogenicity. Vaccine. 2007;25:2120-7.
[100] Wang S, Kennedy JS, West K, Montefiori DC, Coley S, Lawrence J, et al. Cross-subtype antibody and cellular immune responses induced by a polyvalent DNA prime-protein boost HIV-1 vaccine in healthy human volunteers. Vaccine. 2008;26:1098-110.

[101] Connolly NC, Whiteside TL, Wilson C, Kondragunta V, Rinaldo CR, Riddler SA. Therapeutic immunization with human immunodeficiency virus type 1 (HIV-1) peptide-loaded dendritic cells is safe and induces immunogenicity in HIV-1-infected individuals. Clin Vaccine Immunol. 2008 Feb;15(2):284-92.

[102] Gandhi RT, O'Neill D, Bosch RJ, Chan ES, Bucy RP, Shopis J, et al. A randomized therapeutic vaccine trial of canarypox-HIV-pulsed dendritic cells vs. canarypox-HIV alone in HIV-1-infected patients on antiretroviral therapy. Vaccine. 2009;27:6088-94.

[103] Garcia F, Climent N, Assoumou L, Gil C, Gonzalez N, Alcami J, et al. A therapeutic dendritic cell-based vaccine for HIV-1 infection. J Infect Dis. 2011;203:473-8.

[104] Garcia F, Lejeune M, Climent N, Gil C, Alcami J, Morente V, et al. Therapeutic immunization with dendritic cells loaded with heat-inactivated autologous HIV-1 in patients with chronic HIV-1 infection. J Infect Dis. 2005 May 15;191(10):1680-5.

[105] Ide F, Nakamura T, Tomizawa M, Kawana-Tachikawa A, Odawara T, Hosoya N, et al. Peptide-loaded dendritic-cell vaccination followed by treatment interruption for chronic HIV-1 infection: a phase 1 trial. J Med Virol. 2006 Jun;78(6):711-8.

[106] Kloverpris H, Karlsson I, Bonde J, Thorn M, Vinner L, Pedersen AE, et al. Induction of novel CD8+ T-cell responses during chronic untreated HIV-1 infection by immunization with subdominant cytotoxic T-lymphocyte epitopes. AIDS. 2009;23:1329-40.

[107] Kundu SK, Engleman E, Benike C, Shapero MH, Dupuis M, van Schooten WC, et al. A pilot clinical trial of HIV antigen-pulsed allogeneic and autologous dendritic cell therapy in HIV-infected patients. AIDS Res Hum Retroviruses. 1998 May 1;14(7):551-60.

[108] Lu W, Arraes LC, Ferreira WT, Andrieu J-M. Therapeutic dendritic-cell vaccine for chronic HIV-1 infection. Nat Med. 2004;10:1359-65.

[109] Routy J-P, Boulassel M-R, Yassine-Diab B, Nicolette C, Healey D, Jain R, et al. Immunologic activity and safety of autologous HIV RNA-electroporated dendritic cells in HIV-1 infected patients receiving antiretroviral therapy. Clin Immunol. 2010;134:140-7.

[110] Poon B, Safrit J, McClure H, Kitchen C, Hsu J, Gudeman V, et al. Induction of humoral immune responses following vaccination with envelope-containing, formaldehyde-treated, thermally inactivated human immunodeficiency virus type 1. J Virol. 2005;79(8):4927-35.

[111] Girard MP, Osmanov S, Kieny M. A review of vaccine research and development: the human immunodeficiency virus (HIV). Vaccine. 2006;24(19):4062-81.

[112] Girard MP, Osmanov S, Assossou OM, Kieny M-P. Human immunodeficiency virus (HIV) immunopathogenesis and vaccine development: a review. Vaccine. 2011;29:6191-218.

[113] Polo JM, Dubensky TW. Virus-based vectors for human vaccine applications. Drug Discov Today. 2002;7:719-27.

[114] Liu MA. Immunologic basis of vaccine vectors. Immunity. 2010;33:504-15.

[115] Buchbinder SP, Mehrotra DV, Duerr A, Fitzgerald DW, Mogg R, Li D, et al. Efficacy assessment of a cell-mediated immunity HIV-1 vaccine (the Step Study): a double-blind, randomised, placebo-controlled, test-of-concept trial. Lancet. 2008;372:1881-93.

[116] McElrath MJ, De Rosa SC, Moodie Z, Dubey S, Kierstead L, Janes H, et al. HIV-1 vaccine-induced immunity in the test-of-concept Step Study: a case-cohort analysis. Lancet. 2008;372:1894-905.

[117] Sekaly RP. The failed HIV Merck vaccine study: a step back or a launching point for future vaccine development? J Exp Med. 2008 Jan 21;205(1):7-12.

[118] Abbink P, Abbink P, Lemckert A, Ewald B, Lynch D, Denholtz M, et al. Comparative seroprevalence and immunogenicity of six rare serotype recombinant adenovirus vaccine vectors from subgroups B and D. J Virol. 2007;81(9):4654-63.

[119] Barouch DH, Pau MG, Custers JH, Koudstaal W, Kostense S HM, Truitt DM, Sumida SM, Kishko MG, Arthur JC, Korioth-Schmitz B, Newberg MH, Gorgone DA, Lifton MA, Panicali DL, Nabel GJ, Letvin NL, Goudsmit J. Immunogenicity of recombinant adenovirus serotype 35 vaccine in the presence of pre-existing anti-Ad5 immunity. J Immunol. 2004;172(10):6290-7.

[120] Paoletti E, Tartaglia J, Taylor J. Safe and effective poxvirus vectors--NYVAC and ALVAC. Dev Biol Stand. 1994;82:65-9.

[121] Drexler I, Staib C, Sutter G. Modified vaccinia virus Ankara as antigen delivery system: how can we best use its potential? Curr Opin Biotechnol. 2004;15:506-12.

[122] Greenough TC, Cunningham CK, Muresan P, McManus M, Persaud D, Fenton T, et al. Safety and immunogenicity of recombinant poxvirus HIV-1 vaccines in young adults on highly active antiretroviral therapy. Vaccine. 2008;26:6883-93.

[123] Vasan S, Schlesinger SJ, Chen Z, Hurley A, Lombardo A, Than S, et al. Phase 1 safety and immunogenicity evaluation of ADMVA, a multigenic, modified vaccinia Ankara-HIV-1 B'/C candidate vaccine. PLoS One. 2010;5(1):e8816.

[124] Quakkelaar ED, Redeker A, Haddad EK, Harari A, McCaughey SM, Duhen T, et al. Improved innate and adaptive immunostimulation by genetically modified HIV-1 protein expressing NYVAC vectors. PLoS One. 2011;6(2):e16819.

[125] McCormack S, Stohr W, Barber T, Bart P-A, Harari A, Moog C, et al. EV02: a Phase I trial to compare the safety and immunogenicity of HIV DNA-C prime-NYVAC-C boost to NYVAC-C alone. Vaccine. 2008;26:3162-74.

[126] Rerks-Ngarm S, Pitisuttithum P, Nitayaphan S, Kaewkungwal J, Chiu J, Paris R, et al. Vaccination with ALVAC and AIDSVAX to prevent HIV-1 infection in Thailand. N Engl J Med. 2009;361:2209-20.

[127] Barouch DH, Liu J, Li H, Maxfield LF, Abbink P, Lynch DM, et al. Vaccine protection against acquisition of neutralization-resistant SIV challenges in rhesus monkeys. Nature. 2012;Jan 4.

[128] Esslinger C, Romero P, MacDonald HR. Efficient transduction of dendritic cells and induction of a T-cell response by third-generation lentivectors. Hum Gene Ther. 2002;13:1091-100.

[129] Naldini L, Blomer U, Gallay P, Ory D, Mulligan R, Gage FH, et al. In vivo gene delivery and stable transduction of nondividing cells by a lentiviral vector. Science. 1996;272:263-7.

[130] He Y, Zhang J, Donahue C, Falo LD. Skin-derived dendritic cells induce potent CD8(+) T cell immunity in recombinant lentivector-mediated genetic immunization. Immunity. 2006;24:643-56.

[131] Dai B, Yang L, Yang H, Hu B, Baltimore D, Wang P. HIV-1 Gag-specific immunity induced by a lentivector-based vaccine directed to dendritic cells. PNAS. 2009;106:20382-7.

[132] Lemiale F, Asefa B, Ye D, Chen C, Korokhov N, Humeau L. An HIV-based lentiviral vector as HIV vaccine candidate: Immunogenic characterization. Vaccine. 2010;28:1952-61.

[133] Iglesias MC, Mollier K, Beignon A-S, Souque P, Adotevi O, Lemonnier F, et al. Lentiviral vectors encoding HIV-1 polyepitopes induce broad CTL responses in vivo. Mol Ther. 2007;15:1203-10.

[134] Levine BL, Humeau LM, Boyer J, MacGregor R-R, Rebello T, Lu X, et al. Gene transfer in humans using a conditionally replicating lentiviral vector. PNAS. 2006;103:17372-7.

[135] Lemiale F, Korokhov N. Lentiviral vectors for HIV disease prevention and treatment. Vaccine. 2009;27:3443-9.

[136] Walker BD, Ahmed R, Plotkin S. Moving ahead an HIV vaccine: use both arms to beat HIV. Nat Med. 2011;17(10):1194-5.

[137] Hansen SG, Vieville C, Whizin N, Coyne-Johnson L, Sies sD, Drummond D, et al. Effector memory T cell responses are associated with protection of rhesus monkeys from mucosal simian immunodeficiency virus challenge. Nat Med. 2009;15(3):293-9.

[138] Buonaguro L, Devito C, Tornesello M, Schröder U, Wahren B, Hinkula J, et al. DNA-VLP prime-boost intra-nasal immunization induces cellular and humoral anti-HIV-1 systemic and mucosal immunity with cross-clade neutralizing activity. Vaccine. 2007;25(32):5968-77.

[139] Carcelain G, Debre P, Autran B. Reconstitution of CD4+ T lymphocytes in HIV-infected individuals following antiretroviral therapy. Curr Opin Immunol. 2001;13:483-8.

[140] Plana M, Garcia F, Gallart T, Miro JM, Gatell JM. Lack of T-cell proliferative response to HIV-1 antigens after 1 year of highly active antiretroviral treatment in early HIV-1 disease. Immunology Study Group of Spanish EARTH-1 Study. Lancet. 1998;352:1194-5.

[141] Garcia F, Niebla G, Romeu J, Vidal C, Plana M, Ortega M, et al. Cerebrospinal fluid HIV-1 RNA levels in asymptomatic patients with early stage chronic HIV-1 infection: support for the hypothesis of local virus replication. AIDS. 1999 Aug 20;13(12):1491-6.

[142] Smith KY. Selected metabolic and morphologic complications associated with highly active antiretroviral therapy. J Infect Dis. 2002;185 Suppl 2:123-7.

[143] Rinaldo CR. Dendritic cell-based human immunodeficiency virus vaccine. J Intern Med. 2009 Jan;265(1):138-58.

[144] Hel Z, Nacsa J, Tryniszewska E, Tsai W-P, Parks RW, Montefiori DC, et al. Containment of simian immunodeficiency virus infection in vaccinated macaques: correlation with the magnitude of virus-specific pre- and postchallenge CD4+ and CD8+ T cell responses. J Immunol. 2002;169:4778-87.

[145] Day CL, Walker BD. Progress in defining CD4 helper cell responses in chronic viral infections. J Exp Med. 2003;198:1773-7.

[146] Aiuti F, Mezzaroma I. Failure to reconstitute CD4+ T-cells despite suppression of HIV replication under HAART. AIDS Rev. 2006;8(2):88-97.

[147] Yang OO, Sarkis PTN, Trocha A, Kalams SA, Johnson RP, Walker BD. Impacts of avidity and specificity on the antiviral efficiency of HIV-1-specific CTL. J Immunol. 2003;171:3718-24.

[148] Banchereau J, Palucka AK. Dendritic cells as therapeutic vaccines against cancer. Nat Rev Immunol. 2005;5:296-306.

[149] Reis e Sousa C. Dendritic cells as sensors of infection. Immunity. 2001 May;14(5):495-8.

[150] Reis e Sousa C. Dendritic cells in a mature age. Nat Rev Immunol. 2006;6:476-83.

[151] Van Gulck E, Van Tendeloo VF, Berneman ZN, Vanham G. Role of dendritic cells in HIV-immunotherapy. Curr HIV Res. 2010 Jun;8(4):310-22.

[152] Idoyaga J, Steinman RM. SnapShot: Dendritic Cells. Cell. 2011;146:660.

[153] Zhang Z, Wang F. Plasmacytoid dendritic cells act as the most competent cell type in linking antiviral innate and adaptive immune responses. Cell Mol Immunol. 2005;2(6):411-7.

[154] Kadowaki N, Ho S, Antonenko S, Malefyt R, Kastelein R, Bazan F, et al. Subsets of human dendritic cell precursors express different toll-like receptors and respond to different microbial antigens. J Exp Med. 2001;194(6):863-9.

[155] Donaghy H, Gazzard B, Gotch F, Patterson S. Dysfunction and infection of freshly isolated blood myeloid and plasmacytoid dendritic cells in patients infected with HIV-1. Blood. 2003;101(11):4505-11.

[156] Granelli-Piperno A, Golebiowska A, Trumpfheller C, Siegal FP, Steinman RM. HIV-1-infected monocyte-derived dendritic cells do not undergo maturation but can elicit IL-10 production and T cell regulation. Proc Natl Acad Sci U S A. 2004;101:7669-74.

[157] Izquierdo-Useros N, Naranjo-Gomez M, Erkizia I, Puertas MC, Borràs FE, Blanco J, et al. HIV and mature dendritic cells: Trojan exosomes riding the Trojan horse? PLoS Pathog. 2010;6(3):e1000740.

[158] Romani N, Gruner S, Brang D, Kampgen E, Lenz A, Trockenbacher B, et al. Proliferating dendritic cell progenitors in human blood. J Exp Med. 1994 Jul 1;180(1):83-93.

[159] Sallusto F, Lanzavecchia A. Efficient presentation of soluble antigen by cultured human dendritic cells is maintained by granulocyte/macrophage colony-stimulating factor plus interleukin 4 and downregulated by tumor necrosis factor alpha. J Exp Med. 1994;179(4):1109-18.

[160] Lu W, Andrieu JM. In vitro human immunodeficiency virus eradication by autologous CD8(+) T cells expanded with inactivated-virus-pulsed dendritic cells. J Virol. 2001 Oct;75(19):8949-56.

[161] Aline F, Brand D, Bout D, Pierre J, Fouquenet D, Verrier B, et al. Generation of specific Th1 and CD8 T-cell responses by immunization with mouse CD8 dendritic cells loaded with HIV-1 viral lysate or envelope glycoproteins. Microbes Infect. 2007;9(4):536-43.

[162] Huang X-L, Fan Z, Zheng L, Borowski L, Li H, Thomas EK, et al. Priming of human immunodeficiency virus type 1 (HIV-1)-specific CD8+ T cell responses by dendritic cells loaded with HIV-1 proteins. J Infect Dis. 2003;187:315-9.

[163] Fan Z, Huang X, Borowski L, Mellors J, Rinaldo CJ. Restoration of anti-human immunodeficiency virus type 1 (HIV-1) responses in CD8 T cells from late-stage patients on prolonged antiretroviral therapy by stimulation in vitro with HIV-1 protein-loaded dendritic cells. J Virol. 2001;75(9):4413-9.

[164] Huang X-L, Fan Z, Colleton B, Buchli R, Li H, Hildebrand W, et al. Processing and presentation of exogenous HLA class I peptides by dendritic cells from human immunodeficiency virus type 1-infected persons. J Virol. 2005;79(5):3052-62.

[165] Engelmayer J, Larsson M, Lee A, Lee M, Cox W, Steinman R, et al. Mature dendritic cells infected with canarypox virus elicit strong anti-human immunodeficiency virus CD8 and CD4 T-cell responses from chronically infected individuals. J Virol. 2001;75(5):2142-53.

[166] Guerra S, Nájera J, González J, López-Fernández L, Climent N, Gatell J, et al. Distinct gene expression profiling after infection of immature human monocyte-derived dendritic cells by the attenuated poxvirus vectors MVA and NYVAC. J Virol. 2007;81(16):8707-21.

[167] Gudmundsdotter L, Wahren B, Haller B, Boberg A, Edbäck U, Bernasconi D, et al. Amplified antigen-specific immune responses in HIV-1 infected individuals in a double blind DNA immunization and therapy interruption trial. Vaccine. 2011;29(33):5558-66.

[168] Chassin D, Andrieu M, Cohen W, Culmann-Penciolelli B, Ostankovitch M, Hanau D, et al. Dendritic cells transfected with the nef genes of HIV-1 primary isolates specifically activate cytotoxic T lymphocytes from seropositive subjects. Eur J Immunol. 1999 Jan;29(1):196-202.

[169] Kavanagh DG, Kaufmann DE, Sunderji S, Frahm N, Le Gall S, Boczkowski D, et al. Expansion of HIV-specific CD4+ and CD8+ T cells by dendritic cells transfected with mRNA encoding cytoplasm- or lysosome-targeted Nef. Blood. 2006 Mar 1;107(5):1963-9.

[170] Van Gulck ER, Ponsaerts P, Heyndrickx L, Vereecken K, Moerman F, De Roo A, et al. Efficient stimulation of HIV-1-specific T cells using dendritic cells electroporated with mRNA encoding autologous HIV-1 Gag and Env proteins. Blood. 2006 Mar 1;107(5):1818-27.

[171] Van Gulck ER, Vanham G, Heyndrickx L, Coppens S, Vereecken K, Atkinson D, et al. Efficient in vitro expansion of human immunodeficiency virus (HIV)-specific T-cell

responses by gag mRNA-electroporated dendritic cells from treated and untreated HIV type 1-infected individuals. J Virol. 2008 Apr;82(7):3561-73.

[172] Weissman D, Ni H, Scales D, Dude A, Capodici J, McGibney K, et al. HIV gag mRNA transfection of dendritic cells (DC) delivers encoded antigen to MHC class I and II molecules, causes DC maturation, and induces a potent human in vitro primary immune response. J Immunol. 2000;165(8):4710-7.

[173] Garcia F, Routy J-P. Challenges in dendritic cells-based therapeutic vaccination in HIV-1 infection Workshop in dendritic cell-based vaccine clinical trials in HIV-1. Vaccine. 2011;29:6454-63.

[174] Lisziewicz J, Trocio J, Whitman L, Varga G, Xu J, Bakare N, et al. DermaVir: a novel topical vaccine for HIV/AIDS. J Invest Dermatol. 2005 Jan;124(1):160-9.

[175] Allard SD, De Keersmaecker B, de Goede AL, Verschuren EJ, Koetsveld J, Reedijk ML, et al. A phase I/IIa immunotherapy trial of HIV-1-infected patients with Tat, Rev and Nef expressing dendritic cells followed by treatment interruption. Clin Immunol. 2012;142(3):252-6.

[176] Van Gulck E, Vlieghe E, Vekemans M, Van Tendeloo VFI, Van De Velde A, Smits E, et al. mRNA-based dendritic cell vaccination induces potent antiviral T-cell responses in HIV-1-infected patients. AIDS. 2011;26(4):F1-F12.

[177] Angel JB, Routy J-P, Tremblay C, Ayers D, Woods R, Singer J, et al. A randomized controlled trial of HIV therapeutic vaccination using ALVAC with or without Remune. AIDS. 2011;25(6):731-9.

[178] Elsabahy M, Nazarali A, Foldvari M. Non-viral nucleic acid delivery: key challenges and future directions. Curr Drug Deliv. 2011;8(3):235-44.

[179] De Temmerman M-L, Rejman J, Demeester J, Irvine D, Gander B, De Smedt S. Particulate vaccines: on the quest for optimal delivery and immune response. Drug Discov Today. 2011;16(13-14):569-82.

[180] Bachmann MF, Jennings G. Vaccine delivery: a matter of size, geometry, kinetics and molecular patterns. Nat Rev Immunol. 2010;10(11):787-96.

[181] Demento SL, Siefert A, Bandyopadhyay A, Sharp F, Fahmy T. Pathogen-associated molecular patterns on biomaterials: a paradigm for engineering new vaccines. Trends Biotechnol. 2011;29(6):294-306.

[182] Heit A, Schmitz F, Haas T, Busch DH, Wagner H. Antigen co-encapsulated with adjuvants efficiently drive protective T cell immunity. Eur J Immunol. 2007 Aug;37(8):2063-74.

[183] Schlosser E, Mueller M, Fischer S, Basta S, Busch D, Gander B, et al. TLR ligands and antigen need to be coencapsulated into the same biodegradable microsphere for the generation of potent cytotoxic T lymphocyte responses. Vaccine. 2008;26(13):1626-37.

[184] De Haes W, De Koker S, Pollard C, Atkinson D, Vlieghe E, Hoste J, et al. Polyelectrolyte capsules-containing HIV-1 p24 and poly I:C modulate dendritic cells to stimulate HIV-1-specific immune responses. Mol Ther. 2010 Jul;18(7):1408-16.

[185] Steinman RM, Hemmi H. Dendritic cells: translating innate to adaptive immunity. Curr Top Microbiol Immunol. 2006;311:17-58.
[186] De Koker S, De Geest BG, SK. S, R. DR, T. N, Y. VK, et al. Polyelectrolyte microcapsules as antigen delivery vehicles to dendritic cells: uptake, processing, and cross-presentation of encapsulated antigens. Angew Chem Int Ed Engl. 2009;48(45):8485-9.
[187] De Koker S, Lambrecht BN, Willart MA, van Kooyk Y, Grooten J, Vervaet C, et al. Designing polymeric particles for antigen delivery. Chem Soc Rev. 2011;40:320-39.
[188] Trono D, Van Lint C, Rouzioux C, Verdin E, Barre-Sinoussi F, Chun TW, et al. HIV persistence and the prospect of long-term drug-free remissions for HIV-infected individuals. Science. 2010 Jul 9;329(5988):174-80.
[189] Tavernier G, Andries O, Demeester J, Sanders NN, De Smedt SC, Rejman J. mRNA as gene therapeutic: How to control protein expression. J Control Release. 2010 Oct 21;150(3):238-91.
[190] Lori F, Calarota SA, Lisziewicz J. Nanochemistry-based immunotherapy for HIV-1. Curr Med Chem. 2007;14:1911-9.
[191] Rejman J, Tavernier G, Bavarsad N, Demeester J, De Smedt SC. mRNA transfection of cervical carcinoma and mesenchymal stem cells mediated by cationic carriers. J Control Release. 2010 Nov 1;147(3):385-91.
[192] Bettinger T, Carlisle RC, Read ML, Ogris M, Seymour LW. Peptide-mediated RNA delivery: a novel approach for enhanced transfection of primary and post-mitotic cells. Nucleic Acids Res. 2001;29(18):3882-91.
[193] Pascolo S. Vaccination with messenger RNA (mRNA). Handb Exp Pharmacol. 2008(183):221-35.
[194] Roesler E, Weiss R, Weinberger EE, Fruehwirth A, Stoecklinger A, Mostbock S, et al. Immunize and disappear-safety-optimized mRNA vaccination with a panel of 29 allergens. J Allergy Clin Immunol. 2009 Nov;124(5):1070-7.
[195] Weiss R, Scheiblhofer S, Roesler E, Ferreira F, Thalhamer J. Prophylactic mRNA vaccination against allergy. Curr Opin Allergy Clin Immunol. 2010;10:567-74.
[196] Van Tendeloo VF, Van de Velde A, Van Driessche A, Cools N, Anguille S, Ladell K, et al. Induction of complete and molecular remissions in acute myeloid leukemia by Wilms' tumor 1 antigen-targeted dendritic cell vaccination. PNAS. 2010 Aug 3;107(31):13824-9.
[197] Weide B, Carralot JP, Reese A, Scheel B, Eigentler TK, Hoerr I, et al. Results of the first phase I/II clinical vaccination trial with direct injection of mRNA. J Immunother. 2008 Feb-Mar;31(2):180-8.
[198] Gilboa E, Vieweg J. Cancer immunotherapy with mRNA-transfected dendritic cells. Immunol Rev. 2004;199:251-63.
[199] Newman KD, Elamanchili P, Kwon GS, Samuel J. Uptake of poly(D,L-lactic-co-glycolic acid) microspheres by antigen-presenting cells in vivo. J Biomed Mater Res. 2002;60:480-6.

[200] Waeckerle-Men Y, Allmen EU, Gander B, Scandella E, Schlosser E, Schmidtke G, et al. Encapsulation of proteins and peptides into biodegradable poly(D,L-lactide-co-glycolide) microspheres prolongs and enhances antigen presentation by human dendritic cells. Vaccine. 2006 Mar 10;24(11):1847-57.

[201] Fischer S, Uetz-von Allmen E, Waeckerle-Men Y, Groettrup M, Merkle HP, Gander B. The preservation of phenotype and functionality of dendritic cells upon phagocytosis of polyelectrolyte-coated PLGA microparticles. Biomaterials. 2007 Feb;28(6):994-1004.

[202] Waeckerle-Men Y, Scandella E, Uetz-Von Allmen E, Ludewig B, Gillessen S, Merkle HP, et al. Phenotype and functional analysis of human monocyte-derived dendritic cells loaded with biodegradable poly(lactide-co-glycolide) microspheres for immunotherapy. J Immunol Methods. 2004 Apr;287(1-2):109-24.

[203] Kempf M, Mandal B, Jilek S, Thiele L, Voros J, Textor M, et al. Improved stimulation of human dendritic cells by receptor engagement with surface-modified microparticles. J Drug Target. 2003;11:11-8.

[204] Wischke C, Zimmermann J, Wessinger B, Schendler A, Borchert HH, Peters JH, et al. Poly(I:C) coated PLGA microparticles induce dendritic cell maturation. Int J Pharm. 2009 Jan 5;365(1-2):61-8.

[205] Elamanchili P, Diwan M, Cao M, Samuel J. Characterization of poly(D,L-lactic-co-glycolic acid) based nanoparticulate system for enhanced delivery of antigens to dendritic cells. Vaccine. 2004 Jun 23;22(19):2406-12.

[206] Aline F, Brand D, Pierre J, Roingeard P, Severine M, Verrier B, et al. Dendritic cells loaded with HIV-1 p24 proteins adsorbed on surfactant-free anionic PLA nanoparticles induce enhanced cellular immune responses against HIV-1 after vaccination. Vaccine. 2009 May 27;9(4):536-43.

[207] Ataman-Onal Y, Munier S, Ganee A, Terrat C, Durand PY, Battail N, et al. Surfactant-free anionic PLA nanoparticles coated with HIV-1 p24 protein induced enhanced cellular and humoral immune responses in various animal models. J Control Release. 2006 May 15;112(2):175-85.

[208] Tamber H, Johansen P, Merkle HP, Gander B. Formulation aspects of biodegradable polymeric microspheres for antigen delivery. Adv Drug Deliv Rev. 2005;57:357-76.

[209] Kazzaz J, Neidleman J, Singh M, Ott G, O'Hagan DT. Novel anionic microparticles are a potent adjuvant for the induction of cytotoxic T lymphocytes against recombinant p55 gag from HIV-1. J Control Release. 2000;67:347-56.

[210] Lamalle-Bernard D, Munier S, Compagnon C, Charles M-H, Kalyanaraman VS, Delair T, et al. Coadsorption of HIV-1 p24 and gp120 proteins to surfactant-free anionic PLA nanoparticles preserves antigenicity and immunogenicity. J Control Release. 2006;115:57-67.

[211] Johansen P, Martinez Gomez JM, Gander B. Development of synthetic biodegradable microparticulate vaccines: a roller coaster story. Expert Rev Vaccines. 2007;6:471-4.

[212] Walter E, Moelling K, Pavlovic J, Merkle HP. Microencapsulation of DNA using poly(DL-lactide-co-glycolide): stability issues and release characteristics. J Control Release. 1999;61:361-74.
[213] Remaut K, Sanders NN, De Geest BG, Braeckmans K, Demeester J, De Smedt SC. Nucleic acid delivery: Where material sciences and bio-sciences meet. Materials Science and Engineering R. 2007;58:117-61.
[214] Basarkar A, Devineni D, Palaniappan R, Singh J. Preparation, characterization, cytotoxicity and transfection efficiency of poly(DL-lactide-co-glycolide) and poly(DL-lactic acid) cationic nanoparticles for controlled delivery of plasmid DNA. Int J Pharm. 2007;343:247-2
[215]
[216] Donath E, Sukhorukov GB, Caruso F, Davis DA, Mohwald H. Novel hollow polymer shells by colloid-templated assembly of polyelectrolytes. Angewandte Chemie-International Edition. 1998;37:2202-5.
[217] De Koker S, De Geest BG, Cubelier C, Ferdinande L, Deckers W, Hennick WE, et al. In vivo cellular uptake, degradation and biocompatibility of polyelectrolyte microcapsules. Advanced Functional Materials. 2007;17: 3754-63.
[218] De Rose R, Zelikin AN, Johnston APR, Sexton A, Chong SF, Cortez C, et al. Binding, Internalization, and Antigen Presentation of Vaccine-Loaded Nanoengineered Capsules in Blood. Advanced Materials. 2008;20:1-6.
[219] Chong S-F, Sexton A, De Rose R, Kent SJ, Zelikin AN, Caruso F. A paradigm for peptide vaccine delivery using viral epitopes encapsulated in degradable polymer hydrogel capsules. Biomaterials. 2009;30:5178-86.
[220] Zelikin AN, Li Q, Caruso F. Degradable polyelectrolyte capsules filled with oligonucleotide sequences. Angew Chem Int Ed Engl. 2006;45:7743-45.
[221] Selina OE, Belov SI, Vlasova NN, Balysheva VI, Churin AI, Bartkoviak A, et al. Biodegradable microcapsules containing DNA for the new DNA vaccine design. Bioorg Khim. 2009;35:113-21.
[222] Tiera MJ, Qiu X-P, Bechaouch S, Shi Q, Fernandes JC, Winnik FM. Synthesis and characterization of phosphorylcholine-substituted chitosans soluble in physiological pH conditions. Biomacromolecules. 2006;7:3151-6.
[223] Boussif O, Lezoualc'h F, Zanta MA, Mergny MD, Scherman D, Demeneix B, et al. A versatile vector for gene and oligonucleotide transfer into cells in culture and in vivo: polyethylenimine. PNAS. 1995;92:7297-301.
[224] Godbey WT, Wu KK, Mikos AG. Poly(ethylenimine) and its role in gene delivery. J Control Release. 1999;60:149-60.
[225] Itaka K, Harada A, Yamasaki Y, Nakamura K, Kawaguchi H, Kataoka K. In situ single cell observation by fluorescence resonance energy transfer reveals fast intra-cytoplasmic delivery and easy release of plasmid DNA complexed with linear polyethylenimine. J Gene Med. 2004;6:76-84.

[226] Sonawane ND, Szoka FC, Verkman AS. Chloride accumulation and swelling in endosomes enhances DNA transfer by polyamine-DNA polyplexes. J Biol Chem. 2003;278:44826-31.

[227] Behr JP. The proton sponge: A trick to enter cells the viruses did not exploit. Chimia. 1997;51:34-6.

[228] Lori F, Trocio J, Bakare N, Kelly LM, Lisziewicz J. DermaVir, a novel HIV immunisation technology. Vaccine. 2005 Mar 18;23(17-18):2030-4.

[229] Lisziewicz J, Trocio J, Xu J, Whitman L, Ryder A, Bakare N, et al. Control of viral rebound through therapeutic immunization with DermaVir. Aids. 2005 Jan 3;19(1):35-43.

[230] Lisziewicz J. Conference scene--active immunotherapeutics forum: meeting highlights. Immunotherapy. 2009;1:743-8.

[231] Wahren B, Biswas P, Borggren M, Coleman A, Da Costa K, De Haes W, et al. Rational design of HIV vaccine and microbicides: report of the EUROPRISE annual conference. J Transl Med. 2010;8:72.

[232] Felnerova D, Viret J-F, Gluck R, Moser C. Liposomes and virosomes as delivery systems for antigens, nucleic acids and drugs. Curr Opin Biotechnol. 2004;15:518-29.

[233] Alving CR. Liposomes as carriers of antigens and adjuvants. J Immunol Methods. 1991;140:1-13.

[234] Nakanishi T, Kunisawa J, Hayashi A, Tsutsumi Y, Kubo K, Nakagawa S, et al. Positively charged liposome functions as an efficient immunoadjuvant in inducing cell-mediated immune response to soluble proteins. J Control Release. 1999;61:233-40.

[235] Moser C, Metcalfe IC, Viret J-F. Virosomal adjuvanted antigen delivery systems. Expert Rev Vaccines. 2003;2:189-96.

[236] Zheng L, Huang XL, Fan Z, Borowski L, Wilson CC, Rinaldo CR. Delivery of liposome-encapsulated HIV type 1 proteins to human dendritic cells for stimulation of HIV type 1-specific memory cytotoxic T lymphocyte responses. AIDS Res Hum Retroviruses. 1999;15:1011-20.

[237] Steers NJ, Peachman KK, McClain S, Alving CR, Rao M. Liposome-encapsulated HIV-1 Gag p24 containing lipid A induces effector CD4+ T-cells, memory CD8+ T-cells, and pro-inflammatory cytokines. Vaccine. 2009 Nov 16;27(49):6939-49.

[238] Andrieu M, Desoutter J-F, Loing E, Gaston J, Hanau D, Guillet J-G, et al. Two human immunodeficiency virus vaccinal lipopeptides follow different cross-presentation pathways in human dendritic cells. J Virol. 2003;77:1564-70.

[239] Gahery H, Daniel N, Charmeteau B, Ourth L, Jackson A, Andrieu M, et al. New CD4+ and CD8+ T cell responses induced in chronically HIV type-1-infected patients after immunizations with an HIV type 1 lipopeptide vaccine. AIDS Res Hum Retroviruses. 2006;22:684-94.

[240] Pialoux G, Quercia RP, Gahery H, Daniel N, Slama L, Girard P-M, et al. Immunological responses and long-term treatment interruption after human

immunodeficiency virus type 1 (HIV-1) lipopeptide immunization of HIV-1-infected patients: the LIPTHERA study. Clin Vaccine Immunol. 2008;15:562-8.

[241] Cobb A, Roberts LK, Palucka AK, Mead H, Montes M, Ranganathan R, et al. Development of a HIV-1 lipopeptide antigen pulsed therapeutic dendritic cell vaccine. J Immunol Methods. 2011;365:27-37.

[242] Simberg D, Weisman S, Talmon Y, Barenholz Y. DOTAP (and other cationic lipids): chemistry, biophysics, and transfection. Crit Rev Ther Drug Carrier Syst. 2004;21:257-317.

[243] Tresset G. The multiple faces of self-assembled lipidic systems. PMC Biophys. 2009;2(1):3-28.

[244] Rejman J, Bragonzi A, Conese M. Role of clathrin- and caveolae-mediated endocytosis in gene transfer mediated by lipo- and polyplexes. Mol Ther. 2005;12:468-74.

[245] Rejman J, Conese M, Hoekstra D. Gene transfer by means of lipo- and polyplexes: role of clathrin and caveolae-mediated endocytosis. J Liposome Res. 2006;16:237-47.

[246] Zuhorn IS, Kalicharan R, Hoekstra D. Lipoplex-mediated transfection of mammalian cells occurs through the cholesterol-dependent clathrin-mediated pathway of endocytosis. J Biol Chem. 2002;277:18021-8.

[247] Xu Y, Szoka FC. Mechanism of DNA release from cationic liposome/DNA complexes used in cell transfection. Biochemistry. 1996;35:5616-23.

[248] Dow SW, Fradkin LG, Liggitt DH, Willson AP, Heath TD, Potter TA. Lipid-DNA complexes induce potent activation of innate immune responses and antitumor activity when administered intravenously. J Immunol. 1999;163:1552-61.

[249] Jiao X, Wang RYH, Feng Z, Alter HJ, Shih JW-K. Modulation of cellular immune response against hepatitis C virus nonstructural protein 3 by cationic liposome encapsulated DNA immunization. Hepatology. 2003;37:452-60.

[250] Perrie Y, Obrenovic M, McCarthy D, Gregoriadis G. Liposome (Lipodine)-mediated DNA vaccination by the oral route. J Liposome Res. 2002;12:185-97.

[251] Malone RW, Felgner PL, Verma IM. Cationic liposome-mediated RNA transfection. Proc Natl Acad Sci U S A. 1989 Aug;86(16):6077-81.

[252] Zohra FT, Chowdhury EH, Nagaoka M, Akaike T. Drastic effect of nanoapatite particles on liposome-mediated mRNA delivery to mammalian cells. Anal Biochem. 2005;345:164-6.

[253] Zou S, Scarfo K, Nantz MH, Hecker JG. Lipid-mediated delivery of RNA is more efficient than delivery of DNA in non-dividing cells. Int J Pharm. 2010;389:232-43.

[254] Canelle L, Bousquet J, Pionneau C, Hardouin J, Choquet-Kastylevsky G, Joubert-Caron R, et al. A proteomic approach to investigate potential biomarkers directed against membrane-associated breast cancer proteins. Electrophoresis. 2006 Apr;27(8):1609-16.

[255] Martinon F, Krishnan S, Lenzen G, Magne R, Gomard E, Guillet JG, et al. Induction of virus-specific cytotoxic T lymphocytes in vivo by liposome-entrapped mRNA. Eur J Immunol. 1993 Jul;23(7):1719-22.

[256] Dell K, Klein C, Gissmann L. Comparison of DNA- and mRNA-transfected mouse dendritic cells as potential vaccines against the human papillomavirus type 16 associated oncoprotein E7. Antivir Ther. 2008;13:495-509.

[257] Yu H, Babiuk LA, van Drunen Littel-van den Hurk S. Immunity and protection by adoptive transfer of dendritic cells transfected with hepatitis C NS3/4A mRNA. Vaccine. 2007;25:1701-11.

[258] Senior JH, Trimble KR, Maskiewicz R. Interaction of positively-charged liposomes with blood: implications for their application in vivo. Biochim Biophys Acta. 1991;1070:173-9.

[259] Simberg D, Weisman S, Talmon Y, Faerman A, Shoshani T, Barenholz Y. The role of organ vascularization and lipoplex-serum initial contact in intravenous murine lipofection. J Biol Chem. 2003;278:39858-65.

[260] Zuhorn IS, Visser WH, Bakowsky U, Engberts JBFN, Hoekstra D. Interference of serum with lipoplex-cell interaction: modulation of intracellular processing. Biochim Biophys Acta. 2002;1560:25-36.

[261] Bhadra D, Bhadra S, Jain P, Jain NK. Pegnology: a review of PEG-ylated systems. Pharmazie. 2002;57:5-29.

[262] Singh SK, Bisen PS. Adjuvanticity of stealth liposomes on the immunogenicity of synthetic gp41 epitope of HIV-1. Vaccine. 2006;24(19):4161-6.

[263] Rejman J, Oberle V, Zuhorn IS, Hoekstra D. Size-dependent internalization of particles via the pathways of clathrin- and caveolae-mediated endocytosis. Biochem J. 2004;377:159-69.

[264] Burgdorf S, Kurts C. Endocytosis mechanisms and the cell biology of antigen presentation. Curr Opin Immunol. 2008;20:89-95.

[265] Brewer JM, Pollock KGJ, Tetley L, Russell DG. Vesicle size influences the trafficking, processing, and presentation of antigens in lipid vesicles. J Immunol. 2004;173:6143-50.

[266] Ackerman AL, Kyritsis C, Tampe R, Cresswell P. Early phagosomes in dendritic cells form a cellular compartment sufficient for cross presentation of exogenous antigens. Proc Natl Acad Sci U S A. 2003;100(22):12889-94.

[267] Burgdorf S, Kautz A, Bohnert V, Knolle PA, Kurts C. Distinct pathways of antigen uptake and intracellular routing in CD4 and CD8 T cell activation. Science. 2007;316:612-6.

[268] Petros RA, DeSimone JM. Strategies in the design of nanoparticles for therapeutic applications. Nat Rev Drug Discov. 2010;9:615-27.

[269] Engering A, Geijtenbeek TBH, van Vliet SJ, Wijers M, van Liempt E, Demaurex N, et al. The dendritic cell-specific adhesion receptor DC-SIGN internalizes antigen for presentation to T cells. J Immunol. 2002;168:2118-26.

[270] Hattori Y, Kawakami S, Nakamura K, Yamashita F, Hashida M. Efficient gene transfer into macrophages and dendritic cells by in vivo gene delivery with mannosylated lipoplex via the intraperitoneal route. J Pharmacol Exp Ther. 2006;318:828-34.

[271] Lu Y, Kawakami S, Yamashita F, Hashida M. Development of an antigen-presenting cell-targeted DNA vaccine against melanoma by mannosylated liposomes. Biomaterials. 2007;28:3255-62.

[272] Sheng K-C, Kalkanidis M, Pouniotis DS, Esparon S, Tang CK, Apostolopoulos V, et al. Delivery of antigen using a novel mannosylated dendrimer potentiates immunogenicity in vitro and in vivo. Eur J Immunol. 2008;38:424-36.

[273] Bonifaz LC, Bonnyay DP, Charalambous A, Darguste DI, Fujii S-I, Soares H, et al. In vivo targeting of antigens to maturing dendritic cells via the DEC-205 receptor improves T cell vaccination. J Exp Med. 2004;199:815-24.

[274] Connolly NC, Colleton BA, Rinaldo CR. Treating HIV-1 infection with dendritic cells. Curr Opin Mol Ther. 2007;9:353-63.

[275] Gieseler RK, Marquitan G, Hahn MJ, Perdon LA, Driessen WHP, Sullivan SM, et al. DC-SIGN-specific liposomal targeting and selective intracellular compound delivery to human myeloid dendritic cells: implications for HIV disease. Scand J Immunol. 2004;59:415-24.

[276] Tacken PJ, de Vries IJM, Gijzen K, Joosten B, Wu D, Rother RP, et al. Effective induction of naive and recall T-cell responses by targeting antigen to human dendritic cells via a humanized anti-DC-SIGN antibody. Blood. 2005;106:1278-85.

[277] Altin JG, Parish CR. Liposomal vaccines--targeting the delivery of antigen. Methods. 2006;40:39-52.

[278] Altin JG, White FA, Easton CJ. Synthesis of the chelator lipid nitrilotriacetic acid ditetradecylamine (NTA-DTDA) and its use with the IAsys biosensor to study receptor-ligand interactions on model membranes. Biochim Biophys Acta. 2001;1513:131-48.

[279] Faham A, Altin JG. Antigen-containing liposomes engrafted with flagellin-related peptides are effective vaccines that can induce potent antitumor immunity and immunotherapeutic effect. J Immunol. 2010;185:1744-54.

[280] Resh MD. Palmitoylation of ligands, receptors, and intracellular signaling molecules. Sci STKE. 2006;2006(359):re14.

[281] Blander JM, Medzhitov R. Regulation of phagosome maturation by signals from toll-like receptors. Science. 2004;304:1014-18.

[282] Nicholls EF, Madera L, Hancock REW. Immunomodulators as adjuvants for vaccines and antimicrobial therapy. Ann N Y Acad Sci. 2010;1213:46-61.

[283] Baylor NW, Egan W, Richman P. Aluminum salts in vaccines--US perspective. Vaccine. 2002;20 (Suppl 3):18-23.

[284] Blander JM, Medzhitov R. Toll-dependent selection of microbial antigens for presentation by dendritic cells. Nature. 2006 Apr 6;440(7085):808-12.

[285] Ennis FA, Cruz J, Jameson J, Klein M, Burt D, Thipphawong J. Augmentation of human influenza A virus-specific cytotoxic T lymphocyte memory by influenza vaccine and adjuvanted carriers (ISCOMS). Virology. 1999;259:256-61.

[286] Rimmelzwaan GF, Nieuwkoop N, Brandenburg A, Sutter G, Beyer WE, Maher D, et al. A randomized, double blind study in young healthy adults comparing cell mediated

and humoral immune responses induced by influenza ISCOM vaccines and conventional vaccines. Vaccine. 2000;19:1180-7.

[287] Davis ID, Chen W, Jackson H, Parente P, Shackleton M, Hopkins W, et al. Recombinant NY-ESO-1 protein with ISCOMATRIX adjuvant induces broad integrated antibody and CD4(+) and CD8(+) T cell responses in humans. PNAS. 2004;101:10697-702.

[288] Akerblom L, Nara P, Dunlop N, Putney S, Morein B. HIV experimental vaccines based on the iscom technology using envelope and GAG gene products. Biotechnol Ther. 1993;4(3-4):145-61.

[289] Putkonen P, Bjorling E, Akerblom L, Thorstensson R, Lovgren K, Benthin L, et al. Long-standing protection of macaques against cell-free HIV-2 with a HIV-2 iscom vaccine. J Acquir Immune Defic Syndr. 1994;7:551-9.

[290] Agrawal L, Haq W, Hanson CV, Rao DN. Generating neutralizing antibodies, Th1 response and MHC non restricted immunogenicity of HIV-I env and gag peptides in liposomes and ISCOMs with in-built adjuvanticity. J Immune Based Ther Vaccines. 2003;1(1):5.

[291] Cox JC, Sjolander A, Barr IG. ISCOMs and other saponin based adjuvants. Adv Drug Deliv Rev. 1998;32:247-71.

[292] Frazer IH, Quinn M, Nicklin JL, Tan J, Perrin LC, Ng P, et al. Phase 1 study of HPV16-specific immunotherapy with E6E7 fusion protein and ISCOMATRIX adjuvant in women with cervical intraepithelial neoplasia. Vaccine. 2004;23:172-81.

[293] Osterhaus A, de Vries P, Morein B, Akerblom L, Heeney J. Comparison of protection afforded by whole virus ISCOM versus MDP adjuvanted formalin-inactivated SIV vaccines from IV cell-free or cell-associated homologous challenge. AIDS Res Hum Retroviruses. 1992;8(8):1507-10.

[294] Verschoor EJ, Mooij P, Oostermeijer H, van der Kolk M, ten Haaft P, Verstrepen B, et al. Comparison of immunity generated by nucleic acid-, MF59-, and ISCOM-formulated human immunodeficiency virus type 1 vaccines in Rhesus macaques: evidence for viral clearance. J Virol. 1999;73(4):3292-300.

[295] Koopman G, Bogers WMJM, van Gils M, Koornstra W, Barnett S, Morein B, et al. Comparison of intranasal with targeted lymph node immunization using PR8-Flu ISCOM adjuvanted HIV antigens in macaques. J Med Virol. 2007;79(5):474-82.

[296] Morein B, Hu K-F, Abusugra I. Current status and potential application of ISCOMs in veterinary medicine. Adv Drug Deliv Rev. 2004;56:1367-82.

[297] Pulendran B. Modulating vaccine responses with dendritic cells and Toll-like receptors. Immunol Rev. 2004;199:227-50.

[298] Schreibelt G, Tel J, Sliepen KHEWJ, Benitez-Ribas D, Figdor CG, Adema GJ, et al. Toll-like receptor expression and function in human dendritic cell subsets: implications for dendritic cell-based anti-cancer immunotherapy. Cancer Immunol Immunother. 2010;59(10):1573-82.

[299] Espuelas S, Roth A, Thumann C, Frisch B, Schuber F. Effect of synthetic lipopeptides formulated in liposomes on the maturation of human dendritic cells. Mol Immunol. 2005;42:721-9.

[300] Kazzaz J, Singh M, Ugozzoli M, Chesko J, Soenawan E, O'Hagan DT. Encapsulation of the immune potentiators MPL and RC529 in PLG microparticles enhances their potency. J Control Release. 2006 Feb 21;110(3):566-73.

[301] Vandepapeliere P, Horsmans Y, Moris P, Van Mechelen M, Janssens M, Koutsoukos M, et al. Vaccine adjuvant systems containing monophosphoryl lipid A and QS21 induce strong and persistent humoral and T cell responses against hepatitis B surface antigen in healthy adult volunteers. Vaccine. 2008;26:1375-86.

[302] Fischer S, Schlosser E, Mueller M, Csaba N, Merkle HP, Groettrup M, et al. Concomitant delivery of a CTL-restricted peptide antigen and CpG ODN by PLGA microparticles induces cellular immune response. J Drug Target. 2009 Sep;17(8):652-61.

[303] Demento SL, Bonafe N, Cui W, Kaech SM, Caplan MJ, Fikrig E, et al. TLR9-targeted biodegradable nanoparticles as immunization vectors protect against West Nile encephalitis. J Immunol. 2010;185:2989-97.

[304] Li WM, Bally MB, Schutze-Redelmeier MP. Enhanced immune response to T-independent antigen by using CpG oligodeoxynucleotides encapsulated in liposomes. Vaccine. 2001;20:148-57.

[305] Singh M, Ott G, Kazzaz J, Ugozzoli M, Briones M, Donnelly J, et al. Cationic microparticles are an effective delivery system for immune stimulatory cpG DNA. Pharm Res. 2001;18:1476-9.

[306] Johnston D, Zaidi B, Bystryn J-C. TLR7 imidazoquinoline ligand 3M-019 is a potent adjuvant for pure protein prototype vaccines. Cancer Immunol Immunother. 2007;56:1133-41.

[307] Westwood A, Elvin SJ, Healey GD, Williamson ED, Eyles JE. Immunological responses after immunisation of mice with microparticles containing antigen and single stranded RNA (polyuridylic acid). Vaccine. 2006;24:1736-43.

[308] Trumpfheller C, Caskey M, Nchinda G, Longhi MP, Mizenina O, Huang Y, et al. The microbial mimic poly IC induces durable and protective CD4+ T cell immunity together with a dendritic cell targeted vaccine. PNAS. 2008 Feb 19;105(7):2574-9.

[309] Zaks K, Jordan M, Guth A, Sellins K, Kedl R, Izzo A, et al. Efficient immunization and cross-priming by vaccine adjuvants containing TLR3 or TLR9 agonists complexed to cationic liposomes. J Immunol. 2006;176:7335-45.

[310] Bonjardim CA, Ferreira PCP, Kroon EG. Interferons: signaling, antiviral and viral evasion. Immunol Lett. 2009;122:1-11.

[311] Takeuchi O, Akira S. Innate immunity to virus infection. Immunol Rev. 2009;227:75-86.

[312] De Keersmaecker B, Heirman C, Corthals J, Empsen C, van Grunsven LA, Allard SD, et al. The combination of 4-1BBL and CD40L strongly enhances the capacity of dendritic cells to stimulate HIV-specific T cell responses. J Leukoc Biol. 2011 Jun;89(6):989-99.

Chapter 4

Is Anticancer Vaccine Possible: Experimental Application of Produced mRNA Transfected Dendritic Cells Derived from Enriched CD34+ Blood Progenitor Cells

Paula Lazarova, Gunnar Kvalheim and Krassimir Metodiev

Additional information is available at the end of the chapter

1. Introduction

The dendritic cells (DCs) are the most powerful antigen-presenting cells (APC) specialized to induce and regulate immune responses (1,2). The clinical use as cellular adjuvants in vaccination strategies has been aided by the development of methodologies to generate large production of these cells in culture. DCs can be grown ex-vivo from blood monocytes (3,4,5) or enriched CD34+ progenitors (6,7), using combinations of several cytokines/growth factors. Since our laboratory in Oslo routinely uses enriched CD34+ stem cells as stem cell support following high dose radio- and chemotherapy, it was of interest to test if such cells also could be applied for vaccine purposes (8,9), with a long term strategy of combining the two forms of therapy.

There are some publications indicating that CD34+ derived DC may work more efficiently as APC than those derived from monocytes (10), and recent data confirm that vaccine programs using CD34+ cell derived DCs lead to improved clinical results (11).

However, most in vitro culture systems for production of DCs include serum (9,11,12).

Since DCs are able to take up and process serum–derived antigens that are present in the cell cultures, such DC can when injected create unwanted reactions in the patients, in particular when fetal calf serum (FCS) is used. Thus, serum-free culturing condition is preferable, but in most previous culture experiments these conditions resulted in a lower yield of DCs (13,14).

Recently we reported a protocol for producing DCs from monocytes by use of gas-permeable Teflon bags and serum-free medium (15). We have used in the present study this experience and have developed a similar serum-free culture system for CD34+ cell derived DC and investigated the optimal immunological properties of these cells.

2. Materials and methods

2.1. Growth factors, recombinant human cytokines and medium

Flt-3 ligand (Flt-3L), granulocyte-macrophage colony-stimulating factor (GM-CSF), interleukin-4 (IL-4), tumor necrosis factor-alpha (TNF-α) and stem cell factor (SCF) were purchased from CellGenix, Freiburg, Germany. Interferon-alpha (INF- α) was from Roche, Basel, Switzerland. Serum free medium CellGro/SCGM and CellGro/DC medium (CellGenix, Freiburg, Germany) were employed during the culture. To compare the serum free growth conditions with serum containing medium, CellGro/SCGM with 25% human albumin or Dulbecco's Modified Eagle Medium (DMEM) supplemented with 10% FCS were used. Penicillin and Streptomycin was added to all mediums.

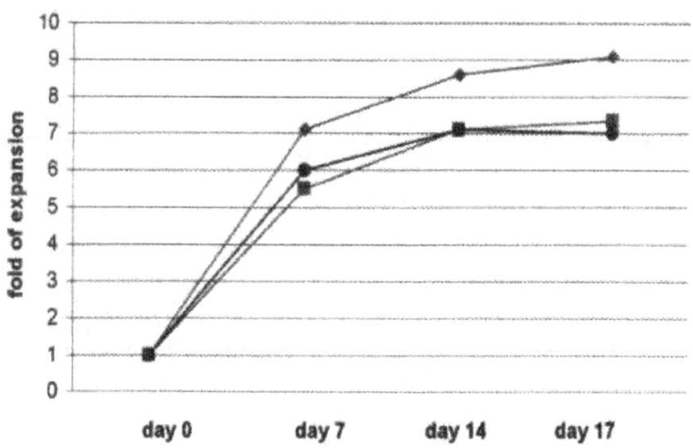

Figure 1. CD34+ cells (three different samples) cultured in serum-free CellGro SCGM/DC medium with added cytokines (as shown in materials and methods). The graphs indicate the fold expansion over time

2.2. CD34+ cell isolation

Leukapheresis-harvested samples were obtained from cancer patients undergoing peripheral blood (PB) stem cell mobilization after informed consent, using a CS 3000 Fenwall Cell Separator (Baxter, Deerfield, IL, USA). The isolation of CD34+cells was carried out using an Isolex 300i magnetic cell selector (Nexell, Irvine, CA, version 2.5CE/2.5CE+) as described earlier (16). The CD34+ samples were frozen in liquid nitrogen using PBS with 10% DMSO and 40% human serum albumin. The purity and viability of thawed CD34+ cells used for DC production was >98% and >95% respectively.

2.3. Generation of CD34+-derived DCs

CD34+ cells were rapidly thawed in a 37ºC water bath and washed once with culture medium. Then cells (0.5-1x10^5/ml) were transferred into VueLife™ FEP Teflon bags

(CellGenix, Freiburg, Germany) with serum containing DMEM/10% FCS medium, serum-free CellGro/SCGM medium or CellGro/SCGM/25% human albumin respectively. The following cytokine cocktail was added: GM-CSF 1000u/ml, IL-4 500u/ml, TNF-α 50ng/ml, Flt-3L 150ng/ml and SCF 50ng/ml. The bags were cultured for 14 days at 37ºC/5% CO_2. To keep a cell concentration of 10^5cells per ml through the entire culture period, re-feeding of the cells with culture medium employing equal concentration of cytokines was performed at weekly intervals. The serum-free medium cultures were from day 7, supplemented with CellGro DC medium instead of CellGro SCGM medium.

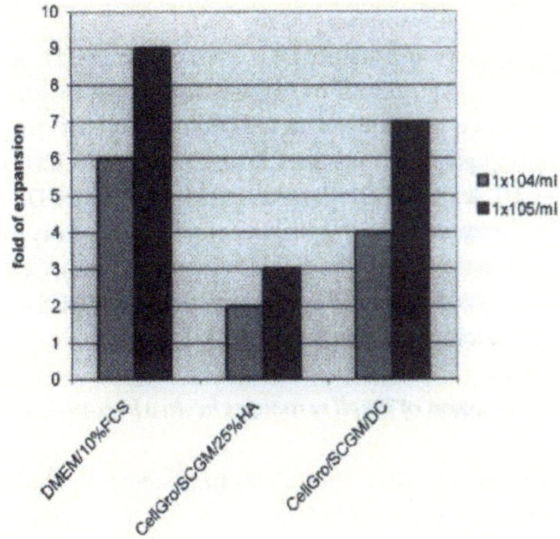

Figure 2. Expansion fold on Day 14. Different initial concentrations of CD34+ cells incubated in different culture medium. Cell concentration 10^5/ml are expanded better than 10^4/ml especially in serum free medium

2.4. Isolation of mRNA from cell line of human prostate cancer origin

Prostate cancer cell line DU 145 obtained from American Type Culture Collection (ATCC), was cultured in RPMI 1640 supplemented with 10% FCS. The method employed for isolation of mRNA from the tumor cell line has been described earlier (15). Briefly, $5x10^7$ cells were washed with cold PBS and transferred to a 1.5 ml microtube. Five hundred microliter ice-cold 2% IGEPAL (polyoxyethylene 9 nonylphenyl ether) (Sigma-Aldrich) was added to lyse the cells. The supernatant containing the cytosol fraction was obtained after centrifugation (10000xG for 1 minute at 4°C) and transferred to a 1.5 ml tube placed on a cooling block (4°C). To the supernatant 80 µl 10% LiDS (Lithium Lauryl Sulfate) (Sigma-Aldrich), 80 ul 5M LiCl (Lithium Chloride) (Sigma-Aldrich) and 0.5 ml Lysis & Binding Solution (Geno Vision) was added. Samples were frozen and stored at –80ºC until use. Isolation and purification of mRNA from the frozen or fresh samples were prepared in a GenoM™-48 Robotic Workstation (Genovision AS, Oslo, Norway) following the procedure as described by the manufacturer (GenoM™-48, Automated mRNA Isolation Handbook, http:// www.qiagen.com /genovision/technical.htm). Denaturing agarose/formaldehyde gel electrophoresis was used to evaluate the quality of mRNA. The prepared mRNA was either used fresh or stored at -80°C until use.

2.5. Transfection of tumor mRNA into immature DCs

Teflon bags containing immature DCs (day14) were concentrated by centrifugation (600xG, 5 min., 4°C), the supernatant was removed using a plasma extractor (FENWAL Laboratories, USA) and the cell pellet was transferred by a syringe to a 50 ml tube. After one additional wash by centrifugation, the DCs were resuspended in cold culture medium to give a final volume of 0.6-0.8 ml and placed in a 4°C cooling block until use. mRNA transfection was performed as described earlier (17) using a BTX ECM 830 square-wave electroporator (Genetronics Inc.,San Diego,CA). Electroporation settings were adjusted to single pulse, 500 volt and 2 ms. The BTX-4mm electroporation cuvette (Genetronics Inc.) was washed twice with sterile DC culture medium. Then mRNA extracted from $5x10^7$ cells (40 µl) was added to the prepared immature DCs and transferred to the electroporation cuvette . After eletroporation, DCs were transferred back into the tube and stored on the cooling block for 1 min. before further incubation and maturation. All mock-mRNA transfected DCs used as control underwent electroporation following the same procedure as described above. The cell processing and electroporation procedure took place in a sterile laminar hood inside the GMP (good manufacturing practice) laboratory facility. In order to assess the transfection efficacy, immature DCs were also electroporated with enhanced green fluorescence protein (EGFP) mRNA as a reporter gene instead of mRNA from tumor. The experimental conditions used and the flow cytometry measurement has been described previously (17).

2.6. Maturation of DCs in sterile VueLife™ FEP Teflon bags

The two cells, mRNA-transfected and mock-transfected DCs, were removed from the tube by a syringe and injected through a sterile sampling site coupler into VueLife™ FEP Teflon bags. In order to mature the DCs, serum-free or serum-containing medium was supplemented with a mixture of the cytokines: 50 ng/ml TNF-α (CELLGenix, Freiburg) and 1000u/ml INF-α (Sigma-Aldrich). The final cell concentration during the incubation at 37°C with 5% CO_2 for 72 hours was $5x10^5$cells per ml.

2.7. Cryopreservation of mature DCs

The bag containing matured DC was centrifuged at 600xG for 10 minutes at room temperature. By the use of plasma extractor the supernatant was removed and the remaining DCs were transferred to a 50 ml tube. Following cell enumeration and sterility testing, cells were transferred into Nunc vials. The cryoprotectant solution was CellGro DC medium with 50% human albumin and 10% DMSO. The final cell concentration was $1x10^7$ cells/ml. Total volume in each Nunc vial was 500 µl. Freezing was performed in a control rate freezer giving a rate of cooling of 1°C/min to -40°C with compensation for heat of fusion, then 1-2°C/min to -90°C. The prepared samples were thereafter transferred to liquid nitrogen and stored until use. The quality control of the frozen DCs consisted of sterility tests, phenotyping and viability testing by trypan blue staining before freezing and after thawing.

2.8. Immunophenotyping of the cells

Immature and mature DCs were phenotyped using the following panel of monoclonal antibodies: fluorescence isothiocyanate (FITC)- or phycoerythrin (PE)- conjugated anti-human CD1a, CD14, CD40, CD33, CD34, HLA DR, CD80 (Becton Dickinson), and CD83, CD86 (Immunotech). Negative controls were isotype-matched irrelevant antibodies (Dakocytomation). Cells were analyzed by flow cytometry using a FACSsort (Becton Dickinson, San Jose, Ca, USA).

2.9. Generation of T-cell responses in vitro by transfected DCs

Autologous-T cells were stimulated four times with weekly intervals in vitro by transfected DCs as described before (15). Briefly, CD34$^-$ PBMC from the same patient were thawed and plated in 6-well plates to get rid of adherent cells. Non-adherent cells containing high numbers of T lymphocytes were collected and used as responder cells. Thawed mRNA-transfected DCs used as stimulator cells were washed and irradiated with 3000 cGy. They were co-incubated in 24-well plates at a ratio 10:1 in serum-free CellGroDC-medium with 20 ng/ml of IL-7 and 100 pg/ml of IL-12. After 7 days incubation at 37°C in 5% CO_2, 1 ml of the suspension from each well was replaced with 1 ml of fresh DC medium containing 20 ng/ml of IL-7. On day 12, 19 and 26 the responder cells were restimulated by new batches of thawed and irradiated transfected DCs as on day 0. On day 14, 21 and 28 the cell cultured were given 1 ml of DC medium containing 20 IU/ml of IL-2. Finally on day 33 the cells were harvested and tested using ELISPOT assay as described below.

2.10. ELISPOT assay

The conditions for the ELISPOT assay have been described previously (15). A 96 well plate (Millipore-MAIP N45) were coated with 75 μl antibodies against human IFN-γ (Mabtech 1-D1K, 1 mg/ml diluted with PBS to a final concentration of 2 μg/ml) and incubated overnight at 4°C. The plate was left at room temperature (RT) for 1 hour and washed six times with PBS, 200 μl/well. Then RPMI-1640 + 1% human albumin was added 100 μl/well and incubated for 1-2 hours at 37°C to block unspecific binding of the antibody. The responder cells and stimulator cells were transferred to the precoated wells in different cell concentrations. As control mock-transfected DC, responder cells alone or medium alone was used. After incubation over night at 37°C, the plates were washed six times with PBS/0.05% Tween. To each well 75 μl of a stock solution of 0.75 μg/ml Biotinylated antibody against human IFN- γ (Mabtech, 7-B6-1-biotin, 1 mg/ml) was added and incubated for 2 hours at RT. Following six repeated washings the plate was incubated for one hour with 75μl per well of Streptavidin-ALP (Mabtech, 3310-8) from a stock solution (diluted 1:1000 in PBS+1%BSA). The plate was again washed 5 times with

PBS/0.05% Tween and one additional time with PBS alone. Then, after adding 75 µl of substrate BCIP/NBT (Sigma B911) to each well the plate was incubated for 4-5 minutes. When spots appeared, water was added to stop the reaction. The number of spots per well was counted under a stereomicroscope and the frequency of reactive T cells was calculated.

3. Results

3.1. Expansion of cells in serum-containing and serum-free medium

CD34+ progenitors were cultured in Teflon bags using serum containing DMEM/10%FCS and serum-free CellGro SCGM/DC medium supplemented with cytokines as described above. Table 1 shows cell expansion and viability on day14. The total cell expansion is 7.9±0.8 fold for CellGro/SCGM/DC medium and 8.3±0.6 fold for DMEM/FCS medium. Both conditions gave high cell viability, but when human albumin was added to the serum-free medium, lower cell expansion and viability was observed.

CD34+ cells proliferate and differentiate very rapidly during the first week, while in the remaining culture period only a minor expansion took place. When different cell concentrations of CD34+ cells were seeded and cultured for 14 days, a cell concentration of $1x10^5$ cells per ml kept through the culture period gave optimal growth conditions. Lower initial cell concentrations ($1x10^4$/ml) in the cultures gave no growth advantages (data not shown).

3.2. Yield and phenotypes of immature and mature DCs

Cultured cells lost their CD34 marker rapidly and no CD34 positive cells could be detected after 7 days of culturing. At day 14, DC purity was 35.9 ± 7.7 % as assessed by expression of CD86 and HLA DR antigens. Figure 2 (A and B) shows the phenotype of DCs in serum free medium on day 14 and 17. The CD86, CD83 and CD80 were up regulated greatly during maturation and the phenotypic profile obtained was comparable to DCs cultured in serum containing medium.

Different transfection parameters with regard to voltages and time of exposure were tested and the most suitable protocol was found to be 500V at 2ms. By the use of these parameters a transfection efficacy of >95% could be achieved and the mean fluorescence levels using EGFP (Enhanced green fluorescent protein) were increased to about 100-fold above background (figure 3). The percentages of surviving DC following mRNA tranfection using propidium iodide staining were 76%. A similar survival was obtained in the mock-transfected DC.

3.3. T-cell responses to thawed transfected DCs

To assess the function of matured DCs we use transfected DCs to stimulate autologous T cells four times weekly. Thereafter the T cells were tested in the ELISPOT assay, which give information of both transfection efficacy, processing and antigen stimulation capacity of transfected DCs. As shown in figure 4, after four times stimulation by thawed transfected DCs in vitro, a significant and specific T-cell response to transfected DCs as compared to the control experiment employing mock-transfected DCs was achieved.

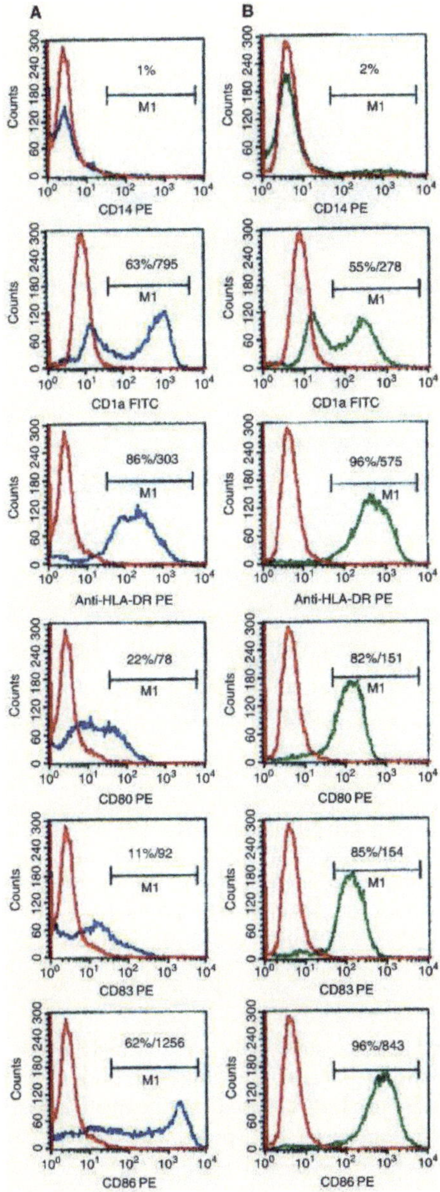

Figure 3. Immunophenotyping profile of: A) Immature DC; B) Mature DC generated from enriched monocytes. Overlay histograms show the expression of relevant antigens of immature (blue) and mature DC (green) versus isotype-matched control (red). The percentage of positive cells and mean fluorescence intensity value is shown too.

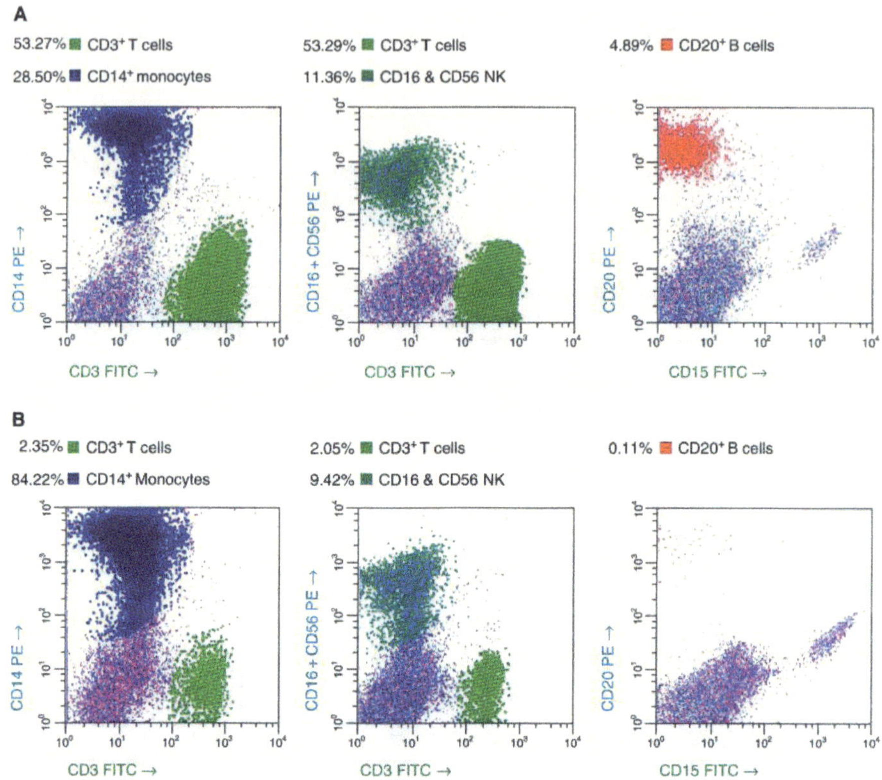

Figure 4. Transfection efficacy of mRNA demonstrated by utilized EGFP mRNA (lower part) compared to non-transfected DC (upper part). Left panels are density plots indicating large cell population gated. Middle panels are density plots showing the viability of cells (non-transfected and EGFP mRNA transfected by application of propidium iodide PI stating FL3). Right panels are histogram plots showing GFP signal in living cells. The green fluorescence intensity is increased about 100-fold in transfected cells than in non-transfected cells.

4. Discussion

In our hospital, enriched CD34+ stem cells are routinely being prepared and used as progenitor stem-cell support to patients receiving high dose therapy (16). In the cases that such patients also are candidates for DC-based vaccine treatment, spared frozen CD34+ cells would be available as a source for DC production thereby avoiding new expensive procedures for production of monocyte-derived DCs (18).

The present study describes the establishment of a clinical ex- vivo culture system for expansion of mature DCs derived from CD34+ cells employing VueLife™ FEP Teflon bags and serum free CellGro/SCGM/CellGro. Most methods applied for production of DC include FCS or pooled human serum. As a foreign protein, FCS is highly unwanted not only because of the danger of disease transmission but also because immune responses against FCS might result in high background responses obscuring the specific T cell immunity. Other studies have indicated that human serum may inhibit DC differentiation and therefore seems not to be a good alternative to replace FCS (13). Serum free conditions have been tested previously (13,14). In these studies cell expansion and DC yield were very low though the phenotype of the DCs were considered not to be affected. In this study we have demonstrated that there is no difference between serum-free and serum-containing medium with regard to ex-vivo expansion of both the total number of cells and the estimated content of matured DCs in the cell products. The addition of serum albumin to our cultures did not result in any growth advantages.

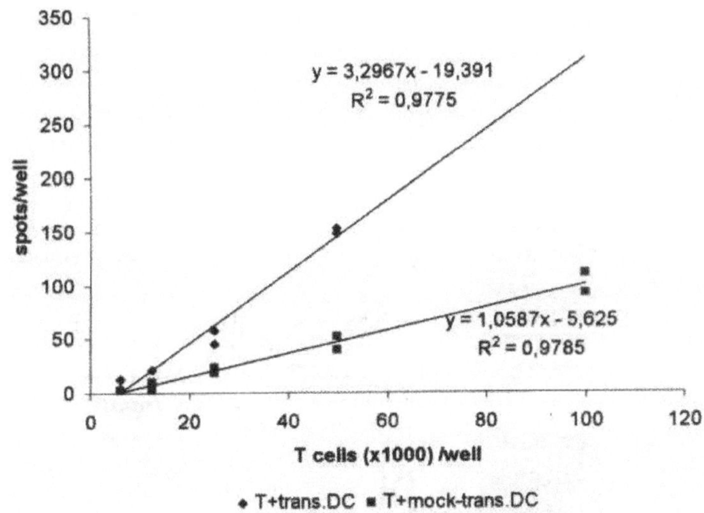

Figure 5. Autologous T cells stimulated with four times ex vivo irradiated transfected DC. ELISPOT assay indicates that stimulated T cells are able to recognize transfected DC specifically by use of mock-transfected DC as conrol

GM-CSF, TNF-α and IL-4 are cytokines that play an import role in DC differentiation (19,20) when serum-containing medium is being employed. However, our experiences and that of others indicate that this cytokine combination alone is not sufficient for ex vivo expansion of DCs from CD34+ cells. As described by others, ex-vivo culturing of CD34+ cells in the presence of SCF and Flt-3 (21) give an efficient expansion of total cell numbers without interfering with DC development. Since these early acting factors does not affect DC differentiation, but sustained the long-term expansion of CFU-DC, we chose to add them to our cultures. In contrast to monocyte- derived DCs, ex-vivo expansion of CD34 derived DCs usually occurred asynchronously over a 2 to 3 weeks period. Since INF-α can efficiently accelerate the course of maturation (22) we also included this cytokine in the cocktail the last 3 days of culture. This resulted in an up regulation of the maturation antigens CD86, CD83 and CD80.

The use of gas permeable bags for ex-vivo production has several advantages when compared to production in culture flasks. The bag system is closed and reduces the risk of contamination. DCs produced in Teflon bags do not attach to the surface and can easily be concentrated by centrifugation without any extra steps. It also facilitates large-scale production, which can be divided into aliquots containing cells with identical properties. We have shown that DCs can efficiently be produced in suspension using gas permeable Teflon bags. When CD34+ progenitors are cultured in flasks, usually the cell concentration is 10^4/ml. In our system we have shown that optimal cell concentration is 10^5/ml, which give a 10-fold reduction in the amount of medium and cytokines used.

DCs have been loaded with several antigens, such as tumor lysate, peptides, proteins, DNA and mRNA. As a source of antigens, the major limitation of using lysate, proteins or peptides isolated from patients' tumor cells is the amount of tumor tissue or the purity of the tumor specimens. The use of nucleic acids, either DNA or RNA, would overcome this practical limitation. As mRNA is a safer alternative due to its limited ability to cause permanent genetic alterations in the host, it appears to be more attractive to be used than DNA transfection (23). For this purpose, a vector-free transfection system based on square-wave electroporation to transfer mRNA into DCs has been developed (17). This method is currently successfully used in the clinic to produce mRNA-transfected monocyte-derived DCs (15). We here demonstrate that this method also resulted in efficient transfection of mRNA into immature CD34+ cell derived DCs without significantly affecting the survival of the cells.

Generally the antigen-stimulating capacity of DCs has been evaluated employing allo-reactive T cells or responses against recall antigens. We have used priming of autologous T cell against antigens encoded by a prostate tumor cell line in order to evaluate the immuno-stimulatory role of the transfected DCs. The ELISPOT assay was used to detect and quantify of single T lymphocyte forming cytokine spots after antigen contact in vitro. The ELISPOT assay is a more stringent system for testing both the efficacy of transfection and the processing and antigen-stimulating capacity of transfected DCs. Our results show that CD34+ cells derived DCs, grown in serum free conditions in clinical scale productions reproducibly are capable of inducing a tumor specific immune response. These results are similar to what was seen in our previous study using monocyte-derived DCs

The finding and results from the present study allows us to proceed with a clinical protocol for application of CD34+ derived DCs for cancer vaccine. Possible attractive candidates for such an approach are relapsed Hodgkin's patients (16) and other patients that have previously been treated with auto transplantation and with spared frozen samples of CD34+ cells.

Experiment	Cell Gro/SCGM&25% HA	DMEM / 10% FCS	Cell Gro / SCGM / DC
	fold / viability	fold / viability	fold / viability
1	1.6 / 61%	9.0 / 97%	8.6 / 94%
2	1.2 / 67%	7.8 / 98%	7.1 / 93%
3	1.8 / 73%	8.8 / 97%	7.1 / 84%

Table 1. Expansion fold and viability on Day 14

Author details

Paula Lazarova[1,2,*], Gunnar Kvalheim[1], Krassimir Metodiev[3]
[1]*Dept. Cellular Therapy, University Rikshospital-Radiumhospital, Oslo, Norway,*
[2]*Clinical laboratory, District Hospital "St. Anna", Varna, Bulgaria,*
[3]*Dept. Preclinical & Clinical Sciences, Medical University, Varna, Bulgaria*

Acknowledgement

We warmly thank the staffs in stem cell laboratory (Radium-Oslo-Norway) for the preparation of frozen CD34+ progenitor cells.

5. References

[1] Banchereau J. and R.M. Steinman. 1998. Dedritic cells and control of immunity. *Nature 392:245.*

[2] Banchereau J., F.Briere, C. Caux, J. Davoust, S. Lebecue, Y. Liu, B. Pulendran and K. Palucka. 2000. Immunobiology of dendritic cells. *Annu. Rev. Immunol. 18:767*

[3] Thurner B., C. Roder, D. Dieckmann, M. Heuer, M. Kruse, A. Glaser, P. Keikavoussi, E. Kampfen, A. Bender, G. Schuler. 1999. Generation of large numbers of fully mature and stable dendritic cells from leukapheresis products for clinical application. *J. Immunological Methods 223:1-15*

[4] Feuerstein B., T.Berger, C. Maczek, C. Roder, D. Schreiner, U. Hirsch, I. Haendle, W. Leisgang, A. Glaser, O. Kuss, T. Diepgen, G. Schuler, B. Thurner. 2000. A method for the production of cryopreserved aliquots of antigen- preloaded, mature dendritic cells ready for clinical use. *J. Immunological Methods 245:15-*

[5] Maria R. Motta, M. Castellani, S. Rizzi, A. Curti, F. Gubinelli, M. Fogli, E. Ferri, C. Cellini, M. Baccarani and R. Lemoli. 2003 Generation of dendritic cells from CD14+ monocytes positively selected by immunomagnetic adsorption for multiple myeloma patients enrolled in a clinical trial of anti- idiotype vaccination. *British J. Haematology, 121: 240-250*

[6] Ramadan G., R. Schmidt and J. Schubert. 2001 In vitro generation of human CD86+ dendritic cells from CD34+ haematopoietic progenitors by PMA and in serum- free medium. *Clinical & Exp. Immunology, 125*

[7] Strunk D., K. Rappersberger, K. Egger, et al. 1996. Generation of human dendritic cells/ Langerhans cells from circulating $CD34^+$ hematopoietic progenitor cells. *Blood 87:1292*

[8] Enomoto M., H Nagayama, K Sato, Y Xu, S Asano and TA Takahashi. 2000. In vitro generation of dendritic cells derived from cryopreserved CD34+ cells mobilized into peripheral blood in lymphoma patients. *Cytotherapy 2:95-104*

[9] Titzer S., O. Christensen, O. Manzke, H. Tesch, J. Wolf, B. Emmerich, C. Carsten, V. Diehl and H. Bohlen. Vaccination of multiple myeloma patients with idiotype-pulsed dendritic cells: immunological and clinical aspects.

* Corresponding Author

[10] Ferlazzo G., A. Wesa, Wie. Wie, and A. Galy. 1999. Dendritic Cells generated either from D34+ progenitor cells or from monocytes differ in their ability to activate antigen-specific CD8+ T cells *J. Immunology, 163:3597-3604*
[11] Banchereau J, AK Palucka, M Dhodapkar, S Burkeholder, N Taquet, A Rolland, S Taquet, S Coquery, KM Wittkowski, N Bhardwaj, L Pineiro, R Steinman, J Fay. 2001. Immune and clinical responses in patients with metastatic melanoma to CD34 (+) progenitor-derived dendritic cell vaccine. Cancer Res. 1; 61(17): 6451-6458
[12] Mackensen A., B. Herbst, J. Chen, G. Kohler, C. Noppen, W. Herr, G. Spagnoli, V. Cerundolo and A. Lindemann. 2000. Phase 1 study in melanoma patients of a vaccine with peptide-pulsed dendritic cells generated in vitro from CD34+ hematopoietic progenitor cells. *Int. J. Cancer, 86:385-392*
[13] Luft T., K. Pang, E. Thomas, C. Bradley, H. Savoia, J. Trapani, and J. Cebon. 1998. A serum-free culture model for studying the differentiation of human dendritic cells from adult CD34+ progenitor cells. *Exp. Hematology, 26:489-500*
[14] Kowalkowski K., M. Alzona, F. Aono, D. Van Epps and M. Vachula. 1998. Ex Vivo Generation of Dendritic Cells from CD34+ Cells in Gas-Permeable containers Under Serum-Free Conditions. *J. Hematotherapy 7: 403-411*
[15] Mu L.J., G. Gaudernack, S. Sæbøe-Larssen, H. Hammerstad, A. Tierens, G. Kvalheim. 2003. A Protocol for Generation of Clinical Grade mRNA-Transfected Monocyte-Derived Dendritic Cells for Cancer Vaccines *Scandinavian J. Immunology* 2, 58: 578-586
[16] Blystad A.K., H. Holte, S. Kvaløy, E. Smeland, J. Delabie, G. Kvalheim. 2001. High-dose therapy in patients with Hodgkin disease: the use of selected CD34+ cells is as safe as unmanipulated peripheral progenitor cells (PBPC). *Bone marrow Transplantation. 28:849-857.*
[17] Sæbøe-Larssen S., E. Fossberg, G. Gaudernack. 2002. mRNA-based electrotransfection of human dendritic cells and induction of T-lymphocyte responses against the telomerase catalytic subunit (hTERT). *J. Immunol. Methods, 1:191*
[18] Kvalheim G. 2002. Clinical use of enriched CD34+ cells. *Blood Therapies in medicine. 2:57-64*
[19] Sallusto F., A. Lanzavecchia, 1994, Efficient presentation of soluble antigen by cultured human dendritic cells is maintained by GM-CSF plus IL-4 and downregulated by TNF-alpha. *J. Exp. Med.*, 179:110919.
[20] Caux C., C. Dezutter-Dambuyant, D. Schmitt, J. Banchereau. 1992. GM-CSF and TNF-alpha cooperate in the generation of dendritic langerhans cells. *Nature 360:258*
[21] Curti A., M. Fogli, M. Ratta, S. Tura, and R.Lemoli 2001. Stem cell factor and FLT3-ligand are strictly required to sustain the long-term expansion of primitive $CD34^{+}$ DR^{-} dendritic cell precursors. *The J. Immunol. 166:*848
[22] Luft T., K. Pang, E. Thomas, P. Hertzog, D.Hart, J. Trapani, and J. Cebon 1998. Type I IFN_s enhance the terminal differentiation of DC. *The J. Immunol. 161:1947-1953*
[23] Boczkowski B., S. K. Nair, J. Nam, H. Lyerly, and E. Gilboa 2000. Induction of tumor immunity and cytotoxic T lymphocyte responses using dendritic cells transfected with messenger RNA amplified from tumor cells. *Cancer Research 60:1028*

Section 2

Immunodeficiency – Mechanisms and Pathophysiology

Chapter 5

Fungal Infections in Immunosuppressed Patients

Luis Enrique Jerez Puebla

Additional information is available at the end of the chapter

1. Introduction

Fungal infections, also called mycoses, are important causes of morbidity and mortality in humans. Some fungal infections are endemic, and these infections are usually caused by fungi that are present in the environment and whose spores enter humans. Other fungal infections are said to be opportunistic because the causative agents cause mild or no disease in healthy individuals but may infect and cause severe disease in immunodeficient persons. The human airway is continuously open to the nonsterile environment where fungal spores have the potential to reach lung tissue and produce disease. In the immunocompromised host, many fungi, including species of fungi typically considered nonpathogenic, have the potential to cause serious morbidity and mortality. Over the last several decades the advent of the human immunodeficiency virus (HIV) epidemic and the increasing use of immunosuppressive drugs for serious medical conditions have dramatically increased the number of persons who are severely immunocompromised. In addition, the range and diversity of fungi that cause disease have broadened. Although *Candida* and *Aspergillus* species continue to be the fungal pathogens that most frequently cause invasive fungal disease in immunocompromised persons overall, infections due to previously uncommon hyaline and dematiaceous filamentous fungi are being reported with increasing frequency. This is significant because, despite marked advances in antifungal therapy, infections caused by opportunistic fungal infections (rare and emerging) continue to be associated with high morbidity, high mortality, and poor patient outcomes. This results from a combination of drug-resistant strains, lack of robust clinical studies evaluating treatments, and severe underlying diseases in the patient [2].

The principal mediators of innate immunity against fungi are neutrophils and macrophages. Patients with neutropenia are extremely susceptible to opportunistic fungal infections. Phagocytes and dendritic cells sense fungal organisms by TLRs and lectin-like receptors called dectins . Neutrophils presumably liberate fungicidal substances, such as reactive oxygen species and lysosomal enzymes, and phagocytose fungi for intracellular killing. Many extracellular fungi elicit strong TH17 responses, which are driven in part by the activation of dendritic cells by fungal products binding to the dectin receptor and resulting production of TH17- inducing cytokines (IL-6, IL-23) from the dendritic cells. The TH17 cells stimulate inflammation, and the recruited neutrophils and monocytes destroy the fungi. *Candida* infections often start at mucosal surfaces, and cell-mediated immunity is believed to prevent spread of the fungi into tissues. TH1 responses are protective in intracellular fungal infections, such as histoplasmosis, but these responses may elicit granulomatous inflammation, which is an important cause of host tissue injury in these infections. Fungi also elicit specific antibody responses that are of protective value [2].

2. Candidiasis

Candidiasis is caused by infection with species of the genus *Candida,* predominantly with *Candida albicans. Candida* species are ubiquitous fungi that represent the most common fungal pathogens that affect humans. The growing problem of mucosal and systemic candidiasis reflects the enormous increase in the number of patients at risk and the increased opportunity that exists for *Candida* species to invade tissues normally resistant to invasion. *Candida* species are true opportunistic pathogens that exploit recent technological advances to gain access to the circulation and deep tissues [3].

The increased prevalence of local and systemic disease caused by these yeasts has resulted in numerous new clinical syndromes, the expression of which depends primarily on the immune status of the host. *Candida* species produce a wide spectrum of diseases, ranging from superficial mucocutaneous disease to invasive illnesses. The clinical manifestations may be acute, subacute or chronic to episodic. Involvement may be localized to the mouth, throat, skin, scalp, vagina, fingers, nails, bronchi, lungs, or the gastrointestinal tract, or become systemic as in septicemia, endocarditis and meningitis. In healthy individuals, Candida infections are usually due to impaired epithelial barrier functions and occur in all age groups, but are most common in the newborn and the elderly. They usually remain superficial and respond readily to treatment. Systemic candidiasis is usually seen in patients with cell-mediated immune deficiency, and those receiving aggressive cancer treatment, immunosuppression, or transplantation therapy. The management of serious and life-threatening invasive candidiasis remains severely hampered by delays in diagnosis and the lack of reliable diagnostic methods that allow detection of both fungemia and tissue invasion by *Candida* species [4].

The first step in the development of a candidal infection is colonization of the mucocutaneous surfaces. All of the factors outlined above are associated with increased colonization rates. The routes of candidal invasion include (1) disruption of a colonized surface (skin or mucosa), allowing the organisms access to the bloodstream, and (2) persorption via the gastrointestinal wall, which may occur following massive colonization with large numbers of organisms that pass directly into the bloodstream [5].

Candida species are the most common cause of fungal infection in immunocompromised persons. Oropharyngeal colonization is found in 30-55% of healthy young adults, and *Candida* species may be detected in 40-65% of normal fecal microbiota [6, 7].

Candida species are yeastlike fungi that can form pseudohyphae and some species can develop true hyphae, as *Candida albicans* do. For the most part, *Candida* species are confined to human and animal reservoirs; however, they are frequently recovered from the hospital environment, including on foods, countertops, air-conditioning vents, floors, respirators, and medical personnel. They are also normal commensals of diseased skin and mucosal membranes of the gastrointestinal, genitourinary, and respiratory tracts [8-10].

Candida species also contain their own set of well-recognized but not well-characterized virulence factors that may contribute to their ability to cause infection. The main virulence factors include the following [11]:

- Surface molecules that permit adherence of the organism to other structures (eg, human cells, extracellular matrix, prosthetic devices)
- Acid proteases and phospholipases that involve penetration and damage of cell envelopes
- Ability to convert to a hyphal form (phenotypic switching)

As with most fungal infections, host defects also play a significant role in the development of candidal infections. Host defense mechanisms against *Candida* infection and their associated defects that allow infection are as follows:

- Intact mucocutaneous barriers - Wounds, intravenous catheters, burns, ulcerations
- Phagocytic cells -Granulocytopenia
- Polymorphonuclear leukocytes - Chronic granulomatous disease
- Monocytic cells -Myeloperoxidase deficiency
- Complement -Hypocomplementemia
- Immunoglobulins -Hypogammaglobulinemia
- Bone marrow transplantation
- Solid organ transplantation (liver, kidney)
- Parenteral hyperalimentation
- Hematologic malignancies
- Foley catheters
- Solid neoplasms
- Recent chemotherapy or radiation therapy
- Corticosteroids
- Broad-spectrum antibiotics
- Burns
- Prolonged hospitalization
- Gastrointestinal tract surgery
- Central intravascular access devices
- Premature birth

- Hemodialysis
- Acute and chronic renal failure

Over 200 species of *Candida* exist in nature; thus far, only a few species have been associated with disease in humans.

- The medically significant *Candida* species include the following [12]:
  - *C albicans,* the most common species identified (50-60%)
  - Candida glabrata (previously known as Torulopsis glabrata) (15-20%)
  - C parapsilosis (10-20%)
  - Candida tropicalis (6-12%)
  - Candida krusei (1-3%)
  - Candida kefyr (< 5%)
  - Candida guilliermondi (< 5%)
  - Candida lusitaniae (< 5%)
  - *Candida dubliniensis,* primarily recovered from patients infected with HIV

C glabrata and *C albicans* account for approximately 70-80% of *Candida* species recovered from patients with candidemia or invasive candidiasis. *C glabrata* has recently become very important because of its increasing incidence worldwide, its association with fluconazole resistance in up to 20% of clinical specimens, and its overall decreased susceptibility to other azoles and polyenes.

C krusei is important because of its intrinsic resistance to ketoconazole and fluconazole (Diflucan); it is also less susceptible to all other antifungals, including itraconazole (Sporanox) and amphotericin B.

Another important *Candida* species is *C lusitaniae;* although not as common as other *Candida* species, *C lusitaniae* is of clinical significance because it may be intrinsically resistant to amphotericin B, although it remains susceptible to azoles and echinocandins.

C parapsilosis is also an important species to consider in hospitalized patients. It is especially common in infections associated with vascular catheters prosthetic devices. Additionally, *in vitro* analyses have shown that echinocandins have a higher minimum inhibitory concentration (MIC) against *C parapsilosis* than other *Candida* species. The clinical relevance of this *in vitro* finding has yet to be determined [13].

C tropicalis has frequently been considered an important cause of candidemia in patients with cancer (leukemia) and in those who have undergone bone marrow transplantation.

The diagnosis of almost any form of *Candida* disease requires an integration of clinical, epidemiological, and laboratory findings. Unfortunately, results from the routine laboratory studies are often nonspecific and not very helpful. Clinicians are required to act definitively and early based on a high index of suspicion. In the past, many patients with life-threatening candidiasis died without receiving antifungal therapy. Systemic candidiasis should be suspected in patients with persistent leukocytosis and either persistent neutropenia or other risk factors and who remain febrile despite broad-spectrum antibiotic therapy. To be effective, antifungal therapy should be provided early and empirically in such high-risk patients. Cultures of nonsterile sites, although not useful for establishing a diagnosis, may demonstrate high degrees of candidal colonization. Always consider positive culture results from sterile sites to be significant and evidence of infection [14].

Candidemia and disseminated candidiasis [14, 15].

- Blood cultures are helpful but yield positive results in only 50-60% of cases of disseminated infection.
- Urinalysis may be helpful and may show either colonization or renal candidiasis.
- The serum (1,3)β-D-glucan detection assay (Glucatell, Fungitell) is a nonculture assay that was approved for use in the United States in May 2004. This assay measures the level of β-glucan (a fungal cell wall component). In a large multicenter study, the assay yielded a high specificity and positive predictive value with highly reproducible results [15].
- Cultures of nonsterile sites, although not useful for establishing a diagnosis, may be useful for initiating antifungal therapy in patients with fever that is unresponsive to broad-spectrum antimicrobials. Therefore, appropriate interpretation is required. Positive results from blood cultures and cultures from other sterile sites always imply the presence of invasive disease. Positive results from sterile sites should always be taken as significant and should always prompt treatment.
- Gastrointestinal, respiratory, and urinary tract cultures that are positive for *Candida* may not always represent invasive disease. However, these should be considered sites of colonization.

- Species identification [14]
  - *C albicans, C dubliniensis,* can be identified morphologically via germ-tube formation (hyphae are produced from yeast cells after 2-3 h of incubation) or biochemical assays.
  - CHROMagar *Candida* allows for the presumptive identification of several *Candida* species by using color reactions in specialized media that demonstrate different colony colors depending on the species of *Candida.*
  - API20C and API32C are biochemical assays that allow for the identification of the different *Candida* species with more precision. These assays evaluate the assimilation of numerous carbon substrates and generate profiles used in the identification of different fungal species.
  - *The C albicans* peptide nucleic acid (PNA) fluorescence in situ hybridization (FISH) test can be used to identify *C albicans in* 24-48 hours when the probe is added to smears that are made directly from the blood culture bottle and followed by hybridization. A newer version of this test now allows for the simultaneous identification of either *C albicans* or *C glabrata* [16, 17].
- Antifungal susceptibility testing [18]
  - In vitro susceptibility testing for *Candida* species is now standardized using the Clinical Laboratory Standards Institute (CLSI) microbroth dilution (CLSI M27-A2, 2002) or the disk diffusion (CLSI M44-P, 2003) methodology. This was formerly

known as the National Committee for Clinical Laboratory Standards (NCCLS) microbroth dilution.

- These methods may be helpful in guiding difficult therapeutic decisions. Most of the difficult decisions involve antifungal-refractory oral or esophageal candidiasis in patients with advanced HIV disease.

- Nonculture *Candida* detection assays [18-20]
  - The *Candida* mannan assay yields a sensitivity of 31-90% (less for non-*albicans Candida* species).
  - The *Candida* heat labile antigen assay yields a sensitivity of 10-71%.
  - The D-arabinitol assay yields a sensitivity of 50% but is not useful for infection with *C krusei* or *C glabrata.*
  - The enolase assay yields a sensitivity of 55-75%, which improves with serial testing.
  - The (1,3)β-D-glucan assay is an amebocyte lysis assay with a sensitivity of 75-100% and a specificity of 88-100%. It is a broad-spectrum assay that detects *Aspergillus, Candida, Fusarium, Acremonium,* and *Saccharomyces* species. β-D-glucan is a cell wall component in a wide variety of fungi and can be detected based on its ability to activate factor G of the horseshoe crab coagulation cascade. The Fungitell assay may be used in the evaluation of invasive fungal infections caused by the fungi mentioned above. The assay does not detect infections caused by *Cryptococcus neoformans* or Zygomycetes.
  - Molecular assays such as the polymerase chain reaction (PCR) assay and DNA probes are still under development and in the early investigational phases, but they appear promising.

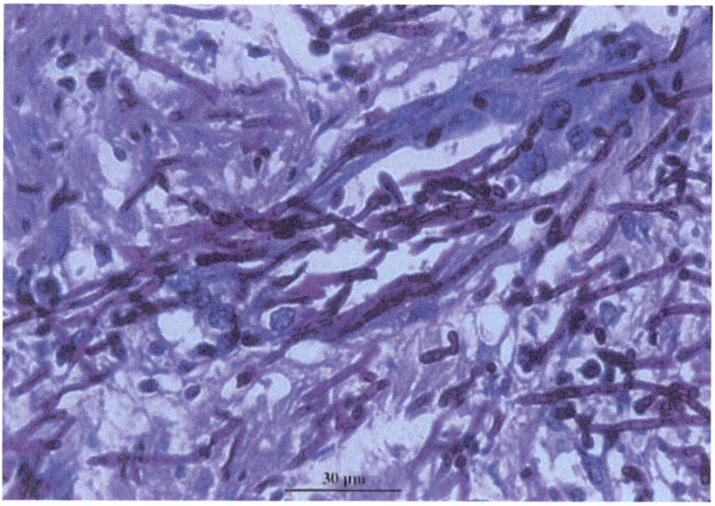

Figure 1. Periodic Acid-Schiff (PAS) stained section of post-mortem oesophagus showing invasion of blood vessel by *C. albicans.* Note blastoconidia and branched pseudohyphae. (Courtesy: www.mycology.adelaide.edu.au)

The treatments used to manage *Candida* infections vary substantially and are based on the anatomic location of the infection, the patients' underlying disease and immune status, the patients' risk factors for infection, the specific species of *Candida* responsible for infection, and, in some cases, the susceptibility of the *Candida* species to specific antifungal drugs. There have been significant changes in the management of candidiasis in the last few years, particularly related to the appropriate use of echinocandins and expanded-spectrum azoles for candidemia, other forms of invasive candidiasis, and mucosal candidiasis [21]. These latest recommendations include the echinocandins caspofungin, micafungin, and anidulafungin, along with voriconazole and posaconazole, as well as lipid formulations of amphotericin B in various situations. Fluconazole is still considered a first-line agent in nonneutropenic patients with candidemia or suspected invasive candidiasis [22].

3. Cryptococosis

Cryptococcus neoformans is an encapsulated yeast. In 1894, Busse, a pathologist, first described the yeast in a paper he presented to the Greifswald Medical Society. Busse isolated the yeast from the tibia of a 31-year-old woman, noted its resistance to sodium hydroxide, and published the case report that same year [23]. The following year, a surgeon named Buschke reported the same isolate from the same patient, thus establishing the early eponym of Busse-Buschke disease [24].

Since the initial reports, researchers have identified the diverse spectrum of host responses to cryptococcal infection. The responses range from a harmless colonization of the airways and asymptomatic infection in laboratory workers (resulting in only a positive skin test finding) to meningitis or disseminated disease. Although virulence in animals and, possibly, humans varies among strains of cryptococci, virulence probably plays a relatively small role in the outcome of an infection. The crucial factor is the immune status of the host. The importance of host immunity to the development of cryptococcosis is the single most critical feature of this infection from diagnosis to prognosis [25, 26]. A major pathological principle in understanding of cryptococcosis is that many individuals are infected with this yeast but their immune system controls the infection with minor and insignificant symptoms. However, like tuberculosis, the yeast can persist in tissue (dormancy) for long periods of time to then reactivate and produce disease during an immunosuppressive event. Furthermore, this reactivation scenario has been supported by recent observations with HIV infection progression to low CD4 counts (50-100 CD4 cells/*ul*) and this immunosuppressive lymphopenia directly linked with higher risk of cryptococcosis as the reduction of cell-mediated immune cells occurs [27].

There are a series of well-known risk factors associated with cryptococcal disease. The two highest risk factors are HIV infection and corticosteroid use. The corticosteroid use as a risk factor incorporates most of the transplant recipients and particularly, the solid organ transplants with their long term corticosteroid exposure and relatively high daily doses (> 20mg/day of prednisone) [28]. Among the other risk factors that require some discussion are the lymphomas/chronic leukemias and the connective tissue diseases in which most of these cases are aided by corticosteroid usage. Diabetes continues to be present in a large number of patients with cryptococcosis [29].

It should be noted, however, that not all patients with cryptococcosis have an underlying disease. In fact, if you exclude HIV- infected patients, approximately 20-30% of patients with disseminated cryptococcosis will present with no apparent underlying diseases or known risk factors [29]. Since the host is classically protected by a vigorous Th_1 response, it is likely that those with no apparent underlying disease but who develop disseminated cryptococcosis do, in fact, have some undetected alterations in their protective immune responses. A small genetic susceptibility study through identification of DNA polymorphisms in certain immune genes has been started [30], but clearly, further comprehensive studies in genetic susceptibility and immune functions will be necessary for us to get a true appreciation for what is really going on in the apparently normal host with disseminated cryptococcosis. In fact, at times, the dysregulated immune systems and heterogenerous populations of patients makes this group of patients (apparently normal hosts)the hardest to manage since they may have late disease (prolonged disease because of delayed diagnosis) with either a high burden of organisms before treatment and/or prone to the development of a very aggressive immune reconstitution inflammatory syndrome (IRIS). In this group of apparently normal hosts with cryptococcosis, it is reasonable to check for underlying HIV infection since it is a treatable illness and also it is probably reasonable to obtain a total CD4 lymphocyte count to identify patients with idiopathic CD4 lymphocytopenia which may require prolonged antifungal suppressive therapy, although present data suggest that this idiopathic syndrome with cryptococcosis actually has a good prognosis [31].

The general theme of immunity for this disease is that prevention of disseminated cryptococcosis is controlled by an efficient cell-mediated immunity. This fact is supported by many *in vitro* studies, animal models and all present cytokine studies in humans [32]. For instance, defective production of interferon gamma and TNF-alpha but not IL-10 occurs in patients who have cryptococcosis which indicates a shifting to a predominant Th_2 host response [33]. Furthermore, during effective treatment at the CNS site of a cryptococcal infection, an up-regulated Th_1 response occurs as measured by higher CSF interferon gamma levels and lower CSF yeast counts [34].

Much of the host issues for diagnosis and initial management of cryptococcosis are based around a deficiency in host responses and the risk groups identify this focus. However, it is essential that clinicians realize that the total management of cryptococcosis must deal with the total immune dysregulation that occurs and not just its early deficiencies. This is emphasized by the many pleomorphic effects of the lingering cryptococcal polysaccharide can have on host immune functions. Thus, even the yeast and its products can modulate the host environment. This immune dysregulation was clearly identified during the AIDS epidemic with cryptococcosis and the use of HAART for HIV infection during cryptococcosis [35, 36].

Cryptococcus neoformans has become a major human pathogen and a common infection in certain immunocompromised hosts [36]. Cryptococcosis, the disease resulting from infection with *C. neoformans,* varies from a localized skin lesion or asymptomatic colonization of the respiratory tree to a widely disseminated life-threatening infection, which may infect all organs of the body. However, *C. neoformans* has a special propensity for invading the central nervous system and cryptococcal meningoencephalitis is the primary clinical presentation for the life-threatening stage of this infection [37].

Although the genus *Cryptococcus* contains more than 50 species, only *C neoformans* and *Cryptococcus gattii* are considered principal pathogens in humans. Previously, *C neoformans* was defined as having two varieties—var *neoformans* and var *gattii.* However, based on the elucidation of the genomic sequences, *C neoformans* and *C gattii* are now considered two distinct species. These two species have 5 serotypes based on antigenic specificity of the capsular polysaccharide; these include serotypes A, D, and AD (*C neoformans*) and serotypes B and C (*C gattii*). *C neoformans* is the most common species in temperate climates throughout the world and is found in aged pigeon droppings. Until recently, *C gattii* was found principally in tropical and subtropical climates. *C gattii* is not associated with birds but grows in the litter around certain species of eucalyptus trees (ie, *Eucalyptus camaldulensis, Eucalyptus tereticornis*) [38].

Worldwide, *C neoformans* serotype A causes most cryptococcal infections in immunocompromised patients, including patients infected with HIV. For unknown reasons, *C. gattii* rarely infects persons with HIV infection and other immunosuppressed patients. Patients infected with *C gattii* are usually immunocompetent, respond slowly to treatment, and are at risk for developing intracerebral mass lesions (eg, cryptococcomas). Naturally occurring cryptococcosis occurs in both animals and humans, but neither animal-to-human transmission nor person-to-person respiratory transmission via the respiratory route has been documented. Transmission via organ transplantation has been reported when infected donor organs were used. *C neoformans* causes the vast majority of cryptococcal infections in immunosuppressed hosts, including patients with AIDS, whereas *C gattii* causes 70%-80% of cryptococcal infections among immunocompetent hosts [39].

C neoformans reproduces by budding and forms round yeastlike cells that are 3-6 μm in diameter. Within the host and in certain culture media, a large polysaccharide capsule surrounds each cell. *C neoformans* forms smooth, convex, yellow or tan colonies on solid media at 20-37°C (68-98.6°F). This fungus is identified based on its microscopic appearance, biochemical test results, and ability to grow at 37°C (98.6°F); most nonpathogenic *Cryptococcus* strains do not grow at this temperature. In addition, *C neoformans* does not assimilate lactose and nitrates or produce pseudomycelia on cornmeal or rice-Tween agar. Most strains of *C neoformans* can use creatinine as a nitrogen source, which may partially explain the growth of the organism in creatinine-rich avian feces. Another useful biochemical characteristic of *C neoformans,* which distinguishes it from nonpathogenic strains, is its ability to produce melanin. The fungal enzyme phenol oxidase acts on certain substrates (eg, dihydroxyphenylalanine, caffeic acid) to produce melanin [40, 41].

C gattii contains genotypes VGI and the more commonly identified VGIIa and VDIIb. *Cryptococcus* species can reproduce via same-sex mating, and VGIIa may have arisen from the same-sex mating of VGIIb and another strain that has yet to be identified [38].

In 1976, Kwon-Chung described the perfect (ie, sexual, teleomorphic) form of *C neoformans,* which was named *Filobasidiella neoformans*. Prior to the identification of *F neoformans,* which is mycelial, *C neoformans* was considered a monomorphic yeast. *F neoformans* results from the mating of suitable strains of serotypes A and D. The perfect state of *C gattii* is *Filobasidiella bacillispora* and results from the mating of serotypes B and C. Some strains of A and D can mate with strains of B and C [42].

Following inhalation, the yeast spores are deposited into the pulmonary alveoli, where they must survive the neutral-to-alkaline pH and physiologic concentrations of carbon dioxide before they are phagocytized by alveolar macrophages. Glucosylceramide synthase (GCS) has been identified as an essential factor in the survival of *C neoformans* in this extracellular environment. Although GCS is a critical factor in extracellular survival of the yeast, the yeast no longer requires GCS to survive the intracellular, more acidic, environment within the macrophage once it is phagocytized by alveolar macrophages. Unencapsulated yeast are readily phagocytosed and destroyed, whereas encapsulated organisms are more resistant to phagocytosis. The cryptococcal polysaccharide capsule has antiphagocytic properties and may be immunosuppressive. The antiphagocytic properties of the capsule block recognition of the yeast by phagocytes and inhibit leukocyte migration into the area of fungal replication [43].

The host response to cryptococcal infection includes both cellular and humoral components. Animal models demonstrate that natural killer cells participate in the early killing of cryptococci and, possibly, antibody-dependent cell-mediated killing. In vitro monocyte-derived macrophages, natural killer cells, and T lymphocytes can inhibit or kill cryptococci. A successful host response includes an increase in helper T-cell activity, skin test conversion, and a reduction in the number of viable organisms in the tissues. In addition to cellular mechanisms, anticryptococcal antibodies and soluble anticryptococcal factors have been described. Antibodies to cryptococcal antigens play a critical role in enhancing the macrophage- and lymphocyte-mediated immune response to the organism. Researchers have used monoclonal antibodies to capsular polysaccharide to passively immunize mice against *C neoformans* [44, 45].

C neoformans infection is usually characterized by little or no necrosis or organ dysfunction until late in the disease. Organ damage may be accelerated in persons with heavy infections. The lack of identifiable endotoxins or exotoxins may be partly responsible for the absence of extensive necrosis early in cryptococcal infections. Organ damage is primarily due to tissue distortion secondary to the expanding fungal burden. Extensive inflammation or fibrosis is rare. The characteristic lesion of *C neoformans* consists of a cystic cluster of yeast with no well-defined inflammatory response. Well-formed granulomas are generally absent. *C neoformans* can cause an asymptomatic pulmonary infection followed later by the development of meningitis, which is often the first indication of disease. If limited to the lungs, *C neoformans* infection may cause pneumonia, poorly defined mass lesions, pulmonary nodules, and, rarely, pleural effusion. Although immune defects are common in patients with meningitis or disseminated infection, patients with disease that is confined to the lungs are usually immunocompetent [46].

Once cryptococcosis is considered in the differential diagnosis of an infectious disease there are very good tools to diagnose it. Histopathology can be relatively distinctive with the capsule around the yeasts identified by alcian blue or mucicarmine stains and a Fontana-Masson stain can identify melanin production. These 5-20um budding or single yeasts can clearly be seen in the low-cost colloidal medium of an initial India ink examination on cerebrospinal fluid that can be positive in up to 80% of HIV-infected patients with cryptococcal meningoencephalitis and with careful examination can be positive in 50% of non-HIV infected patients. This is generally related to burden of yeasts and frequently patients with AIDS and disseminated cryptococcosis will have a large burden of yeasts in CSF that can range between 10^6-10^7CFU of yeasts/ml. The India ink examination has difficulty in identifying yeasts when their concentrations drop to 10^3 CFU of yeasts/ml or lower. There are some clinical cases and this is more commonly reported in the lung where the histopathology has some difficulty in detecting small capsules. However, it is still likely that a capsule is present since an acapsular mutant is uniformly avirulent. There are a series of non -specific stains which might identify this yeast and particularly calcofluor and Gomori's methenamine silver stains which represent classic fungal stains will identify this yeast in tissue. There are culture, molecular, and antibody methods to distinguish *C. neoformans* from *C. gattii* but at present except for epidemiological purposes it is not clear that separating an isolate into specific species is a necessary requirement of the laboratory to help clinical management of the patient [47, 48].

The serologies of cryptococcosis for diagnosis have been very well studied. Serum cryptococcal antibodies are not particularly helpful in diagnosing and deciding treatment for cryptococcosis and therefore are not used clinically. These antibodies, however, are useful for epidemiological studies of exposure and their presence may actually suggest a good prognostic sign. On the other hand, the detection of cryptococcal capsular polysaccharide antigen in serum or CSF has performed extraordinarily well in diagnosis for many years . It is one of the premier diagnostic tests in all of medical mycology. There is also some correlation between antigen load and burden of viable yeasts in the host prior to treatment so the height of the antigen titer may have some prognostic features. There are primarily two types of commercial tests, latex agglutination and ELISA systems. The sensitivity and specificity of these tests are above 90% and although there are occasional false positives or false negatives, these results can frequently be sorted out with careful repeat testing or confirmatory culture results. Therefore, in areas where this fungus is endemic, any subacute or chronic meningitis case should have a CSF cryptococcal polysaccharide antigen test performed. It is rapid and accurate. Despite its diagnostic utility and possessing some general prognostic features on initial titer, the cryptococcal antigen test is not very precise for use in following therapy. It is a large molecule with many immunological effects but the exact kinetics of its elimination from the body are variable and not precisely predictive of success. All clinicians would like to see the antigen eliminated from the host with successful therapy but treatment decisions cannot be directly linked to the quantitative antigen measurement. The term isolated cryptococcal polysaccharidemia describes a condition in very high-risk patients primarily those with HIV infection who have a positive cryptococcal antigen titer and no positive cultures or prominent symptoms. In these patients the incidence of eventually developing cryptococcosis is very high and in most patients an examination of CSF is warranted and even if negative, administration of empiric antifungal therapy should be considered [49, 50].

The use of the cryptococcal antigen in a high prevalence area such as sub-Saharan Africa as a screening device has great appeal if it could be cheap and easily performed. There is now a Lateral Flow Test being studied and marketed which has the great potential to be cheap and could use finger stick blood or urine. It is very low tech as a simple dipstick test and has an easy storage requirement. There are now prospective data that in those HIV-infected patients that have a negative cryptococcal antigen test are unlikely to develop cryptococcosis over the next year. A positive cryptococcal antigen test will need a lumbar puncture work up to rule out CNS disease and even with negative CNS disease but a positive test, it probably supports antifungal treatment until HAART returns improved host immunity. This simple Lateral Flow Test could have a profound effect on new management strategies for the vast number of patients with this disease. It simply needs to be integrated into the health care systems in resource-limited environments. All these issues are being examined at present [51].

Finally, the yeast is relatively easy to culture on standard media with growth in 2-10 days and it can be isolated from blood culture systems. Although quantitative CSF yeast counts have excellent predictive value for therapeutic outcome in research studies, they have yet to be incorporated into clinical practice. In fact, future strategies should consider measurement of the rate of yeast decline in CSF as a judge to success of induction therapy and its length [52, 53].

The demonstration of encapsulated yeast cells in CSF, biopsy tissue, blood or urine should be considered significant, even in the absence of clinical symptoms. Positive sputum specimens should be considered potentially significant, even though *Cryptococcus* may also occur in respiratory secretions as a saprophyte. Basically, all patients with a positive microscopy for cryptococci, from any site should be investigated for disseminated disease, especially by culture and antigen detection.

In patients who are co-infected with HIV and *C neoformans,* the therapeutic goal may differ from that in patients with cryptococcal infection uncomplicated by HIV infection. For cryptococcal infections in patients with concomitant HIV infection who have a CD4 count of less than 200 cells/μL, the therapeutic goal is to control the acute infection, followed by life-long suppression of *C neoformans*. For patients infected with HIV who have successfully completed an initial course of therapy, remain free of symptoms of cryptococcal disease, and reconstitute their CD4 count to more than 200 CD4 cells/μL for more than 6 months, some authorities suggest that suppressive therapy may be discontinued. However, if the patient's CD4 count falls to less than 200 cells/μL, suppressive therapy should be reinstituted [54].

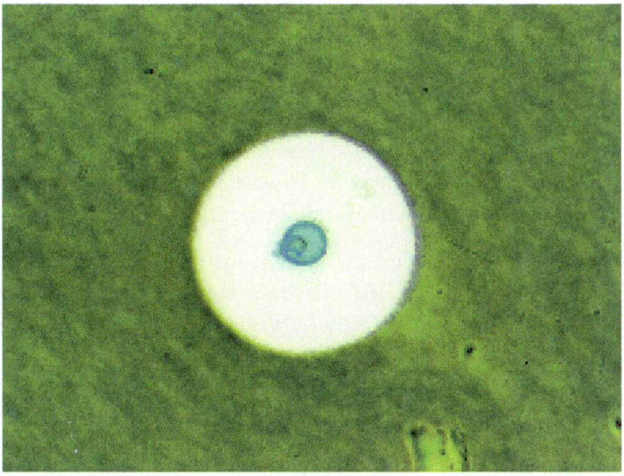

Figure 2. India ink preparation of CSF showing a typical yeast cell of *C. neoformans* surrounded by a characteristic wide gelatinous capsule. (Courtesy: www.mycology.adelaide.edu.au)

4. Pneumocystosis

Pneumocystis is a genus of unicellular fungi found in the respiratory tracts of many mammals and humans. Distinct genomic variability exists between host-specific members of the genus. The organism was first described in 1909 by Chagas and then a few years later by Delanöes, who ultimately named the organism in honor of Dr. Carini after isolating it from infected rats. Years later, Dr. Otto Jirovec and his group isolated the organism from humans, and the organism responsible for PCP was renamed after him [55].

The taxonomic classification of the *Pneumocystis* genus was debated for some time. It was initially mistaken for a trypanosome and then later for a protozoan. In the 1980s, biochemical analysis of the nucleic acid composition of *Pneumocystis* rRNA and mitochondrial DNA identified the organism as a unicellular fungus rather than a protozoan. Subsequent genomic sequence analysis of multiple genes including elongation factor 3, a component of fungi protein synthesis not found in protozoa, further supported this notion.

The organism is found in 3 distinct morphologic stages, as follows:

- The trophozoite (trophic form), in which it often exists in clusters
- The sporozoite (precystic form)
- The cyst, which contains several intracystic bodies (spores)

Pneumocystis organisms are commonly found in the lungs of healthy individuals. Most children are believed to have been exposed to the organism by age 3 or 4 years, and its occurrence is worldwide [56].

Pneumocystis carinii pneumonia (PCP), as the condition is commonly termed (although the causative organism has been renamed *Pneumocystis jiroveci,* is the most common opportunistic infection in persons with HIV infection. *Pneumocystis* first came to attention as a cause of interstitial pneumonia in severely malnourished and premature infants during World War II in Central and Eastern Europe. Before the 1980s, fewer than 100 cases of PCP were reported annually in the United States, occurring in patients who were immunosuppressed (eg, cancer patients receiving chemotherapy and solid-organ transplant recipients receiving immunosuppressants). In 1981, the Centers for Disease Control and Prevention reported PCP in 5 previously healthy homosexual men residing in the Los Angeles area [57].

P jiroveci is now one of several organisms known to cause life-threatening opportunistic infections in patients with advanced HIV infection worldwide. Well over 100,000 cases of PCP were reported in the first decade of the HIV epidemic in the United States in people with no other cause for immunosuppression.

While officially classified as a fungal pneumonia, PCP does not respond to antifungal treatment. Although a histopathologic demonstration of the organism is required for a definitive diagnosis (see Histologic Findings), treatment should not be delayed [58].

Treatment of PCP may be initiated before the workup is complete in severely ill high-risk patients. Treatment of PCP depends on the degree of illness at diagnosis, determined on the basis of the alveolar-arterial gradient. Antibiotics are primarily recommended for treatment of mild, moderate, or severe PCP. Trimethoprim-sulfamethoxazole (TMP-SMX) has been shown to be as effective as intravenous pentamidine and more effective than other alternative treatment regimens. Corticosteroids are used as adjunctive initial therapy only in patients with HIV infection who have severe PCP. Preventive measures (eg, smoking cessation and chemoprophylaxis) can play an important role in disease management [59].

4.1. Transmission of Pneumocystis

Animal studies have suggested that *Pneumocystis* organisms are communicable; airborne transmission has been reported. Human evidence of this is provided by molecular analysis of *Pneumocystis* isolates obtained from groups of patients involved in hospital outbreaks [60, 61].

Further evidence of human transmission has been found in cases of recurrent pneumonia in which the genotype of *Pneumocystis* organisms in the same person differed in prior episodes. Despite this, barrier precautions are not required for patients hospitalized with *P carinii* pneumonia (PCP) except to protect other patients with depressed immunity.

4.2. Development of PCP

Disease occurs when both cellular immunity and humoral immunity are defective. Once inhaled, the trophic form of *Pneumocystis* organisms attach to the alveoli. Multiple host immune defects allow for uncontrolled replication of *Pneumocystis* organisms and development of illness. Activated alveolar macrophages without $CD4^+$ cells are unable to eradicate *Pneumocystis* organisms. Increased alveolar-capillary permeability is visible on electron microscopy.

Physiologic changes include the following:

- Hypoxemia with an increased alveolar-arterial oxygen gradient
- Respiratory alkalosis
- Impaired diffusing capacity
- Changes in total lung capacity and vital capacity

There have been reports of PCP occurring as part of the immune reconstitution syndrome [62, 63].

4.3. Risk factors for PCP

PCP is caused by infection with *P jiroveci*. The following groups are at risk for PCP [64, 65]:

- Persons with HIV infection whose $CD4^+$ cells fall below 200/μL and who are not receiving PCP prophylaxis (In addition, in patients with HIV infection, findings of other opportunistic infections [eg, oral thrush] increases the risk of PCP, regardless of $CD4^+$ count).
- Persons with primary immune deficiencies, including hypogammaglobulinemia and severe combined immunodeficiency (SCID).
- Persons receiving long-term immunosuppressive regimens for connective-tissue disorders, vasculitides, or solid-organ transplantation (eg, heart, lung, liver, kidney)
- Persons with hematologic and nonhematologic malignancies, including solid tumors and lymphomas
- Persons with severe malnutrition

Before the widespread use of prophylaxis for *P carinii* pneumonia (PCP), the frequency of *Pneumocystis* infection in lung transplant patients alone was as high as 88%. Now, with the routine use of prophylaxis, PCP is very rare in solid-organ transplant patients and has significantly decreased in patients infected with HIV. Prior to the widespread use of highly active antiretroviral therapy (HAART), PCP occurred in 70-80% of patients with HIV infection. The frequency of PCP is decreasing with the use of PCP prophylaxis and HAART. PCP is still the most common opportunistic infection in patients with HIV infection. Patients with HIV infection are more prone to PCP recurrence than patients not infected with HIV. In developing regions of the world, the prevalence of PCP was once thought to be much lower, but studies have shown that the lower reported incidence is likely a failure to accurately diagnose PCP. An accurate diagnosis requires access to modern medical care, which is not available worldwide [66].

Currently, the frequency of documented *Pneumocystis* infection is increasing in Africa, with *Pneumocystis* organisms found in up to 80% of infants with pneumonia who have HIV infection. In sub-Saharan Africa, tuberculosis is a common co-infection in persons with PCP [67].

A lactic dehydrogenase (LDH) study is performed as part of the initial workup. LDH levels are usually elevated (>220 U/L) in patients with *P carinii* pneumonia (PCP). They are elevated in 90% of patients with PCP who are infected with HIV. The study has a high sensitivity (78-100%); its specificity is much lower because other disease processes can result in an elevated LDH level. LDH levels appear to reflect the degree of lung injury. They should decline with successful treatment. Consistently elevated LDH levels during treatment may indicate therapy failure and a worse prognosis [68].

Quantitative PCR for pneumocystis may become useful in distinguishing between colonization and active infection, but these assays are not yet available for routine clinical use [69].

In one study, patients with positive quantitative PCR but negative immunofluorescence for pneumocystis had a higher 1-year mortality but only in the context of systemic inflammatory conditions. There was no significant difference for patients with solid-organ or hematologic malignancy [70].

β-D-Glucan (BDG) is a cell-wall component of many fungi, including candida, aspergillus, and pneumocystis (but not the zygomycetes). It has been shown to be a sensitive test to detect PCP in a meta-analysis of 12 studies assessing the sensitivity, specificity and overall accuracy of the test [71].

5. Aspergilosis

Aspergillus species are ubiquitous molds found in organic matter. Although more than 100 species have been identified, the majority of human illness is caused by *Aspergillus fumigatus* and *Aspergillus niger* and, less frequently, by *Aspergillus flavus* and *Aspergillus clavatus*. The transmission of fungal spores to the human host is via inhalation [72].

Aspergillus may cause a broad spectrum of disease in the human host, ranging from hypersensitivity reactions to direct angioinvasion. *Aspergillus* primarily affects the lungs, causing 4 main syndromes, including allergic bronchopulmonary aspergillosis (ABPA), chronic necrotizing *Aspergillus* pneumonia (or chronic necrotizing pulmonary aspergillosis [CNPA]), aspergilloma, and invasive aspergillosis. However, in patients who are severely immunocompromised, *Aspergillus* may hematogenously disseminate beyond the lung, potentially causing endophthalmitis, endocarditis, and abscesses in the myocardium, kidney, liver, spleen, soft tissue, and bone. *Aspergillus* is second to *Candida* species as a cause of fungal endocarditis. *Aspergillus* -related endocarditis and wound infections occur in the context of cardiac surgery [73].

ABPA is a hypersensitivity reaction to *A fumigatus* colonization of the tracheobronchial tree and occurs in conjunction with asthma and cystic fibrosis (CF). Allergic fungal sinusitis may also occur alone or with ABPA. Bronchocentric granulomatosis and malt worker's lung are 2 hypersensitivity lung diseases that are caused by *Aspergillus* species, but they are rare [74].

An aspergilloma is a fungus ball (mycetoma) that develops in a preexisting cavity in the lung parenchyma. Underlying causes of the cavitary disease may include treated tuberculosis or other necrotizing infection, sarcoidosis, CF, and emphysematous bullae. The ball of fungus may move within the cavity but does not invade the cavity wall; however, it may cause hemoptysis [75].

CNPA is a subacute process usually found in patients with some degree of immunosuppression, most commonly that associated with underlying lung disease, alcoholism, or long-term corticosteroid therapy. Because it is uncommon, CNPA often remains unrecognized for weeks or months and can cause a progressive cavitary pulmonary infiltrate [74].

Invasive aspergillosis is a rapidly progressive, often fatal infection, associated with significant mortality, with a rate of 30-95%, that occurs in patients who are severely immunosuppressed, including those who are profoundly neutropenic, those who have received bone marrow or solid organ transplants, and patients with advanced AIDS or chronic granulomatous disease. This infectious process is characterized by invasion of blood vessels, resulting in multifocal infiltrates, which are often wedge-shaped, pleural-based, and cavitary. Dissemination to other organs, particularly the central nervous system, may occur [76].

Aspergillus causes a spectrum of disease, from colonization to hypersensitivity reactions to chronic necrotizing infections to rapidly progressive angioinvasion, often resulting in death. Rarely found in individuals who are immunocompetent, invasive *Aspergillus* infection almost always occurs in patients who are immunosuppressed by virtue of underlying lung disease, immunosuppressive drug therapy, or immunodeficiency [73].

Aspergillus hyphae are histologically distinct from other fungi in that the hyphae have frequent septae, which branch at 45° angles. The hyphae are best visualized in tissue with silver stains. Although many species of *Aspergillus* have been isolated in nature, *A fumigatus* is the most common cause of infection in humans. *A flavus* and *A niger* are less common. Likely, this relates to the ability of *A fumigatus,* but not most other *Aspergillus* species, to grow at normal human body temperature. Human host defense against the inhaled spores begins with the mucous layer and the ciliary action in the respiratory tract. Macrophages and neutrophils encompass, engulf, and eradicate the fungus. However, many species of *Aspergillus* produce toxic metabolites that inhibit macrophage and neutrophil phagocytosis. Corticosteroids also impair macrophage and neutrophil function. Underlying immunosuppression (eg, HIV disease, chronic granulomatous disease, pharmacologic immunosuppression) also contributes directly to neutrophil dysfunction or decreased numbers of neutrophils. In individuals who are immunosuppressed, vascular invasion is much more common and may lead to infarction, hemorrhage, and necrosis of lung tissue. Persons with CNPA typically have granuloma formation and alveolar consolidation. Hyphae may be observed within the granulomata [77].

Because *Aspergillus* infection may cause colonization, allergy, or invasive infection, its manifestations are quite variable and are best considered based on the disease process. Allergic bronchopulmonary aspergillosis is defined by several abnormalities, including asthma, eosinophilia, a positive skin test result for *A fumigatus,* marked elevation of the serum immunoglobulin E (IgE) level to greater than 1000 IU/dL, fleeting pulmonary infiltrates, central bronchiectasis, mucoid impaction, and positive test results for *Aspergillus* precipitins (primarily immunoglobulin G [IgG], but also immunoglobulin A and immunoglobulin M, antibodies). Minor criteria for diagnosis include positive *Aspergillus* radioallergosorbent assay test results and culture findings for *Aspergillus* in sputum [74].

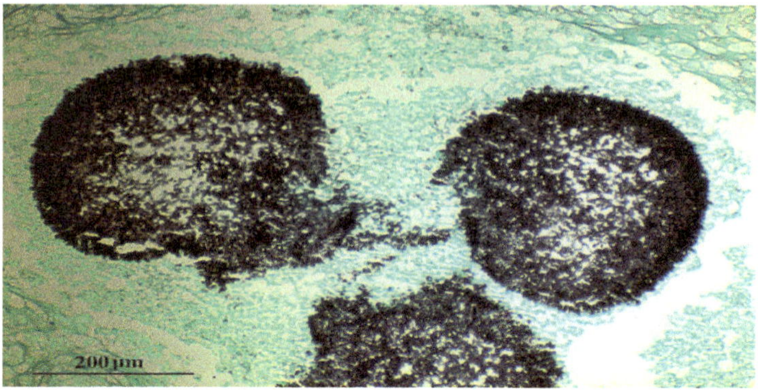

Figure 3. Grocott's methenamine silver (GMS) stained tissue section of lung showing fungal balls of hyphae of *Aspergillus fumigatus*. (Courtesy: www.mycology.adelaide.edu.au)

Diagnostic criteria for ABPA in persons with CF were revised by the Cystic Fibrosis Foundation. ABPA is considered a definite diagnosis requiring treatment if the following are noted: (1) clinical deterioration, including cough, wheeze, increased sputum production, diminished exercise tolerance, or diminished pulmonary function; (2) total serum IgE level greater than 1000 IU/mL or a greater than 2-fold rise from baseline; (3) positive serology results for *Aspergillus* (*Aspergillus* precipitins or *Aspergillus* -specific IgG or IgE); and (4) new infiltrates on chest radiographs or CT scans. Treatment for ABPA is also recommended in patients with CF who have new radiographic findings and symptoms and a change in baseline IgE level to greater than 500 IU/mL [79].

Definitive diagnosis of invasive aspergillosis or chronic necrotizing *Aspergillus* pneumonia depends on the demonstration of the organism in tissue [76].

In the appropriate clinical setting of pulmonary infiltrates in a patient who is neutropenic or immunosuppressed, visualization of the characteristic fungi using Gomori methenamine silver stain or Calcofluor or a positive culture result from sputum, needle biopsy, or bronchoalveolar lavage (BAL) fluid should result in the prompt institution of therapy. This is especially important after bone marrow transplantation because a positive *Aspergillus* culture result from sputum has a 95% positive predictive value for invasive disease. However, a negative fungus result from culture of sputum or BAL fluid does not exclude pulmonary aspergillosis because *Aspergillus* is cultured from sputum in 8-34% of patients and from BAL fluid in 45-62% of patients eventually found by biopsy or autopsy to have invasive disease [80].

An assay to detect galactomannan, a major component of the *Aspergillus* cell wall, is available. Patients who are at high risk, such as those who have received stem cell transplants or who have prolonged neutropenia, may be screened for the development of invasive *Aspergillus* infection by monitoring serum galactomannan levels weekly.The presence of an elevated galactomannan level in BAL fluid may also be helpful in the diagnosis of pulmonary aspergillosis in patients in whom compatible radiographic changes are present and BAL testing is performed in the suspicious area. A meta-analysis and systematic review determined that the measurement of BAL-galactomannan levels may help in diagnosing invasive aspergillosis early [81, 82].

A study by Luong et al of 150 BAL samples from lung transplant recipients concluded that real-time polymerase chain reaction (PCR) assays could be useful in diagnosis of invasive aspergillosis in high-risk populations. Pan-*Aspergillus* PCR combined with BAL galactomannan testing was 97% specific and 93% sensitive for invasive pulmonary aspergillosis. Species-specific real-time PCR assays for *A fumigatus* and for *A terreus* could be used to rule out or identify the common *A fumigatus* and the amphotericin B-resistant *A terreus* [83].

Histopathology and silver staining for persons with invasive aspergillosis demonstrates the characteristic septate hyphae, branching at acute angles, and acute inflammatory infiltrate and tissue necrosis with occasional granulomata and blood vessel invasion. The airways of patients with ABPA contain mucus filled with degenerating eosinophils and typical fungal hyphae. ABPA may occur on a background of chronic eosinophilic pneumonia and bronchiolitis, granulomatous bronchitis, bronchocentric granulomatosis, and, occasionally, BOOP [84].

Selection of therapy also needs to consider the certainty of the diagnosis. Voriconazole, itraconazole, the investigational azoles with anti-mould activity, and amphotericin B all possess a reasonably broad-spectrum of activity against *Aspergillus* and the related hyaline moulds. Their activity does, however, vary for the agents of zygomycosis, with posaconazole being the azole with the most reliable activity against this class of fungi. The echinocandin glucan synthesis inhibitors (caspofungin, FK463, and anidulafungin) possess a narrower spectrum of activity and should only be used if the infection is known to be due to *Aspergillus* spp [85, 86].

6. Zygomycosis

Zygomycosis is an infection caused by fungi in the orders Mucorales and Entomophthorales. The Mucorales order contains 2 families exist—Mucoraceae and Cunninghamellaceae. Mucormycosis is another common name applied to this same group of diseases. This designation reflected the predominance of the Mucorales in causing disease in humans. However, this term ignored the role of the Entomophthorales (*Conidiobolus* species and *Basidiobolus* species). The currently accepted designation is zygomycosis, reflecting all disease processes caused by the members of the class Zygomycetes. During the past decade, the Zygomycetes have emerged as common causes of invasive fungal infections [87].

The pathogens that cause zygomycosis are commonly found in the environment on fruit, on bread, and in soil and are common components of decaying organic debris. These organisms are ubiquitous and generally saprophytic, rarely causing disease in immunocompetent hosts, but they are the third-most-common cause of invasive fungal infection in immunocompromised patients, especially stem cell transplant recipients and patients with underlying hematologic malignancies [88].

Fungi are ubiquitous in the natural world, often found in association with plants, mammals, and insects. Accordingly, humans are continually exposed to multiple genera of fungi via various routes, including the respiratory and gastrointestinal routes, which allow the possibility of colonization. Depending on the interaction between host mucosal defense mechanisms and fungal virulence factors, colonization may be transient or persistent, or local disease may ensue [89].

Overall, *Rhizopus* species from the Mucoraceae family are the most commonly identified etiologic agents of zygomycosis in humans. Of the *Rhizopus* species, the most common agent associated with zygomycosis is *Rhizopus arrhizus* (*Rhizopus oryzae*), followed by *Rhizopus rhizopodiformis*. Other causes include *Mucor* species, *Cunninghamella bertholletiae, Apophysomyces elegans, Absidia* species, *Saksenaea* species, *Rhizomucor pusillus, Entomophthora* species, *Conidiobolus* species, and *Basidiobolus* species [90].

Zygomycosis caused by *R arrhizus* is acute and rapidly fatal despite early diagnosis and treatment. These organisms have a particular predilection for invading major blood vessels, with ensuing ischemia, necrosis, and infarction of adjacent tissues, resulting in the production of black pus. Persons at particular risk include those with granulocytopenia and acidosis. For unknown reasons, the Zygomycetes have a propensity to affect patients with acidosis, particularly those with diabetes. They also infect patients with acidosis secondary to renal insufficiency, diarrhea, and aspirin intake. Patients who are receiving glucocorticoids or deferoxamine and those who have undergone splenectomy also are at risk [90].

The overall mortality rate associated with zygomycosis is approximately 50% and has remained at this level for the past 50 years. Rhinocerebral zygomycosis carries a mortality rate of approximately 85%. Mortality rates are very high because, by the time zygomycosis is suspected and diagnosed, it has frequently spread diffusely and caused extensive tissue destruction. However, the risk of mortality varies depending on the characteristics of the host, the type of infection, the site of infection, and the use of surgical intervention. In general, antifungal therapy and surgical management independently decrease the likelihood of death [91].

Zygomycosis manifests as a spectrum of diseases, depending on the portal of entry and the predisposing risk factors of the patient. The 5 major clinical forms include rhinocerebral zygomycosis, pulmonary zygomycosis, abdominopelvic and gastric (gastrointestinal) zygomycosis, primary cutaneous zygomycosis, and disseminated zygomycosis [91].

Most persons who develop zygomycosis are immunocompromised, although 15-20% of patients have no evidence of any underlying condition at the time of the diagnosis.Thus, sporadic cases in immunocompetent hosts are not uncommon. The most common risk factors include the following [91, 92] :

- Stem cell transplantation
- Poorly controlled diabetes mellitus, either type 1 or type 2
- Hematologic malignancy (eg, leukemias, lymphomas)
- Solid organ transplants
- Steroid use
- Metabolic acidosis
- Deferoxamine therapy
- Severe and prolonged neutropenia
- Intravenous drug use
- Renal failure
- Peritoneal dialysis
- Burns
- Penetrating trauma (rare)

Unfortunately, findings from laboratory studies are nonspecific for zygomycosis. Diagnosis requires a high index of suspicion, a host with appropriate risk factors, and evidence of tissue invasion with the characteristic appearance of broad nonseptate hyphae with right-angle branches. No serologic tests are available, and blood cultures are of no benefit [93].

7. Conclusion

Opportunistic fungal infections of the body which occur almost exclusively in debilitated patients whose normal defence mechanisms are impaired. The organisms involved are cosmopolitan fungi which have a very low inherent virulence. The increased incidence of these infections and the diversity of fungi causing them, has paralleled the emergence of Acquired Immune Deficiency Syndrome (AIDS), more aggressive cancer and post-transplantation chemotherapy and the use of antibiotics, cytotoxins, immunosuppressives, corticosteroids and other macro disruptive procedures that result in lowered resistance of the host allowing fungi to invade tissues and produce pathological changes that can cause death. Compromised immunity is the most important predisposing factor for clinically significant fungal infections. Neutrophil deficiency as a result of bone marrow suppression or damage is frequently associated with such infections. Different fungi infect humans and may live in extracellular tissues and within phagocytes. Therefore, the immune responses to these microbes are often combinations of the responses to extracellular and intracellular bacteria. However, less is known about antifungal immunity than about immunity against bacteria and viruses. This lack of knowledge is partly due to the paucity of animal models for mycoses and partly due to the fact that these infections typically occur in individuals who are incapable of mounting effective immune responses. Improved diagnostic methods have been developed for an early diagnostic of opportunistic mycosis in order to control the disease and save more lives.

Author details

Luis Enrique Jerez Puebla
Parasitology Department, Institute Pedro Kourí (IPK), Havana, Cuba

Acknowledgement

To the others professionals of the Mycology Laboratory of "Pedro Kourí" that aided to me in that period.

8. References

[1] Pappas PG. Invasive candidiasis. *Infect Dis Clin North Am.* 2006;20(3):485-506.
[2] Romani L. Cell-mediated immunity to fungi: a reassessment. *Medical Mycology.* 2008; 46:515-29.
[3] Pappas PG, Kauffman CA, Andes D, Benjamin DK Jr, Calandra TF, Edwards JE Jr, et al. Clinical practice guidelines for the management of candidiasis: 2009 update by the Infectious Diseases Society of America. *Clin Infect Dis.* 2009; 48(5):503-35.
[4] Maródi L, Johnston RB Jr. Invasive Candida species disease in infants and children: occurrence, risk factors, management, and innate host defense mechanisms. *Curr Opin Pediatr.* 2007;19(6):693-7.
[5] Guery BP, Arendrup MC, Auzinger G, Azoulay E, Borges Sá M, Johnson EM, et al. Management of invasive candidiasis and candidemia in adult non-neutropenic intensive care unit patients: Part I. Epidemiology and diagnosis. *Intensive Care Med.* Jan 2009;35(1):55-62.
[6] de Repentigny L, Lewandowski D, Jolicoeur P. Immunopathogenesis of oropharyngeal candidiasis in human immunodeficiency virus infection. *Clin Microbiol Rev.* 2004; 17(4):729-59.
[7] Pfaller MA, Pappas PG, Wingard JR. Invasive fungal pathogens: current epidemiological trends. *Clin Infect Dis.* 2006; 43 (Suppl 1):S3-S14.
[8] Pappas PG, Kauffman CA, Andes D, Benjamin DK Jr, Calandra TF, Edwards JE Jr, et al. Clinical practice guidelines for the management of candidiasis: 2009 update by the Infectious Diseases Society of America. *Clin Infect Dis.* 2009; 48(5):503-35.
[9] Sobel JD. Vulvovaginal candidosis. *Lancet.* 2007; 369(9577):1961-71.
[10] Malani AN, Kauffman CA. Candida urinary tract infections: treatment options. *Expert Rev Anti Infect Ther.* 2007;5(2):277-84.
[11] Yang YL. Virulence factors of Candida species. *J Microbiol Immunol Infect.* 2003; 36(4):223-8.
[12] Vazquez JA, Sobel JD. Candidiasis. In: Clinical Mycology, Dismukes WE, Pappas PG, and Sobel JD, eds. *Oxford Univers.* 2003:143-87.
[13] Eiland EH, Hassoun A, English T. Points of concern related to the micafungin versus caspofungin trial. *Clin Infect Dis.* 2008; 46(4):640-1.

[14] Alexander BD, Pfaller MA. Contemporary tools for the diagnosis and management of invasive mycoses. *Clin Infect Dis.* 2006; 43:S15-S27.

[15] Odabasi Z, Mattiuzzi G, Estey E, et al. Beta-D-glucan as a diagnostic adjunct for invasive fungal infections: validation, cutoff development, and performance in patients with acute myelogenous leukemia and myelodysplastic syndrome. *Clin Infect Dis.* Jul 15 2004; 39(2):199-205.

[16] Shepard JR, Addison RM, Alexander BD, et al. Multicenter evaluation of the Candida albicans/Candida glabrata peptide nucleic acid fluorescent in situ hybridization method for simultaneous dual-color identification of *C. albicans* and *C. glabrata* directly from blood culture bottles. *J Clin Microbiol.* Jan 2008; 46(1):50-5.

[17] João Inácio, Orfeu Flores, and Isabel Spencer-Martins. Efficient identification of clinically relevant Candida yeast species by use of an Assay combining panfungal loop-mediated isothermal DNA amplification with hybridization to species-specific oligonucleotide probes. *J Clin Microbiol.* 2008; 46: 713-20.

[18] Espinel-Ingroff A, Canton E, Gibbs D, Wang A. Correlation of Neo-Sensitabs tablet diffusion assay results on three different agar media with CLSI broth microdilution M27-A2 and disk diffusion M44-A results for testing susceptibilities of *Candida* spp. and *Cryptococcus neoformans* to amphotericin B, caspofungin, fluconazole, itraconazole, and voriconazole. *J Clin Microbiol.* 2007;45(3):858-64.

[19] Odabasi Z, Mattiuzzi G, Estey E, et al. Beta-D-glucan as a diagnostic adjunct for invasive fungal infections: validation, cutoff development, and performance in patients with acute myelogenous leukemia and myelodysplastic syndrome. *Clin Infect Dis.* Jul 15 2004; 39(2):199-205.

[20] Shepard JR, Addison RM, Alexander BD, et al. Multicenter evaluation of the *Candida albicans/Candida glabrata* peptide nucleic acid fluorescent in situ hybridization method for simultaneous dual-color identification of *C. albicans* and *C. glabrata* directly from blood culture bottles. *J Clin Microbiol.* 2008; 46(1):50-5.

[21] Kett DH, Shorr AF, Reboli AC, et al. Anidulafungin compared with fluconazole in severely ill patients with candidemia and other forms of invasive candidiasis: Support for the 2009 IDSA treatment guidelines for candidiasis. *Crit Care.* 2011; 15(5):R253.

[22] Pappas PG, Rex JH, Sobel JD, et al. Guidelines for treatment of candidiasis. *Clin Infect Dis.* 2004; 38(2):161-89.

[23] Busse O. Ueber parasitare zelleninschlusse und ihre zuchtung. *Zentralbl. Bakterial.* 1894; 16:175-80.

[24] Buschke A. Ueber eine durch Coccidien Hervergerufene Krankheit des menschen. *Deutsche Med. Wochenschr.* 1895;21 (3):14.

[25] Chayakulkeeree M, Perfect JR. Cryptococcosis. *Infect Dis Clin North Am* 2006; 203:507-44.

[26] Heitman J, Kozel T, Kwon-Chung KJ, Perfect JR. *Cryptococcus neoformans*: from Human pathogen to Model Yeast. *American Society of Microbiology* 2011, 1-620.

[27] Crowe SM, Carlin JB, Stewart KI, Lucas CR, Hoy JF. Predictive value of CD4 lymphocyte numbers for the development of opportunistic infections and malignancies in HIV-infected persons. *J Acquir Immune Defic Syndr* 1991; 4:770-6.

[28] Husain S, Wagener MM, Singh N. *Cryptococcus neoformans* infection in organ transplant recipients: variables influencing clinical characteristics and outcome. *Emerg Infect Dis* 2001; 73:375-81.
[29] Pappas PG, Perfect JR, Cloud GA et al. Cryptococcosis in Human Immunodeficiency Virus-negative patients in the era of effective azole therapy. *Clin Infect Dis.* 2001; 335:690-9.
[30] Meletiadis J, Walsh TJ, Choi EH et al. Study of common functional genetic polymorphisms of FCGR2A, 3A and 3B genes and the risk for cryptococcosis in HIV-uninfected patients. *Med Mycol* 2007; 456:513-8.
[31] Zonios DI, Falloon J, Huang CY, Chaitt D, Bennett JE. Cryptococcosis and idiopathic CD4 lymphocytopenia. *Medicine Baltimore.* 2007; 862:78-92.
[32] Shoham S, Levitz SM. The immune response to fungal infections. *Br J Haematol.* 2005; 12:569-82.
[33] Brouwer AE, Siddiqui AA, Kester MI et al. Immune dysfunction in HIV-seronegative, *Cryptococcus gattii* meningitis. *J Infect* 2007; 543:165-8.
[34] Siddiqui AA, Brouwer AE, Wuthiekanun V et al. IFN-gamma at the site of infection determines rate of clearance of infection in cryptococcal meningitis. *J Immunol* 2005; 1743:1746-50.
[35] Shelburne SA, Visnegarwala F, Darcourt J et al. Incidence and risk factors for immune reconstitution inflammatory syndrome during highly active antiretroviral therapy. *AIDS* 2005; 194:399-406.
[36] Sungkanuparph S, Filler SG, Chetchotisakd P, Pappas PG, Nolen TL, Manosuthi W, et al. Cryptococcal immune reconstitution inflammatory syndrome after antiretroviral therapy in AIDS patients with cryptococcal meningitis: a prospective multicenter study. *Clin Infect Dis.* 15 2009; 49(6):931-4.
[37] Sungkanuparph S, Filler SG, Chetchotisakd P, Pappas PG, Nolen TL, Manosuthi W, et al. Cryptococcal immune reconstitution inflammatory syndrome after antiretroviral therapy in AIDS patients with cryptococcal meningitis: a prospective multicenter study. *Clin Infect Dis.* Sep 15 2009; 49(6):931-4.
[38] D'Souza CA, Kronstad JW, Taylor G et al. Genome Variation in *Cryptococcus gattii,* an Emerging Pathogen of Immunocompetent Hosts. *MBio.* 2011; 2:342-10.
[39] Mirza SA, Phelan M, Rimland D et al. The changing epidemiology of cryptococcosis: an update from population-based active surveillance in 2 large metropolitan areas, 1992-2000. *Clin Infect Dis* 2003; 366:789-94.
[40] Perfect JR. Cryptococcus neoformans: a sugar-coated killer with designer genes. *FEMS Immunol Med Microbiol* 2005; 453:395-404.
[41] Perfect, J.R. and Casadevall, A. Cryptococcosis. *Infect Dis Clin North Am.* 2002; 16, 837–74.
[42] Heitman J, Kozel T, Kwon-Chung KJ, Perfect JR. Cryptococcus neoformans: from Human pathogen to Model Yeast. *American Society of Microbiology*, 2011; 1-620.
[43] Rittershaus regulator of pathogenicity of *Cryptococcus neoformans.* PC, Kechichian TB, Allegood JC, Merrill AH Jr, Hennig M, Luberto C. Glucosylceramide synthase is an essential. *J Clin Invest.* 2006;116(6):1651-9

[44] Mitchell AP. Cryptococcal virulence: beyond the usual suspects. *J Clin Invest.* Jun 2006; 116(6):1481-3.

[45] Casadevall A, Perfect JR. Animal models and veterinary aspects of cryptococcosis. In: Casadevall A, Perfect JR, editors. *Cryptococcus neoformans*. ASM Press, 1998;325-50.

[46] Brouwer AE, Siddiqui AA, Kester MI et al. Immune dysfunction in HIV-seronegative, *Cryptococcus gattii* meningitis. *J Infect.* 2007; 543:165-8.

[47] Friedman GD, Jeffrey Fessel W, Udaltsova NV, Hurley LB. Cryptococcosis: the 1981-2000 epidemic. *Mycoses.* 2005;48(2):122-5.

[48] Ro JY, Lee SS, Ayala AG. Advantage of Fontana - Masson stain in capsule - deficient cryptococcal infection. *Arch Pathol Lab Med.* 1987; 111:53-7.

[49] Goldman DL, Khine H, Abadi J et al. Serologic evidence for *Cryptococcus neoformans* infection in early childhood. *Pediatrics.* 2001; 107:65-6.

[50] Perfect JR. *Cryptococcus neoformans*. In Mandell; Douglas, Bennett's Principles and Practice of Infectious Diseases. 2005: 2997-3012.

[51] Jarvis JN, Lawn SD, Vogt M, Bangani N, Wood R, Harrison TS. Screening for cryptococcal antigenemia in patients accessing an antiretroviral treatment program in South Africa. *Clin Infect Dis.* 2009; 487:856-62.

[52] Bicanic T, Muzoora C, Brouwer AE et al. Independent association between rate of clearence of infection and clinical outcome of HIV-associated cryptococcal meningitis: analysis of a combined cohort of 262 patients. *Clin Infect Dis.* 2009; 49: 702-9.

[53] Brouwer AE, Rajanuwong A, Chierakul W et al. Combination antifungal therapies for HIV-associated crytpococcal meningitis: feasibility and power of quantitative CSF cultures to determine fungicidal activity. *Lancet* 2004; 363:1764-7.

[54] Kaplan JE, Masur H, Holmes KK. Guidelines for preventing opportunistic infections among HIV-infected persons--2002. Recommendations of the U.S. Public Health Service and the Infectious Diseases Society of America. *MMWR Recomm Rep.* 2002; 51:1-52.

[55] Cushion MT, Stringer JR. Has the name really been changed? It has for most researchers. *Clin Infect Dis.* 2005; 41(12):1756-8.

[56] Slogrove AL, Cotton MF, Esser MM. Severe Infections in HIV-Exposed Uninfected Infants: Clinical Evidence of Immunodeficiency. *J Trop Pediatr.*2010; 56(2):75-81.

[57] Fujii T, Nakamura T, Iwamoto A. Pneumocystis pneumonia in patients with HIV infection: clinical manifestations, laboratory findings, and radiological features. *J Infect Chemother.* 2007; 13(1):1-7.

[58] Hui M, Kwok WT. *Pneumocystis carinii* pneumonia in Hong Kong: a 10 year retrospective study. *J Med Microbiol.* 2006; 55:85-8.

[59] Safrin S, Finkelstein DM, Feinberg J, et al. Comparison of three regimens for treatment of mild to moderate *Pneumocystis carinii* pneumonia in patients with AIDS. A double-blind, randomized, trial of oral trimethoprim-sulfamethoxazole, dapsone-trimethoprim, and clindamycin-primaquine. ACTG 108 Study Group. *Ann Intern Med.* 1996; 124(9):792-802.

[60] Schmoldt S, Schuhegger R, Wendler T, et al. Molecular evidence of nosocomial *Pneumocystis jirovecii* transmission among 16 patients after kidney transplantation. *J Clin Microbiol.* 2008;46(3):966-71.

[61] de Boer MG, Bruijnesteijn van Coppenraet LE, Gaasbeek A, et al. An outbreak of *Pneumocystis jiroveci* pneumonia with 1 predominant genotype among renal transplant recipients: interhuman transmission or a common environmental source?. *Clin Infect Dis*. 2007; 44(9):1143-9.

[62] Mori S, Polatino S, Estrada-Y-Martin RM. Pneumocystis-associated organizing pneumonia as a manifestation of immune reconstitution inflammatory syndrome in an HIV-infected individual with a normal CD4+ T-cell count following antiretroviral therapy. *Int J STD AIDS*. 2009;20(9):662-5.

[63] Kolditz M, Halank M, Bandt D, Spornraft-Ragaller P, Höffken G. Early recurrence of Pneumocystis jiroveci pneumonia in two HIV-infected patients: linking infection relapse and immune reconstitution syndrome. *Respirology*. 2009; 14(6):910-2.

[64] Mori S, Cho I, Sugimoto M. A followup study of asymptomatic carriers of *Pneumocystis jiroveci* during immunosuppressive therapy for rheumatoid arthritis. *J Rheumatol*. 2009;36(8):1600-5.

[65] Ritter ML, Pirofski L. Mycophenolate mofetil: effects on cellular immune subsets, infectious complications, and antimicrobial activity. *Transpl Infect Dis*. 2009; 11(4):290-7.

[66] Abouya YL, Beaumel A, Lucas S, et al. Pneumocystis carinii pneumonia. An uncommon cause of death in African patients with acquired immunodeficiency syndrome. *Am Rev Respir Dis*. 1992; 145(3):617-20.

[67] Murray JF. Pulmonary complications of HIV-1 infection among adults living in Sub-Saharan Africa. *Int J Tuberc Lung Dis*. 2005; 9(8):826-35.

[68] Grover SA, Coupal L, Suissa S, et al. The clinical utility of serum lactate dehydrogenase in diagnosing pneumocystis carinii pneumonia among hospitalized AIDS patients. *Clin Invest Med*. 1992; 15(4):309-17.

[69] Alanio A, Desoubeaux G, Sarfati C, Hamane S, Bergeron A, Azoulay E, et al. Real-time PCR assay-based strategy for differentiation between active *Pneumocystis jirovecii* pneumonia and colonization in immunocompromised patients. *Clin Microbiol Infect*. 2011; 17(10):1531-7.

[70] Botterel F, Cabaret O, Foulet F, Cordonnier C, Costa JM, Bretagne S. Clinical Significance of Quantifying *Pneumocystis jirovecii* DNA by Using Real-Time PCR in Bronchoalveolar Lavage Fluid from Immunocompromised Patients. *J Clin Microbiol*. 2012; 50(2):227-31.

[71] Onishi A, Sugiyama D, Kogata Y, Saegusa J, Sugimoto T, Kawano S, et al. Diagnostic Accuracy of Serum 1,3-ß-D-Glucan for *Pneumocystis jiroveci* Pneumonia, Invasive Candidiasis, and Invasive Aspergillosis: Systematic Review and Meta-Analysis. *J Clin Microbiol*. 2012; 50(1):7-15.

[72] Bennett, JE. *Aspergillus* species,. In G. L. Mandell, J. E. Bennett, and R. Dolin (ed.), Mandell, Douglas and Bennett's Principles and Practice of Infectious Diseases, 4th edition ed. Churchill Livingstone, New York. 1995; 2306-10.

[73] Virnig C, Bush RK. Allergic bronchopulmonary aspergillosis: a US perspective. *Curr Opin Pulm Med*. 2007; 13(1):67-71.

[74] Ader F, Bienvenu AL, Rammaert B, Nseir S. Management of invasive aspergillosis in patients with COPD: rational use of voriconazole. *Int J Chron Obstruct Pulmon Dis*. 2009; 4(2):279-87.

[75] Smith NL, Denning DW. Underlying conditions in chronic pulmonary aspergillosis including simple aspergilloma. *Eur Respir J*. 2011; 37(4):865-72.

[76] Naidich DP, Rom WN. Pulmonary aspergilloma and AIDS. A comparison of HIV-infected and HIV-negative individuals. *Chest*. 1997; 111(3):612-8.

[77] Magill SS, Chiller TM, Warnock DW. Evolving strategies in the management of aspergillosis. *Expert Opin Pharmacother*. 2008; 9(2):193-209.

[78] Stevens DA, Moss RB, Kurup VP, Knutsen AP, Greenberger P, Judson MA, et al. Allergic bronchopulmonary aspergillosis in cystic fibrosis--state of the art: Cystic Fibrosis Foundation Consensus Conference. *Clin Infect Dis*. 2003;37 Suppl 3:S225-64.

[79] Ader F, Bienvenu AL, Rammaert B, Nseir S. Management of invasive aspergillosis in patients with COPD: rational use of voriconazole. *Int J Chron Obstruct Pulmon Dis*. 2009; 4(2):279-87.

[80] Agarwal R. Allergic bronchopulmonary aspergillosis. *Chest*. 2009; 135(3):805-26.

[81] Pfeiffer CD, Fine JP, Safdar N. Diagnosis of invasive aspergillosis using a galactomannan assay: a meta-analysis. *Clin Infect Dis*. 2006; 42(10):1417-27.

[82] Becker MJ, Lugtenburg EJ, Cornelissen JJ, Van Der Schee C, Hoogsteden HC, De Marie S. Galactomannan detection in computerized tomography-based broncho-alveolar lavage fluid and serum in haematological patients at risk for invasive pulmonary aspergillosis. *Br J Haematol*. 2003; 121(3):448-57.

[83] Luong ML, Clancy CJ, Vadnerkar A, et al. Comparison of an *Aspergillus* real-time polymerase chain reaction assay with galactomannan testing of bronchoalvelolar lavage fluid for the diagnosis of invasive pulmonary aspergillosis in lung transplant recipients. *Clin Infect Dis*. 2011; 52(10):1218-26.

[84] Virnig C, Bush RK. Allergic bronchopulmonary aspergillosis: a US perspective. *Curr Opin Pulm Med*. 2007; 13(1):67-71.

[85] Herbrecht R, Denning DW, Patterson TF, Bennett JE, Greene RE, Oestmann JW, et al. Voriconazole versus amphotericin B for primary therapy of invasive aspergillosis. *N Engl J Med*. 2002; 347(6):408-15.

[86] Marr KA, Boeckh M, Carter RA, Kim HW, Corey L. Combination antifungal therapy for invasive aspergillosis. *Clin Infect Dis*. 2004; 39(6):797-802.

[87] Kontoyiannis DP, Wessel VC, Bodey GP, et al. Zygomycosis in the 1990s in a tertiary-care cancer center. *Clin Infect Dis*. 2000; 30(6):851-6.

[88] Rippon JW. Zygomycosis. In: Wonsiewicz M, ed. *Medical Mycology. The Pathogenic Fungi and the Pathogenic Actinomycetes*. 3rd ed. Philadelphia, Pa: W.B. Saunders; 1998:681-713.

[89] Greenberg RN, Scott LJ, Vaughn HH, et al. Zygomycosis (mucormycosis): emerging clinical importance and new treatments. *Curr Opin Infect Dis*. 2004;17(6):517-25.

[90] Petrikkos G, Skiada A, Sambatakou H, et al. Mucormycosis: ten-year experience at a tertiary-care center in Greece. *Eur J Clin Microbiol Infect Dis*. 2003; 22(12):753-6.

[91] Ibrahim AS, Edwards JE, Filler SG. Zygomycosis. In: Dismukes WE, Pappas PG, Sobel JD, eds. *Clinical Mycology*. First ed. New York: Oxford University Press; 2003:241-251.

[92] Kauffman CA. Zygomycosis: reemergence of an old pathogen. *Clin Infect Dis*. 15 2004;39(4):588-90.
[93] Gonzalez CE, Rinaldi MG, Sugar AM. Zygomycosis. *Infect Dis Clin North Am*. 2002;16(4):895-914,

Chapter 6

Pattern of Clinical Presentations in Immunocompromised Patient

Umezurike Hughes Okafor

Additional information is available at the end of the chapter

1. Introduction

Immunodeficiency (or immune deficiency) is a state in which the immune system's ability to fight infectious disease is compromised or entirely absent. Most cases of immunodeficiency are acquired (secondary) but some people are born with defects in their immune system (Primary) immunodeficiency.

The following conditions and diseases that are associated with primary immunodeficiency disorder include, Combined variable immunodeficiency disease, Ataxia-telangiectasia, Chediak-Higashi syndrome, Complement deficiencies, DiGeorge syndrome, Hypogammaglobulinemia, Job syndrome, Leukocyte adhesion defects, Bruton disease, Congenital agammaglobulinemia, Selective deficiency of IgA, Wiscott-Aldrich syndrome etc

As for acquired immunodeficiency, in 2006, UNAIDS and the World Health Organization estimated that approximately 39.5 million people were living with HIV. That year alone, there were 4.3 million new infections, with the majority occurring in sub-Saharan Africa. HIV targets T cells, and in particular, T helper cells, which are critical to fighting infections caused by fungi and parasites. This is why people with advanced, untreated AIDS develop unusual infections such as *Pneumocystis carinii* pneumonia and *Toxoplasmosis gondii.*

Since transplanted organs such as kidneys, hearts, livers, and lungs are foreign bodies, recipients' immune systems must be permanently suppressed to prevent them from attacking and destroying the organs. More than 19,000 transplants are performed in the United States each year. Each month, approximately 3,700 people are added to the U.S. national transplant waiting list, and each day, 77 people receive organ transplants. The breakthrough in transplant technology occurred in 1983 when cyclosporine, a powerful immunosuppressive drug, became licensed. However, even with cyclosporine, transplanted organs typically only last around 10 years before needing to be replaced. Research efforts to induce bodies to tolerate transplanted organs without using immunosuppressive drugs are ongoing. But until a breakthrough in understanding immunologic tolerance or a way to grow replacement organs occurs, newly immunocompromised organ-transplant recipients will occur each year.

In addition, cancer chemotherapies typically cause immunosuppression. Since cancer cells are cells that multiply uncontrollably, the goal of cancer therapy is to kill them without killing too many normal cells. Unfortunately, the cells involved in immunity are frequently adversely affected by chemotherapy, thus rendering the patient vulnerable to infections.

Autoimmune disorders are typically treated with immunosuppressive drugs such as corticosteroids, 6-mercaptopurine, and azathioprine to keep the immune system from attacking the body. For example, Crohn's disease is an autoimmune disease in which the immune system attacks the body's gastrointestinal system, causing intense pain, bleeding, and obstructions. Another treatment is infliximab, which stops the body's inflammatory response. But these treatments only alleviate pain and suffering, they don't cure the underlying immune disorder.

Also splenectomy, diabetes mellitus, cancer, increasing age, chronic diseases and strenuous exercise had been associated with various degrees of impairment in immune functions

The immune System`s primary function is to fight off infection. When the immune system is suppressed or dysfunctional the ability to combat infection is reduced. A person who has an immunodeficiency of any kind is said to be immunocompromised. These immunocompromised patients are more vulnerable to infections including infection with organisms that don't normally cause disease. In addition, they are more likely to develop severe and sometimes life-threatening illness following infection.

Many patients admitted into the Medical Unit especially Intensive Care Unit (ICU) have varying degrees of immunosuppression. In some, immunosuppression is easily apparent, especially when caused directly by underlying disease (such as haematological malignancy) or treatment (such as drugs used to prevent organ rejection or as a side effect of cancer chemotherapy). In others, immunosuppression is less apparent and is induced by the underlying disease, for example following traumatic injury or sepsis, or as a response to therapies provided during intensive care such as steroids.

Immunosuppression itself does not cause pathology but does leave the patient prone to infection and other disease conditions. There is no good clinical test to measure the degree of immunosuppression; the clinician must simply maintain a high index of suspicion. The consequences of immune suppression in most patients highlight the importance of infection prevention and control, as well as surveillance measures to ensure that appropriate treatment is implemented safely and quickly. Thus there is need to understand the pattern of clinical presentations of patients with immune dysfunction to avoid delay in making diagnosis and hence intervention.

Immunocompromised patients are prone to various infectious and non infectious disorders. The infectious disease is the commonest presentations of these patients because of the weakening of the patient's immune state. The severity of the infection depends on the degree of the immunosuppression. Some organs like respiratory pathways are more liable to infections in these patients for obvious anatomical reasons; however all organs are at risk of developing infection.

Also there are various non infectious manifestation in patients with immunosuppression. These may be directly or indirectly related to the degree of immune suppression in the patient. Patients have presented with various degrees of impaired kidney function, liver disease, cardiorespiratory dysfunction, psychosocial, dermatological and neurological disorders that are not directly related to infections.

Immunocompromised patients also can present with features not directly related to immunosupression. For example obesity in patients on steroid therapy, and hepatic disease associated with severe combined immunodeffiency disease.

Clinical presentations in immunocompromised differs among patients. The presentations are determined by the severity of the immunosupression, the severity of the infection and other comorbid condition. Furthermore the organ involved and the type of the associated clinical state play important role in determining the presentation of the patient. There are many uncommon presentations that have been reported in these patients. However poor response to treatment of infection, incomplete recovery from illness, certain types of infections and malignancies are common presentations seen in immunocompromised patients.

The clinical setting is extremely important in recognizing immunosuppression. Immune dysfunction induced by therapeutic intervention will be evident from the history, but immune impairment due to underlying disease may be more difficult to recognize. Inherited immune deficiencies often have characteristic patterns of disease distribution and may be associated with other clinical abnormalities (such as cardiac anomalies).

The various organs/systems in the body have differing impact by the resultant effect of immunosuppression. This results from either the direct impact of the immunosupression or diseases resulting from the immunosupression.

These manifestations will be discussed according to the impact on various systems and organs..

2. Gastrointestinal tract in immunocompromised

The primary function of the gastrointestinal tract is digestive, absorption and assimilation of nutrients. It has the largest surface area among all organs. With such large surface area and its close proximity to the external environment it necessitates that it evolved a large compliment of both innate and acquired immune mechanism. The gastrointestinal associated lymphoid tissue constitutes the largest immune compartment in the body. It is estimated that the GIT contains about 60% of the total body lymphocyte. The immune cells in the GIT are organized into distinct anatomic and functional sub compartments..

The gastrointestinal tract associated lymphoid tissue, can be divided into three sectors. The first is represented by the pharyngeal tonsils, the appendix, and the large aggregates of nodules known as Peyer patches located at intervals throughout the small intestine. The second sector includes the lymphocytes and plasma cells that populate the basement membrane (lamina propria) of the small intestine, the area of loose connective tissue above the supporting tissue of the mucosal lining extending into the villi. The third sector comprises lymphocytes that lie between the epithelial cells in the mucosa. The interaction between these cells of the lymphatic system and the threatening agent is the basis of defense in the gastrointestinal tract. The gastrointestinal tract also posses other protective measures which include tight epithelial junctions, the digestive enzymes, the acidic gastric fluid, the lysozyme and the high flow of the gastrointestinal fluid.

However the gastrointestinal tract is particularly at risk of infectious and non infectious injuries because of the following reasons – because of their close proximity to the external environment and continuous exposure to myriad of food and other infectious and non infectious antigens, the mucosa is maintained in physiologic inflammatory state characterized by presence of proinflammatory cytokines, marked expression of CCR5 and CXCR4 chemokine receptor that promotes HIV entry into the mucosa cells.

In immunocompromised patients the normal defenses are disrupted, leading to a wide range of clinical and pathogenic consequences. This usually leads to various disease conditions that can be classified into one of several general categories: infections, mucosal injury and ulceration, biliary tract diseases, diverticular disease, pancreatitis, and malignancy

The infections may be bacterial, viral, fungal, or parasitic and may infect one or more gut segments between the mouth and anus. The viral infections that had been reported in these patients include cytomegalovirus, herpes simplex, human papilloma virus, ebstein barr virus and rota virus. The bacterial infections include cloctridium dificile, salmonella spp, shigella spp, *H. pylori,* eiserichia coli, campylobacter spp, *Yersinia enterocolitica,* mycobacterium tuberculosis, mycobacterium avium intracellurale complex. The parasitic infections include cryptosporidium, microsporidium, entamoeba histolytica, giardia lamblia, *Strongyloides stercoralis. The fungal infections include histoplasma capsulatum, candida albicans, candida tropicalis, mucormyces spp. The gastrointestinal infections have varying presentations but the commonest presentation is diarrhea.*

Mucosal injuries and ulceration of the gastrointestinal tract has been reported in patients with immunodeficiency. Many factors had been associated with ulcer formation and propagation in these patients. Some of these factors include stress, impairment of native cytoprotection of the gastrointestinal mucosa, drugs and infections especially helicobacter pylori. Complications that had resulted from gastrointestinal mucosa injury and ulceration include perforation, penetration, peritonitis and gastrointestinal bleeding.

Diverticular disease had been reported in immunocompromised patients especially in post transplant patients on immunosuppressive therapy. The clinical presentation varies from asymptomatic to peritonitis. Complicated diverticulitis which was reported in 1.1% of renal transplant patients can presents as intestinal perforation, abscess, phlegmon or fistula.

Acute pancreatitis in immunocompromised patients are not common. It has been associated with alcohol ingestion, billiary stones, malignancy, hepatitis B and cytomegalovirus infection. Acute pancreatitis markedly increase the morbidity and mortality associated with immunodeficiency. The clinical presentation is usually atypical.

There is increase in prevalence of both common and uncommon gastrointestinal malignancies in patients with immune deficiency. Decreased immune surveillance, continuous mucosa inflammation, gastrointestinal infections, ingestion of carcinogens including medications are some of the factors suspected to be responsible for the heightened prevalence of malignancy in these patients. Also cigarette smoking, sclerosing cholangitis, crohns syndrome and splenectomy had been reported as risk factor for the development of gastrointestinal malignancy in these patients. The gastrointestinal malignancies that have been associated with immunosuppression include Kaposi sarcoma, colorectal carcinoma, post transplant lymphoproliferative lymphoma, gastric mucosa associated lymphoma. The malignancies are initially asymptomatic however acute abdomen from perforation or obstruction and gastrointestinal bleeding are the usual though late presentations.

The commonly experienced gastrointestinal (digestive) complications; include oral lesions, esophageal lesions, diarrhea, and anorectal diseases (disease that affects the anus and/or rectum). The oral lesions are aphthous ulcer, oral thrush (candidiasis), oral wart, oral hairy leukoplakia, Kaposi sarcoma.

The oesophageal lesions include oesophageal candidiasis, oesopheal herpes simplex, cytomegalovirus, aphthous ulcer, malignancy, and reflux oesophagitis manifesting as dysphagia, odynophagia, and sensation of food sticking in the throat.

The anorectal lesions which are usually seen in immunocompromised patients with AIDS include herpes simplex infection, gonorhoea, syphilis, anal wart(condylomata) and Chlamydia.

Diarhoea is a common clinical presentation in immunocompromised patients independent of the cause. This has been attributed to gastrointestinal infections, malabsorption, medications etc.

3. Hepato billiary system in immunocompromised

The hepatobilliary system is usually considered part of the digestive system however they have both digestive and non digestive functions. The liver acts as a detoxifier by processing potentially harmful agents into safe chemicals. It is also responsible for metabolism of glucose, fat and protein. It manufactures and controls the release of bile.

The bile plays an important role in breaking down of fats, the source of cellular energy. It is necessary for the absorption of many vitamins and other fat related substances. It also participates in the excretion of many product of metabolism including bilirubin, bile acid and medications.

The hepatobilliary system receives dual blood supply, from the portal and systemic circulation. Hence in immunocompromised patient the hepatobilliary system is exposed to many infectious and non infectious antigens. This predisposes the patient to many disease conditions relating/affecting the system.

Immunodeficiency states resulting from AIDS, cytotoxic chemotherapy, radiation, organ transplantation and common variable immunodeficiency disorders have been associated with hepatobilliary disease. These disorders that have been reported in immunocompromised patients include infectious hepatitis, granulomatous hepatitis, alcoholic liver disease, cholangiopathy, hepatocellular carcinoma, schistosomiasis, haemangioma and hepatic adenoma. Nodular regenerative hyperplasia of the liver has also been reported in patients with combined variable immunodeficiency syndrome.

There are various clinical manifestations relating to this system in these patients. In a study of patients with common variable immunodeficiency syndrome with nodular regenerative hyperplasia 39% of the patients were asymptomatic but had deranged liver functions, 46% had jaundice, 46% had hepatomegaly, 23% had pruritus, 15% had ascitis, 15% had oesophageal varices. Also jaundice and hepatomegaly is a common presentation in immunocompromised patients resulting from opportunistic and conventional infections of either hepatobilliary or other systems. Other manifestations include portal hypertension, cirrhosis, primary and secondary malignancies of the liver and billiary tree, and hepatic failure.

4. Respiratory system in immunocompromised

The immune system in the airways consists of both innate and specific immunity. Innate immunity consists of mechanical defenses, antimicrobial molecules generated in the airways, and phagocytic defenses provided by the resident alveolar macrophages and the polymorphonuclear leukocytes (PMNs) that are recruited into the lung in response to infection. The specific immunity are usually initiated by the dendritic cell that act as the antigen presenting cell. They migrate to the regional lymphoid tissue to initiate the primary response with generation of memory B and T cells.

This sophisticated immune defense system effectively protects the host from infections and other immunodeficiency related diseases of the respiratory tract. However this function is impaired in immunocompromised individuals thus exposing them to many diseases of the airways.

Patients with compromised immune function suffer from a wide variety of infectious and non infectious lung insults. Infections are the most common cause of both acute and chronic lung diseases in immunocompromised patients however noninfectious diseases are not uncommon.

Pulmonary infections decisively contribute to morbidity and mortality in immunocompromised patients. The prevalence of both the common infections implicated in community acquired pneumonia and some uncommon infections including opportunistic infections are increased in immunocompromised patients. Among the infections encountered are streptococcus pneumoniae, klebsiella pneumonia, haemophilus influenza, pseudomonas aeruginosa, actinobacter spp, fusobacterium nucleatum, bacteroids melaninogenicus, bacteroids fragilis, mycobacterium tuberculi, mycobacterium avium intracellurale, pneumocystis carinii (jirovecii), norcadia spp, coccidomyces spp, aspergilus spp, *Rhodococcus equi* etc. The infections usually present as pneumonia, suppurative lung disease, interstitial lung disease and obstructive lung diseases

The spectrum of noninfectious lung injury and response in the immunosuppressed host includes interstitial edema, interstitial fibrosis, diffuse idiopathic pneumonia, acute respiratory distress syndrome, obliterative bronchiolitis, alveolar hemorrhage, pulmonary embolism, radiation pneumonitis, drug toxicity, progression or recurrence of neoplastic disorders, chemotherapy, transfusion and transplant related lung injuries. The clinical manifestations of various non infectious complications in immunocompromised patients are non specific and may mimic infections.

Clinical approach to respiratory tract diseases in immunocompromised patients are classified into five categories. The first situation is defined by a slow progression of the disease, the absence of fever (or mild fever), and diffuse opacities. Pulmonary oedema, pulmonary localisation of the underlying disease, or toxic treatment induced pneumonitis are usually the cause. Non-specific pneumonitis may also be responsible, particularly in bone marrow transplant recipients.

The second situation, defined by a rapid progression of the condition, fever, and diffuse opacities, usually indicates an opportunistic pneumonia but, in a few cases, a hypersensitivity drug induced pneumonitis (for example, to methotrexate) or a localisation of the underlying disease—for example, in cases of vasculitis or collagen vascular disease—may be the cause. In the absence of new extrapulmonary symptoms, *Pneumocystis carinii* must be considered. In contrast, the presence of new extrapulmonary symptoms or signs suggests an association or another opportunistic infection such as cytomegalovirosis, cryptococcosis, toxoplasmosis, or tuberculosis.

In the third situation the clinical feature is that of bacterial pneumonia or sepsis with ARDS. The pathogens responsible are usually*Streptococcus pneumoniae* or *Haemophilus influenzae* and, to a lesser degree, *Legionella* spp.

The fourth situation with rapid to moderate progression of the condition, fever, nodules or round infiltrates evolving towards dissemination and/or cavitation is highly suggestive of fungal pneumonia. However, legionellosis, tuberculosis and even pulmonary infarction or specific localisation of vasculitis may also result in similar manifestations.

The last situation is certainly the most complex. The clinician is confronted with focal pulmonary infiltrates which do not respond to antibiotics. Opportunistic agents such as *Mycobacteria* spp, *Nocardia* spp, or *Rhodococcus equi*, organising pneumonia or tumour may be the cause.

5. Skin in immunocompromised

Skin, once thought to be an inert structure, plays a vital role in protecting the individual from the external environment. The epidermis impedes penetration of microbial organisms, chemical irritation, and toxins, absorbs and blocks solar and ionized radiation, and inhibits water loss.

The stratum corneum, the outermost layer of the epidermis that results from the terminal differentiation of the keratinocytes, forms the primary layer of protection from the external environment. This layer of anucleated keratinocytes is composed of highly cross-linked proteinaceous cellular envelopes with extracellular lipid lamellae consisting of ceramides, free fatty acids, and cholesterol. The free fatty acids create an acidic environment that inhibits colonization by certain bacteria such as Staphylococcus aureus, providing further protection.

Apart from the physical barriers the skin also contain other innate immunomodulating substances and cells. This include cathelicidins, cytokines. neuropeptides, eicosanoids, reactive oxygen species and langhern cell which has phagocytic properties, and act as antigen presenting cell. The skin is consistently exposed to host of injuries because of their size and exposure to the environment. These coordinated protective barriers, cells and substances maintain the integrity of the skin.

In immunodeficiency state there is alteration in this innate immune state in the skin. This thus predisposes the skin to many injuries – infectious and non infectious. Dermatological manifestations are important healthcare concerns in patients with immunodeficiency state. About 25% of patients with immunodeficiency had been reported with dermatological injuries.

Subsequent invasion of the skin by various bacterial, viral, fungal, and parasitic agents spur infectious skin lesions, whereas non-infectious skin conditions mainly emerge from adverse drug reactions or certain inflammatory or malignant aetiologies. Thus microbial infections, inflammatory conditions, and neoplasms are the three main causes for the development of dermatological findings in immunocompromised patients.

There have been several reports detailing the high frequency of dermatological manifestations in HIV infected patients, 96% in India, 70% in Taiwan, 65.3% in France, 65.3% in Tanzania, 34% in Thailand, 32.6% in Iran. The dermatological manifestations in these patients may be as a result of primary dermatological infection, metastastic infection with primary in another organ or systemic infection.

There are many organisms that are associated with infection of or manifestations in the skin in patients with immunodeficiency. The infections could be as a result of conventional or opportunistic infection. These infections include viral, bacterial, fungal and parasitic. The organisms that have been associated with dermatological infections or manifestation in immunocompromised patients are herpes simplex virus, varicella zoster virus, cytomegalovirus and pappiloma virus, staphylococcus spp, streptococcus spp, pseudomonas spp, atypical mycobacterium spp, the fungal infections including malasezia furfur, candidiasis, norcadia spp, Cryptococcus neoformans, Aspergillus species, Paecilomyces, Rhizopus species, Candida tropicalis, and scabies.

The commonly reported dermatological lesions in immunocompromised patients include dermatitis, seborrheic dermatitis, folliculitis, dermatophytes including pityriasis versicolor, wart, Kaposi sarcoma, herpes zoster, acne vulgaris, urticaria, pruritus, psoriasis, malasma and erythema multiforme. Other Skin lesions including pustules, gangrenous cellulitis, erythematous subcutaneous nodules, hemorrhagic bullae, petechiae, ecchymoses, and ecthyma gangrenosum had also been reported in immunocompromised patients.

Cutaneous manifestations often are accompanied by fever, defined as an isolated temperature of 38.3°C (101°F), that cannot be attributed to exogenous causes, such as blood products, or a temperature above 38°C (100.4°F) that persists for more than 1 hour.

6. Central nervous system in immunocompromised

Immune responses in the CNS are common, despite its perception as a site of immune privilege. These responses can be mediated by resident microglia and astrocytes, which are innate immune cells without direct counterparts in the periphery. Furthermore, CNS immune reactions often take place in virtual isolation from the innate/adaptive immune interplay that characterizes peripheral immunity. However, microglia and astrocytes also engage in significant cross-talk with CNS-infiltrating T cells and other components of the innate immune system.

Microglia are key players of the immune response in the central nervous system (CNS) and being the resident innate immune cells, they are responsible for the early control of infections and for the recruitment of cells of the adaptive immune system required for pathogen clearance. The innate and adaptive immune responses triggered by microglia include the release of proinflammatory mediators. Although an efficient immune response is required for the defense against invading pathogens, an inflammatory response in the CNS may also lead to tissue injury and neurodegeneration. Engagement of Toll-like receptors (TLRs), a major family of pattern recognition receptors that mediate innate immunity but also link with the adaptive immune response, provides an important mechanism by which microglia are able to sense both pathogen and host derived ligands within the CNS.

Patients with immunodeficiency are at risk of a wide range of neurologic diseases including infections, neoplasms, and drug-related complications of therapy

CNS infections caused by infective agents are rare in immunocompetent host, but more frequent in immunocompromised patients. The spectrum of causative organisms may vary greatly, depending on the underlying malignancy, its treatment and various other factors. Infections that had been reported to cause neurological diseases in immunocompromised patients are as detailed below;

Viral – herpes simplex virus, JC virus, cytomegalovirus, varicella zoster virus.
Bacterial – staphylococcus spp, pneumococcus, haemophilus spp, mycobacterium tuberculosis, mycobacterium Avium/ Intracellulare Complex, Listeria spp, norcadia spp.
fungal – *Cryptococcus neoformans, Aspergillus fumigatus, Zygomycetes (Mucor and Rhizopus), Candida albicans,* Coccidioides spp
Parasitic - toxoplasmosis, strongyloides.

Development of neurologic manifestations depends on a variety of factors, including therapy with drugs like antiretroviral drugs and the patient's overall degree of immunosuppression. Heavily immunocompromised patients like those after allogeneic stem cell transplantation (SCT) or previous T cell depleting treatment regimens (e.g. with fludarabine or alemtuzumab) are at highest risk for cerebral infections. . The infections can cause global or focal cerebral dysfunction, subhemispheric impairment, spinal cord injury and occasionally, peripheral nerve injury.

Thus, in the immunosuppressed patient with neurological involvement there are three inter-related areas to consider. First, has whatever caused the immunosuppression either directly or indirectly affected the nervous system? Second, are such problems due to an infection of the nervous system? And last, are there any medical complications that might produce a neurological disturbance? In assessing immunosuppressed patients, the clinician must remember that more than one of these factors may be involved in the neurological presentation.

Clinical presentations in these patients may include headache, signs and symptoms of increased intracranial pressure, and lateralizing signs appropriate to the area(s) of involvement. These symptoms can include behavioral, cognitive, and personality changes. Focal symptoms include hemiparesis, aphasia, and visual field defects. Ataxia, seizures, and cranial nerve palsies can also occur but are not as common.

Meningoencephalitis is a common presentation however the classical symptoms and signs may be absent in these patients.. Also cerebral toxoplasmosis, cerebral lymphoma and cerebral vascular accident in immunocompromised patients may have similarities in their clinical presentations. The nature of neurological manifestation in patients with impaired immune state also varies with the cause and the degree of the immunosuppression. There is need for high index of suspicion to avoid delay or misdiagnosis that may lead to delay in intervention.

7. Musculoskeletal system in immunocompromised

The immune cells and mediators had been implicated in some musculoskeletal diseases. The bone marrow is the source of various haematological cells including the primordial immune cells. The bone marrow also harbours matured and maturing immune cells. However the physiological activities of both innate and acquired immunity in the musculoskeletal system are poorly documented.

There is increased prevalence of musculoskeletal diseases especially infections in immunocompromised patients. Musculoskeletal syndromes that occur in HIV-infected patients include manifestations of drug toxicity, reactive arthritis, Reiter's syndrome, infectious arthritis, and myositis. Post transplant patients have developed myopathies and various bony and joint disorders. Myopathy and myositis have been reported in patients with diabetes mellitus and some primary immune deficiency disorders.

Some other musculoskeletal disorders in patients with immunodeficiency include some syndromes with arthritis or myositis as one of the components eg Reiters syndrome, Dermatomyositis, Sjogrens syndrome, Polyomyositis and Psoriasis.

The hallmark of the presentation is pain in the muscle, swelling of muscle, occasionally associated with fever and muscle atrophy. Arthralgia, swelling of the joint and when intervention is delayed distortion of the joint. Patient may develop cellulitis with or without abscess formation and osteomyelitis. There is need for prompt diagnosis and intervention as delay may lead to rapid spread of the infection in these patients.

8. Urogenital system in immunocompromised

The urogenital tract contain both cellular and non cellular innate immune components. This ensure the sterility of the urinary tract and part of the genital tract. In immunodeficiency state the urogenital tract are exposed to higher prevalence of both common and rare infections. The urogenital diseases that have been reported in immunocompromised patients include urinary tract infection, epididymitis, prostatitis, extensive condylomata of the urethra, renal abscess and other renal related diseases.

The occurrence of urinary tract infection and its clinical impact is determined, as with any infectious disease, by the interaction between the virulence of the infecting organism and the host defense mechanisms that can be mobilized. In the case of urinary tract infections, an anatomically and functionally intact kidney and urinary tract are the primary host defenses, with phagocytic function and immune mechanisms coming into play to limit the consequences of those infections.

Defects in the immune system determine the clinical manifestations and severity of urinary tract infections (UTI) and the rates of complication. However they only have an indirect role in influencing susceptibility to infection. Of all the categories of immunocompromised hosts, the renal transplant patient is the one most susceptible to the direct and indirect consequences of urinary tract infections. The rates of UTI in diabetics, renal transplant, recipients, neutropenic patients, and patients with AIDS are primarily determined by the degree and duration of urinary tract manipulation, and the higher perineal prevalence of potential pathogens that result from frequent hospitalization and antimicrobial use.

Urogenital tract infection has a different clinicoradiological presentation in immunocompromised patients, with predominance of systemic symptoms, multiple parenchymatous renal foci, and lower frequency of lesions of the collecting system. In the context of immunosuppression, Urogenital tract infection behaves as a severe bacterial infection, with bacteremia and visceral metastatic foci.

Many patients are asymptomatic. Symptoms that may occur include dysuria, urinary frequency and incontinence, flank pain, and fever. Confusion and delirium are often attributed to UTI, although without high fever or sepsis. Uncomplicated UTI is unlikely to cause serious central nervous dysfunction. The clinical signs and follow up of these infections were straight forward in half of the cases. However, in some patients, the infection is fulminant with progression to an abscess despite the use of antibiotics or is unusual because of the pathogens isolated.

Mycobacterial agents causing UTIs are less frequent in immunocompetent individuals; they are more common and severe in immunocompromised individuals. Extra pulmonary tuberculosis (EPTB) represents a progressively greater proportion of new cases and the genitourinary tract is the most common site of EPTB. The most common causative organism of kidney and urinary tract tuberculosis is the Mycobacterium tuberculosis, and occasionally Mycobacterium bovis can also be responsible. Mycobacterium tuberculosis (MTB) has an important impact on kidney transplant recipients, particularly during the first year after surgery. Tuberculosis of the urinary tract is easily overlooked. Symptoms that sometimes occur include back, flank and suprapubic pain, hematuria, frequency, and nocturia. These might also suggest conventional bacterial urinary tract infection. Symptoms such as fever, weight loss, and night sweats also are not unusual.

A variety of renal syndromes have been reported in patients with immunosupression. These can be either acute or chronic kidney disease including electrolyte abnormalities. Renal impairment from opportunistic infections and drugs used in these patients has also been reported. A broad spectrum of renal diseases affecting glomerular, tubular and interstitial tissues had been documented in immunocompromised patients especially HIV infected patients. Most of the renal manifestations represent complications of concurrent infections in a severely immunocompromised host, or side effects of the plethora of treatments required to manage these patients. The renal related presentations except for hypertension and oedema are consistent with clinical presentations in renal disease in immunocompetent patients, however severity varies with the degree of immunosuppression. Hypertension and oedema were reported as not common in immunocompromised patients. The renal disease in these patients deteriorates faster without intervention thus the need for early diagnosis and prompt intervention.

9. Conclusion

Immunocompromised patients are predisposed to a variety of clinical syndromes. The manifestations depend on the cause of immunosuppression, the degree of immunosupression, the endemic infections, the system or organ with predominant injury, and other associated diseases like Malignancies and infiltrative diseases. It is noteworthy that these patients may have atypical presentations. Thus there is need for surveillance and high index of suspicion of injuries/diseases in these patients to ensure early diagnosis and intervention.

Author details

Umezurike Hughes Okafor
Enugu State University Teaching Hospital, Parklane, Enugu, Nigeria

10. References

Ayaz A, Biviji MD, Guy D. et al. musculoskeletal manifestation of human immunodeficiency virus. Am Acad Ortho Surgeons; 10(3): 833-838

Ana Rañó, Carlos Agustí, Natividad Benito et al. Prognostic Factors of Non-HIV Immunocompromised Patients with Pulmonary Infiltrates. CHEST (2002); 122 (1): 253-261

C Dougan, I Ormerod. A neurologist's approach to the immunosuppressed patient. J Neurol Neurosurg Psychiatry 2004;75:i43-i49 doi:10.1136/jnnp.2003.035071

Dawn McGuire. Neurologic Manifestations of HIV .HIV InSite Knowledge Base Chapter June 2003

Elizabeth Boskey Immunocompromised. www/ *About.com (2010)*

Figueiredo AA, Lucon AM, Júnior RF, Ikejiri DS, Nahas WC, Srougi M. Urogenital tuberculosis in immunocompromised patients. Int Urol Nephrol. 2009;41(2):327-33. Epub 2008 Jul 22.

Foroughi et al. Prevalence of dermatologic manifestations among people living with HIV/AIDS in Imam Khomeini Hospital in Tehran, Iran. Journal of AIDS and HIV Research Vol. 4(2), pp. 56-59, February 2012

Fred A. Lopez, Charles V. Sanders. Recognizing Cutaneous Signs of Infection in Immunocompromised Patients. Hematol Oncol. 2003;6(3): 1 – 4

Immune Deficiency Foundation. *Primary Immunodeficiency Diseases.* Family Handbook; Baxter. Fourth Edition. 2007 : Chapter XI.

J. Harold Helderman, Simin G. Gastrointestinal complications of transplant immunosuppression. J Am Soc Nephrol 13: 277–287, 2002

Javier Munoz, Philip Kuriakose. Rash in an Immunocompromised Patient. JAMA. (2012);307(6):612-613. .

Kahn LH. The growing number of immunocompromised. Bulletin of the Atomic Scientists (2008): www/thebulletin.org

Nancy Lane. Rheumatologic and musculoskeletal manifestation of HIV. HIV inSite Knowledge Base chapter 1998.

Nick Murphy, Tony Whitehouse, Mark Cook. Immunocompromised; PACT (2010): 1 –57

Ping Zhang, Gregory J. Bagby, Kyle I. Happel, Caroline E. Raasch, Steve Nelson. Alcohol Abuse, Immunosuppression, and Pulmonary Infection Current Drug Abuse Reviews, 2008, Vol. 1, No. 1

Ranjan K , Sharma M . An Approach to the Detection of Mycobacteria in Clinically Suspected Cases of Urinary Tract Infection in Immunocompromised Patients . WebmedCentral. Bacteriology 2010;1(9):WMC00616

Tolkoff-Rubin NE, Rubin RH. Urinary tract infection in the immunocompromised host. Lessons from kidney transplantation and the AIDS epidemic. Infect Dis Clin North Am. 1997 Sep;11(3):707-17.

Wolfson JS, Sober AJ, Rubin RH. Dermatologic manifestations of infections in immunocompromised patients. Medicine (Baltimore). 1985 Mar;64(2):115-33

Chapter 7

Chemokine Receptors as Therapeutic Targets in HIV Infection

Cleo G. Anastassopoulou

Additional information is available at the end of the chapter

1. Introduction

Acquired immunodeficiency syndrome (AIDS) evolved into a pandemic in less than a decade since the first reports of a new set of symptoms that included severe opportunistic infections and unusual neoplasms, particularly Kaposi's sarcoma, in homosexual men [1]. Nearly 30 years since the discovery of the causative agent [2, 3], human immunodeficiency virus (HIV) cannot still be eradicated, nor is there sight of a safe and effective prophylactic vaccine in the horizon. Infection with either virus type invariably leads to AIDS; however, the less pathogenic HIV-2 stains have been geographically restricted mainly to West Africa, whilst the more virulent HIV-1 strains have spread around the globe causing the AIDS pandemic [4]. The worst afflicted region is sub-Saharan Africa, where in a few countries more than one in five adults is infected with the virus; at the same time, the epidemic is spreading most rapidly in Eastern Europe and Central Asia, where the number of people living with HIV increased by 250% between 2001 and 2010 [5]. Worldwide, an estimated 34 million people, including 3.4 million children, were living with HIV at the end of 2010, while the related deaths and new infections were 1.8 and 2.7 million, respectively [5].

Despite these frightening numbers, which are indicative of a growing epidemic far from the UNAIDS vision of zero AIDS-related deaths and zero new infections, considerable progress has undoubtedly been noted in basic and clinical research in the field of HIV/AIDS [6]; we now understand most aspects of HIV pathogenesis and have identified targets suitable for therapeutic intervention. The introduction of combination antiretroviral therapy (ART) in 1996 revolutionized patient care and brought about a significant reduction in AIDS-related morbidity and mortality; HIV infection has been transformed into a chronic condition that is generally controllable with lifelong treatment, at least in the developed world where treatment is available. At the forefront of current anti-HIV research, CCR5 inhibitors represent a novel drug class that broadens the therapeutic options of patients, which are currently limited by chronic toxicities or by the presence of resistance to conventional antiretrovirals targeting ever mutating virus-encoded structures.

This chapter focuses on describing the scientific rationale that led to the development of coreceptor inhibitors as a new class of host-targeted antiretroviral agents. This description entails a revision of the biology of coreceptor usage during HIV entry into target cells and viral tropism during the course of infection. The various approaches undertaken to pharmaceutically target the most commonly used coreceptor, CCR5, will then be described, with a special focus on small molecule CCR5 inhibitors (also termed "CCR5 antagonists") and their mechanism of action. The current status of the small molecule CCR5 inhibitor pipeline, with emphasis on the generation of resistance, including *in vitro* and *in vivo* HIV escape pathways and mechanisms, will be presented, while implications as well as future perspectives for the clinical use of CCR5 inhibitors will be discussed.

2. The HIV entry process and the coreceptors

2.1. Discovery of the HIV coreceptors

CD4 had been known to be the principal cell surface receptor for HIV-1, and also for HIV-2 and simian immunodeficiency virus (SIV), since 1984 [7, 8]. It had also been known for almost as long, however, that the presence of the CD4 antigen alone was not sufficient to allow for HIV entry. To infect $CD4^{+}$ cells, HIV-1 strains of different biological phenotypes, namely macrophage (M)-tropic and T-cell line (T)-tropic, were supposed to utilize different auxiliary co-factors [9], the identity of which remained elusive until early 1996. At that time, a member of the seven-transmembrane (7-TM) spanning family of chemokine receptors initially termed "fusin", was identified as the coreceptor for T-tropic HIV-1 variants [10]; the term was changed to C-X-C chemokine receptor type 4 (CXCR4) once its natural ligand was discovered to be stromal derived factor-1 (SDF-1)/CXCL12 [11, 12]. CXCR4 had been previously identified as an orphan receptor called leukocyte-derived seven-transmembrane domain receptor (LESTR), but it only received attention after its isolation as an HIV-1 coreceptor [13].

The knowledge that the β-chemokines macrophage inflammatory protein (MIP)-1α/CCL3, MIP-1β/CCL4 and regulated upon activation normal T-cell expressed and secreted (RANTES)/CCL5 exhibited antiviral activity against M-tropic HIV-1 isolates *in vitro* [14], provided the basis for the discovery of C-C chemokine receptor type 5 (CCR5) as the entry co-factor for these strains by five groups simultaneously [15-19]. The virus thus uses chemokine receptors, mainly CCR5 and CXCR4, to enter susceptible cells, while the cognate chemokine ligands act as natural entry inhibitors. Other chemokine receptors may also function as HIV coreceptors; nonetheless, infection of primary cells via alternative coreceptors is rare and the process can normally be fully blocked by CCR5 or CXCR4 inhibitors [20-22]. Hence, at present, CCR5 and CXCR4 are considered as the only HIV coreceptors of physiological significance.

2.2. Physiological roles of the main coreceptors

CCR5 and CXCR4 are two structurally related, heptahelical chemokine receptors that belong to different classes [C-C and CXC, respectively, based on the position of the two conserved cysteine (Cys) residues in their N-termini (Nt)] of the superfamily of G protein-coupled receptors (GPCRs) (reviewed in [13, 23-25]). About half of the drug targets in the pharmaceutical industry are GPCRs, which also, not coincidentally, comprise the largest family of cell-surface receptors [26]. GPCRs become activated by chemokines, small (8-10 kDa) soluble protein ligands that are either promiscuous or specific for a given receptor. Once activated by such extracellular signals, GPCRs undergo conformational changes that trigger the intracellular signal transduction cascade; these series of events begin with the rapid phosphorylation by G protein-coupled receptor kinases (GRKs) predominantly on serine (Ser) and threonine (Thr) residues within the C-tail and third intracellular loop and continue with the activation of heterotrimeric G proteins [27]. In this mode, chemokines and their receptors control cell migration associated with routine immune surveillance, inflammation and development [28].

CCR5, in particular, appears to play a role in the initiation of adaptive immune responses and the trafficking of effector cells to sites of infection and inflammation as indicated by its expression profile on several effector T cell subsets and antigen-presenting cells, including macrophages, immature dendritic cells and Langerhans cells (reviewed in [22, 29, 30]). Nonetheless, the lack of expression of this gene due to a deletion polymorphism known as "delta32" does not appear to have any deleterious effects; in fact, heterozygosity for the *CCR5Δ32* allele is generally associated with delayed disease progression, and homozygosity with incomplete protection from HIV transmission (reviewed in [31]). The observation that its congenital absence does not lead to any overt pathology suggested that CCR5 might be a valid target for pharmacological blockade.

CXCR4, on the other hand, and its single known ligand SDF-1/CXCL12 are both highly conserved [13]; they play an essential role during embryonic development and in several major processes in the adult, including hematopoiesis, leukocyte trafficking in the adaptive immune system, and vascularization [22]. CXCR4 knockout mice show hematopoietic and cardiovascular defects during embryogenesis and die *in utero*; mice lacking SDF-1/CXCL12 are characterized by deficient B-lymphopoiesis and myelopoiesis and abnormal neuronal and cardiovascular development [13]. Clinically tested CXCR4 inhibitors AMD3100, which lacked oral bioavailability, and AMD070 caused significant leukocytosis (reviewed in [22]). The non-cyclam antagonist AMD070 (or AMD11070) is currently in Phase II clinical trials as an HIV cell-entry inhibitor [32]. The development of AMD3100 (by AnorMED) for use in the treatment of HIV infection was terminated, but further studies led to a new indication for this drug; AMD3100 (now Plerixafor, Genzyme) has been approved by the US Food and Drug Administration (FDA) for autologous transplantation in patients with non-Hodgkin's lymphoma and multiple myeloma [32]. The fact that Plerixafor is well tolerated in the developed organism minimizes the concerns of antagonizing such a crucial receptor/ligand axis in mature individuals. CXCR4 antagonists could be used in combination with antiretrovirals targeting other steps of the viral life cycle; they could also be administered simultaneously with CCR5 antagonists, even as one compound with high affinity for both receptors, as suggested recently [32]. Down-modulating the expression of CXCR4 may certainly be beneficial for some HIV patients [13]. The pharmacologic targeting of CXCR4 may additionally have therapeutic utility for the treatment of acute viral infections of the central nervous system (CNS) [33]. The rest of this chapter focuses on issues related to the development of CCR5 inhibitors.

2.3. The coreceptors in HIV entry

Conformationally masked by carbohydrate structures and variable amino acid loops that enable it to evade the humoral immune response, the envelope glycoprotein (Env) on virions is organized into trimers of noncovalently associated surface gp120 and transmembrane gp41 heterodimers (reviewed in [34]). The interaction of HIV with host cell surface receptors trigger the fusogenic potential of Env and allow the virus to enter into its target cells by fusion, presumably at the plasma membrane [35]. The process has long been assumed to occur at the cell surface for such pH-independent viruses as HIV [36], although recent studies support the notion that HIV enters disparate cell types through fusion with endosomes [37, 38]. A schematic of the first steps of the HIV entry process, according to the presently accepted molecular mechanism, is shown in Figure 1.

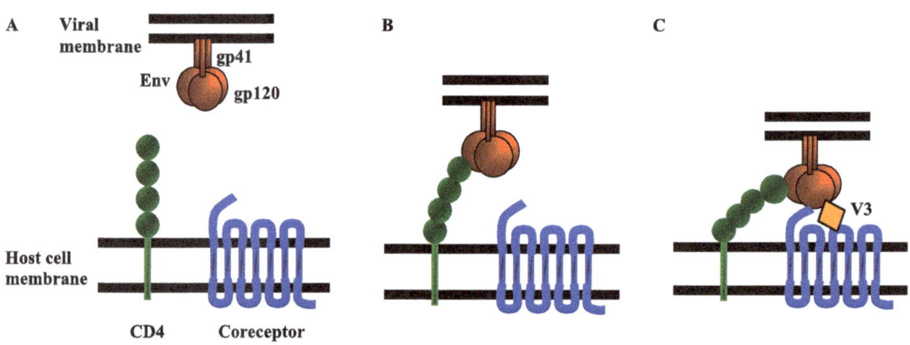

Figure 1. Schematic diagram of the first steps of the HIV entry process. (**A**) HIV entry into target cells is mediated through the interaction of the viral envelope glycoprotein (Env) with host cell surface receptors. (**B**) Surface gp120 first contacts CD4 and then (**C**) a chemokine receptor, typically CCR5 or CXCR4, triggering molecular rearrangements in the gp41 that result in membrane fusion and the initiation of infection.

HIV entry begins with the high affinity binding of gp120 to the host cell CD4, which induces a major conformational change in Env that exposes or creates a binding site on gp120 for the coreceptor, typically either CCR5 or CXCR4. Current structural models suggest that the gp120 "bridging sheet", formed between the constant C1, C2, and C4 domains of gp120 after CD4 binding, interacts with the tyrosine (Tyr)-sulfated coreceptor N-terminus (Nt), while the V3 crown interacts principally with the second extracellular loop (ECL2) region of the coreceptor [39-42]. Coreceptor engagement of CD4-bound gp120 induces additional reconfigurations, leading to the insertion of the gp41 fusion peptide (FP) into the host cell membrane and the formation of a pre-fusion complex. This pre-fusion intermediate is then refolded into an energetically favorable six-helix bundle that brings the two membranes in close proximity so that fusion can occur; the viral core is thereby released into the cytoplasm and a new cycle of infection is initiated.

Our understanding of HIV entry has provided invaluable insights into viral tropism and pathogenesis and led to the development of novel classes of antiretroviral agents that inhibit specific stages of the process. CCR5 inhibitors interrupt the viral replication cycle by preventing CCR5 binding and aborting fusion.

3. Coreceptor use and HIV tropism

3.1. Classification systems of HIV biological phenotype

Before the identification of the coreceptors, three biological properties were the criteria used to classify the phenotype of HIV variants: (i) the preference for specific target cells (cellular tropism) that distinguished between macrophage (M)-tropic and laboratory T-cell line (T)-tropic viruses; (ii) cytopathology, which distinguished between syncytium-inducing (SI) and non-syncytium-inducing (NSI) strains based on the capacity or not to form syncytia (i.e., giant multinucleated cells) through cell fusion in the MT-2 cell line; and (iii) replicative capacity, which mainly considered the *in vitro* growth kinetics of viral strains in culture and distinguished between slow/low (S/L) and rapid/high viruses (R/H) (reviewed in [43]).

The above dichotomies may be explained by the more precise, newly adopted classification system that is based on coreceptor usage; accordingly, viruses that use CCR5 alone or CXCR4 alone for cell entry are currently termed R5 and X4, correspondingly, while variants that can use either coreceptor with comparable efficiency are termed R5X4 [44]. A more appropriate designation for the latter is R5+X4 or D/M (Dual/Mixed), particularly when tropism has not been determined at the clonal level, since many R5X4 isolates are in fact mixtures of R5 plus X4 or, less commonly, either R5 plus dual (R5X4), or even R5 plus dual (R5X4) plus X4, clones [22]. The term R5X4 should thus be reserved for clones that are genuinely capable of using both coreceptors.

3.2. Determinants of HIV biological phenotype and coreceptor tropism assessment

The determinants of coreceptor choice, and thus of biological phenotype, have been mapped to the surface gp120 subunit of Env and primarily to the V3 domain. Swapping the V3 region alone often suffices to switch the coreceptor tropism of a viral clone from R5 to X4 and vice versa [45]. Furthermore, the charge of the V3 region appears to be an important parameter affecting biological phenotype and, tropism, although it alone cannot be used as a marker for phenotype prediction; in general, however, higher net charges ($\geq +5$) characterize X4 variants compared to the lower V3 region net charges ($\leq +4$) of R5 variants typically associated with acute infection (reviewed in [43]). The increase of the overall positive charge of the V3 region that may switch the viral phenotype results from the introduction of basic amino acid residues at one of the two positions 11 and/or 25 of the V3 [46, 47], a property that may not be shared by the uncommon subtype C CXCR4-using strains (reviewed in [48]).

Simple genotypic approaches undertaken for predicting coreceptor usage include the detection of positively charged amino acids at positions 11 and 25 (often referred to as the "11/25 rule") and the determination of the total charge of V3, with the cut-off set at +5; heteroduplex tracking assays and various bioinformatics approaches are additional genotypic methods for determining HIV tropism (reviewed in [49-51]). Predictive algorithms of coreceptor usage have been developed based on genetic sequences in the V3 region, but also taking into account genotypic correlates outside the V3, structural information and clinical data [48]. Apart from these genotypic tools, different phenotypic assays have been developed to assess HIV tropism. These phenotypic methods, which are reviewed elsewhere [49-52], include the original MT-2 assay or coreceptor usage assays using reporter cell lines, and cell-based assays that use different methodologies to generate *env*-recombinant or pseudotyped viruses with distinct detection systems. The Trofile assay (Monogram Biosciences, Inc., South San Francisco, CA; now Laboratory Corporation of America [LabCorp]) is the most widely used phenotypic test in clinical practice. In the new era of CCR5 inhibitors, an accurate determination, and perhaps quantification, of coreceptor usage is necessary for the successful clinical management of HIV-infected individuals.

3.3. HIV phenotypes, tropism and disease course

Regardless of the route of HIV transmission, R5 viruses seem to prevail in the vast majority of primary and early stage HIV infection cases, whilst the X4 phenotype evolves *in vivo* in approximately 40-50% of (subtype B or D) infected subjects, usually 5–7 years after infection (reviewed in [43, 53]). Recent transmitted/founder virus genetic studies confirmed that only R5 (and typically a single R5 virus isolate) and in a few instances R5X4, but not X4 HIV-1, are initially transmitted [54, 55]. Consequently, a "gatekeeper" that nearly always selects transmission of R5 over X4 HIV may well exist. The suppression of X4 transmission has been suggested to result not from one powerful gatekeeper, but from an aggregate of multiple functional gatekeepers, the localization and precise molecular mechanisms of which remain to be determined (reviewed in [56]). CCR5 thus has a pivotal role in viral transmission, but infection by X4 (or R5X4) viruses is not impossible as indicated by the few known cases of HIV acquisition by *CCR5-Δ32* homozygotes; the lower pre-AIDS viral loads and slower disease progression of *CCR5-Δ32* heterozygotes, in whom the CCR5 expression levels on target cells are lower, underscore the importance of the CCR5 coreceptor in the early asymptomatic stages of the infection [31, 53].

The emergence of X4 viruses in a proportion of cases correlates with accelerated disease progression [43, 53]. The virological or immunological basis of the selection mechanism is still debated; in other words, it is still unclear whether disease progression is accelerated as a direct consequence of the emergence or predominance of X4 isolates, or, conversely, whether the declining competence of the host immune system permits the outgrowth of viral strains with increased replicative capacity [43]. The pathogenicity of X4 viruses seems to be greater than that displayed by R5 strains both *in vitro* and probably *in vivo*, as suggested by experiments in macaques [22]. R5 viruses alone can also cause severe damage to the immune system; X4 viruses are never detected in about half of HIV-infected subjects who do progress to AIDS [22, 53]. These late-emerging, R5 viral strains, which have reduced sensitivity to entry inhibitors and increased ability to cause $CD4^+$ T-lymphocyte loss, also possess an improved ability to utilize relatively low levels of CD4 and CCR5 expressed on macrophages (reviewed in [57]). Correlations between increased gp120 net charge, enhanced viral fitness, and augmented cell attachment were disclosed as well for these R5 HIV-1 variants that emerge in an opportunistic manner during severe immunodeficiency [58].

Different $CD4^+$ T cell subpopulations are targeted by the phenotypic variants of HIV: replication of R5 viruses is favored in activated, memory/effector T cells, whereas X4 viruses may additionally infect intrathymic T progenitor cells and naïve T cells in the peripheral lymphoid system [39, 43]. Of note is the massive depletion in the gut-associated lymphoid tissue (GALT) of CCR5-expressing memory $CD4^+$ T cells as a consequence of acute HIV infection (reviewed in [59]). The engagement by gp120 of integrin $\alpha_4\beta_7$, the gut homing receptor, facilitates infection of $CD4^+$ T cells in the earliest stages of transmission [60]. HIV replicates intensively first in the GALT and then systemically in all lymphoid tissues, where it establishes stable viral reservoirs (in the form of latently infected resting $CD4^+$ T cells at the cellular level) that constitute major impediments to virus eradication [59]. The switch in coreceptor usage at the peak of viral diversity expands virus accessibility to circulating naïve $CD4^+$ T cells, thereby increasing viral burden and leading to rapid $CD4^+$ T cell depletion [61, 62]. The regenerative capacity of the immune system is also affected by the X4 emergence or predominance since chronic immune activation is then exacerbated. T cell homeostasis is disrupted, eventually leading to the collapse of the immune system [43].

4. The development of CCR5 inhibitors as anti-HIV therapeutics – Focus on small molecules

As discussed above, the first clues regarding the potential therapeutic utility of targeting CCR5 came from the observation of the naturally occurring blockade of the coreceptor due to the CCR5Δ32 polymorphism. Recently, the first successful allogeneic stem cell transplantation has been reported in an HIV-positive, acute myeloid leukemia patient from Berlin with a *CCR5Δ32* homozygous donor [63]. Investigators claimed to have "cured" this HIV-infected patient as indicated by the functional reconstitution of his T cell immunity without any signs of viral rebound after the discontinuation of ART [64]. The long-term effects of stem cell transplantation remain nevertheless unknown. Even though it would obviously be impractical to follow such a therapeutic approach in the millions of HIV-infected subjects worldwide, the proof-of-principle case of "the Berlin patient" demonstrates that a functional cure, i.e. a permanent suppression of viral replication in the absence of ART, may be within reach, under certain circumstances, at present; a true sterilizing cure with complete eradication of the virus continues to be the ultimate goal of therapy [6].

Towards this goal, there has been hope that CCR5 inhibitors will make an impact on controlling the epidemic by enhancing our therapeutic arsenal against HIV.

It should be noted, however, that the development of these host-targeting agents raises additional safety concerns that lie beyond the typical pharmacological concerns associated with the development of any antiretroviral drug, such as efficacy, safety and tolerability, bioavailability, drug-drug interactions, and the emergence of escape mutants (reviewed in [22, 65]). These safety concerns stem from the disruption of the physiological functions of the coreceptor as well as from the potential escape of R5 viruses by switching coreceptor use to CXCR4, or the breakthrough of X4 viruses following the suppression of R5 strains [22, 65]. The latter virological concern will be discussed in the next section on the generation of resistance to CCR5 inhibitors. The absence of any apparent immunological deficits of significance among individuals with naturally occurring loss-of-function mutations (i.e., *CCR5Δ32* homozygotes) provides some reassurance that pharmacological blockade of CCR5 will be relatively benign [66]. Redundancy in the chemokine network presumably allows other chemokine receptors to subsume the function of CCR5 [67]. However, the abrupt pharmacological blockade of a receptor in mature individuals may have different consequences than the congenital absence of the receptor where the immune system has had years to adapt to its loss [22, 67]. Corroborating the results of previous studies in mice (reviewed in [67]), studies in humans have shown that *CCR5Δ32* heterozygotes have a six-fold increased risk for severe West Nile virus (WNV) infection and a five-fold increased risk of mortality [68]. A meta-analysis of the four patient cohorts in the United States confirmed that CCR5 deficiency is a strong and consistent risk factor for symptomatic WNV infection [69]. An additional association between the lack of functional CCR5 due to the CCR5Δ32 deletion and tick-borne encephalitis has also been reported [70]. Overall, however, currently available data suggest that pharmacological blockade of CCR5 is likely to be largely well tolerated; stringent safety studies will nevertheless be required to monitor the long-term safety of CCR5 blockade, with particular attention paid to the consequences of infection by certain pathogens, effects on responses to immunization, and the emergence of opportunistic infections and malignancies [22, 65].

Several different approaches have been undertaken to pharmaceutically target CCR5, including the use of chemokine analogues, anti-CCR5 antibodies, gene knockdown and knockout strategies, and small molecule coreceptor inhibitors. The development of coreceptor inhibitors for use in prevention, including topical microbicides, is discussed elsewhere [22, 67].

4.1. Chemokine analogues

Chemokine analogues engineered to enhance their natural anti-HIV properties were the first generation of CCR5 inhibitors (reviewed in [22, 71, 72]). RANTES, an N-terminally truncated variant of RANTES/CCL5 was the first such engineered analogue, but it was found to exhibit only modest anti-HIV activity. Its identification nonetheless helped establish the concept that the agonist activity on coreceptors is not a component of the anti-

HIV mechanism of native chemokines. Further N-terminal modifications led to the generation of chemokine analogues such as AOP-RANTES [73] and PSC-RANTES [74], which have improved potency due to their mechanism of action; they induce receptor sequestration that results in the internalization and physical removal of the coreceptor from the cell surface, effects that are more profound and prolonged compared to those of native chemokines [22]. The clinical development of chemokine analogues as anti-HIV therapeutics is complicated by the fact that as proteins, chemokines would not be expected to be orally bioavailable and their production costs would be prohibitively high; moreover, chemokine analogues are unlikely to show suitable pharmacokinetics after injection because they readily bind to and form aggregates on cell surface proteoglycans [22]. The potential adverse effects due to the possible inflammatory activity mediated through CCR5 activation is another concern associated with their use.

4.2. Anti-CCR5 antibodies

Most anti-CCR5 monoclonal antibodies (MAbs) have been described as chemokine antagonists that inhibit the receptor via steric blockade (reviewed in [22]). Many rodent anti-CCR5 MAbs with anti-HIV activity have been identified and extensively characterized. PRO 140 (Progenics pharmaceuticals) is a humanized monoclonal antibody, currently available only for parenteral administration; PRO 140 received fast-track approval by the FDA. The efficacy, tolerability and toxicity profiles of PRO 140 have been assessed by several preclinical and clinical studies, which showed promising results (reviewed in [75]). Of note is the evidence of activity shown by PRO 140 against escape mutants with cross-class resistance to small molecule CCR5 inhibitors [76]; however, as a complex biological molecule requiring parenteral administration, PRO 140 faces a different set of development challenges compared to the orally bioavailable small molecule compounds [77]. Human CCR5mAb004 antibody also performed well in early clinical trials [22]. Currently available data further suggest that anti-CCR5 MAbs act synergistically with other CCR5 inhibitors and have different resistance profiles. Their typically long circulatory half-lives do not necessitate frequent dosing, suggesting that the lack of oral bioavailability may not be a serious limitation in their development as anti-HIV drugs.

4.3. Gene knockdown and knockout strategies

CCR5 expression in HIV-1 target cells can be suppressed by RNA-based gene modulation technologies such as RNA interference (RNAi), or completely eliminated by such techniques as zinc finger nuclease (ZFN)-mediated gene disruption. RNAi refers to the sequence-specific degradation of messenger RNA (mRNA) that follows the cellular introduction of homologous, short-interfering RNA (siRNA), a technique that has emerged as a powerful tool to probe the function of genes of known sequence *in vitro* and *in vivo* [78, 79]. RNAi has been shown to decrease the replication of HIV-1 in lymphocytic cells using siRNA targeting both viral (e.g., Tat, Gag and Rev) and host proteins, including CD4 and CCR5 (reviewed in [80]). The numerous challenges associated with converting RNAi from a laboratory technique to an anti-HIV therapeutic have been reviewed elsewhere [22]. Recent advances in the development of RNAi-based therapeutics for HIV-1 are presented by Zhou and Rossi [81]. Zinc-finger nucleases (ZFNs) are artificial restriction enzymes engineered by fusing a zinc finger DNA-binding domain to a DNA-cleavage domain; the generated double-stranded DNA break is repaired by the endogenous DNA repair machinery of the cell, potentially leading to the permanent disruption of the gene's open reading frame [82]. CCR5 gene knockout in T cells or hematopoietic stem/progenitor cells (HSC) by ZFNs effectively suppresses the replication of CCR5-tropic strains of HIV-1 in animal models (reviewed in [83]). ZFNs are currently being evaluated in a phase I clinical trials using *ex vivo* expanded T cells; HSC targeted therapies are under development as well.

4.4. Small molecule CCR5 inhibitors

Small molecule CCR5 inhibitors (Table 1) prevent HIV-1 from entering its target cells, mainly $CD4^+$ T cells and macrophages, by blocking the CD4-dependent binding of the viral surface envelope glycoprotein (gp120) to the most commonly used coreceptor CCR5 (reviewed in [22, 67, 72, 77]).

The identification of the first such molecule, TAK-779, in 1999 [84] was followed by several reports on additional CCR5 inhibitors with improved potency and more favorable pharmacological properties (Table 1). The development of these compounds has been principally pursued for the treatment of HIV-1 infection, although, theoretically, they could also be used as preventive agents [98]. Maraviroc (MVC, Selzentry; Pfizer, Inc., Figure 2A) was the first, and so far only, small molecule CCR5 inhibitor to be approved for treating HIV-1 infection by the US FDA and by the European Agency for the Evaluation of Medicinal Products (reviewed in [99]). MVC is licensed for administration in both treatment-naïve (i.e., yet to receive any ART) and in treatment-experienced patients with R5 HIV-1. Other investigational compounds have also entered clinical trials, but a number of them were discontinued due to observed side effects (Table 1). The development of Vicriviroc (VCV, Schering-Plough Research Institute; now Merck Research Laboratories, Figure 2B) was abandoned because it did not meet primary efficacy endpoints in late stage (Phase III in treatment-experienced subjects and Phase II in treatment-naïve individuals) clinical trials. Additional compounds are in preclinical or clinical development (reviewed in [77]). Previously designated as TBR-652 or TAK-652 (Figure 2C), cenicriviroc is a small-molecule CCR5 antagonist licensed by the Takeda Pharmaceutical Company to Tobira Pharmaceuticals; cenicriviroc has pharmacokinetic data supportive of once daily dosing and a favorable tolerability profile in single-dose studies in healthy volunteers. PF-232798 (Figure 2D), a second-generation small-molecule oral CCR5 antagonist with potency similar to MVC and the potential for once daily dosing, has demonstrated activity against a laboratory-generated MVC-resistant R5 virus. INCB9471 (Incyte, Wilmington, DE, USA) is yet another small-molecule oral CCR5 inhibitor that showed promising results in a Phase IIa trial in treatment-naïve and treatment-experienced patients with once daily dosing over 14 days [77].

Drug	Other names	Key features	Manufacturer	Current status	References
TAK-779	N/A	(Nonpeptidic) quaternary ammonium anilide that prevents gp120 and CC-chemokines, but not anti-CCR5 MAbs, from binding to CCR5	Takeda	Preclinical only	[84]
Cenicriviroc	TBR-652, TAK-652	Orally bioavailable, improved potency TAK-779-derivative; also blocks CCR2	Takeda; now Tobira	Phase II completed	[85, 86]
AD101	SCH-350581	Piperidino-piperazine-based compound structurally related to, but more potent than SCH-C; also blocks MAbs mainly against the ECL2 of CCR5	Schering-Plough	Preclinical only	[87, 88]
SCH-C	SCH-351125	Oximino-piperidino-piperidine amide that also blocks MAbs mainly against the ECL2 of CCR5; unable to exert its antiviral effects when residue 198 in TM helix 5 of CCR5 is methionine (Met) as in rhesus macaques [89]	Schering-Plough	Discont-inued; hERG K^+ channel blockade & CNS side effects	[90-92]
Vicriviroc (VCV)	SCH-D, SCH-417690, VVC	Piperazino-piperidine-based compound; improved potency & pharmacokinetics, reduced tendency for hERG channel blockade compared to SCH-C	Schering-Plough; now Merck	Discont-inued from Phase III; primary efficacy points unmet	[93, 94]
Aplaviroc (AVC)	AK602/ONO4128/873140, GW873140, APL	Spirodiketopiperazine-based compound; it preserves RANTES and MIP-1β binding to $CCR5^+$ cells and their functions	Glaxo SmithKline	Discont-inued from Phase IIb/III; idiosyncratic hepatotoxicity	[95]
Maraviroc (MVC, Selzentry)	UK-427,857	Spirodiketopiperazine with favorable pharmacological properties	Pfizer	Approved for clinical use	[96, 97]

hERG K^+, human ether-a-go-go related gene potassium channel; **MAb**, monoclonal antibody; **N/A**, not applicable.

Table 1. Nomenclature, characteristics, and developmental status of selected small molecule CCR5 inhibitors

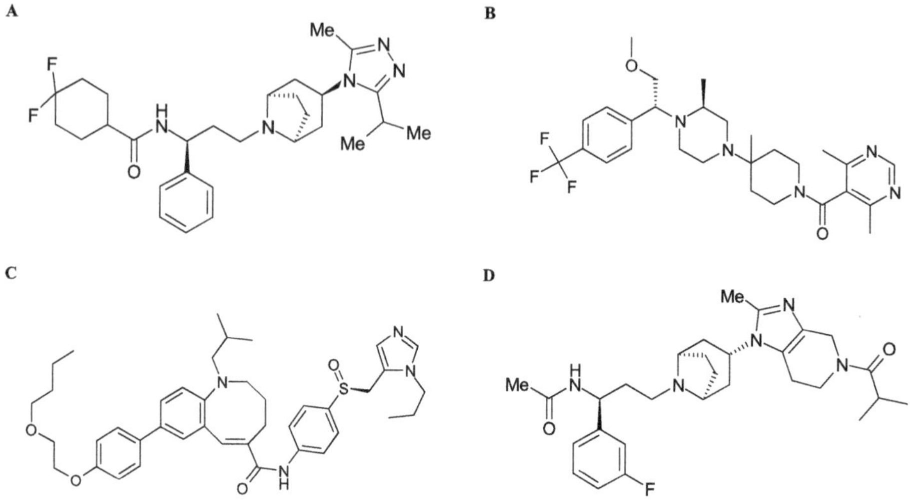

Figure 2. Chemical structures of selected small molecule CCR5 inhibitors. A. Maraviroc (MVC, Selzentry), B. Vicriviroc (VCV), C. Cenicriviroc (TBR-652), D. PF-232798.

Binding site. The binding site of small molecule CCR5 inhibitors does not overlap with the binding site for HIV gp120. In the absence of a high-resolution structure of a gp120-coreceptor complex, biochemical studies of CCR5 have revealed the importance of its N-terminus (Nt) and second extracellular loop (ECL2) in binding gp120 and mediating viral entry (reviewed in [34]). Small molecule CCR5 inhibitors, on the other hand, are believed to bind within a cavity between the transmembrane (TM) helices on the extracellular surface of the coreceptor, as suggested by site-directed mutagenesis experiments and molecular modeling of CCR5 on the basis of the available crystal structure of bovine rhodopsin that is characterized by a similar TM topology [100, 101]. More specifically, the binding "pocket" of such molecules as TAK-779, AD101, and SCH-C is thought to be located between TM helices 1-3, and 7; other TM helices, particularly helix 6, contribute to some compound-specific variations [102, 103]. Simultaneous administration of multiple antagonists showed that, indeed, they bind to a common site on CCR5 [104]. A key set of aromatic and aliphatic residues that serve as a hydrophobic core for this ligand binding pocket has also been identified, while a glutamic acid (Glu) in helix 7, E283, appears to be critical for high affinity interaction; this residue probably acts as the counterion for a positively charged nitrogen atom common to TAK-779, AD101, and SCH-C [105].

The binding of all small molecule CCR5 antagonists to a broadly similar site within the TM helices of the coreceptor renders cross-resistance within this drug class possible, but not necessarily inevitable since compound-specific variations with respect to properties such as structure, shape, and electrostatic potential, do exist [106]; hence, despite the insensitivity of AD101 escape mutants to all other tested CCR5 inhibitors, including SCH-C, aplaviroc (AVC), MVC and VCV [107-109], a MVC-resistant variant has been reported to retain its sensitivity to SCH-C and AVC [110]. Susceptibility to other classes of licensed drugs that target different stages of the viral life cycle, or even different steps of the same stage of the viral life cycle such as viral entry, should be maintained. Accordingly, clinical resistance to Enfuvirtide (ENF, Fuzeon/T-20) was not found to affect viral sensitivity to the fusion inhibitor T-1249 or to coreceptor inhibitors [111].

Mechanism of action. Small molecule (molecular weight 500-600 D) CCR5 inhibitors act via a similar, allosteric (from the Greek "*allos*"+"*stereos*" meaning "other"+"shape," respectively) mechanism; in other words, they induce or stabilize a conformation of the coreceptor that renders it unrecognizable by the wild-type virus. The results of recent biochemical studies support the noncompetitive and allosteric nature of the mechanism of action of small molecule antagonists of CCR5 [104]. The difference in binding sites between the two ligands also supports the allosteric modulation of the HIV-1 gp120 binding site by this class of drugs; as mentioned above, CCR5 inhibitors bind within the TM helices in the extracellular facet of the coreceptor, whereas HIV gp120 targets the extracellular domains of CCR5 and, more specifically, the negatively-charged Tyr-sulfated amino terminus (Nt) and the ECL2 between TM helices 4 and 5 [103].

Moreover, the action of some CCR5 inhibitors may be blocked by the introduction of certain mutations into CCR5 despite the binding of the inhibitor to the coreceptor; namely, the antiviral effects of SCH-C are blocked, although its antagonism of the signaling by RANTES/CCL5 persists, when residue 198 in the TM helix 5 of CCR5 is methionine (Met) as in rhesus macaques [89]. This observation led to the hypothesis that the I198M substitution may be involved in the induction of a CCR5 conformation that is incompatible with HIV-1 infection. It should be noted, however, that not all CCR5 inhibitors are modulated in the same manner by this amino acid change. I198M has been shown not to block the antiviral effects of AD101, whereas another mutation, F113A, may block the inhibitory action of AD101, but not of SCH-C, via a similar mechanism [89]. Further subtle differences exist in the stabilized or induced conformations by the binding of these small molecules to the TM pocket of CCR5 and, therefore, in the mechanism of action of these compounds. For instance, although most CCR5 inhibitors antagonize potently the three natural ligands of the coreceptor, AVC only antagonizes MIP-1α/CCL3 efficiently and much less potently the other two ligands (MIP-1β/CCL4, and RANTES/CCL5) [95].

Displacement binding assays and dissociation kinetics demonstrated that TAK779 and MVC inhibit CCL3 and gp120 binding to CCR5 by a noncompetitive and allosteric mechanism, supporting the view that these compounds bind to regions of CCR5 distinct from the gp120- and CCL3-binding sites [112]. MVC is predicted to insert deeply in the CCR5 TM cavity where it can occupy three different binding sites, whereas CCL3 and gp120 lie on distinct, yet overlapped regions of the CCR5 ECL2 [113]. TAK779 and MVC were found to be full and weak inverse agonists for CCR5, respectively, indicating that they stabilize distinct CCR5 conformations with impaired abilities to activate G-proteins [112]. The finding that the TM cavity remains accessible for MVC in CCL3-bound and gp120-bound CCR5 [113], provides an explanation for the enhancement by TAK779 and MVC of the dissociation of preformed ligand-CCR5 complexes with an efficiency that correlates with their ability to act as inverse agonists [112]. The identification of residues mandatory for gp120 binding in the predicted CCR5 dimer interface suggests that receptor dimerization might represent a target for new CCR5 entry inhibitors [113].

AK530 and AK317, two CCR5 inhibitors containing spirodiketopiperazine scaffolds, lodge in a hydrophobic cavity located between the upper TM domain and the ECL2 of CCR5 [114]. The interaction profile of the inhibitors with ECL2 residues S180 and K191 was found to be an important determinant of antiviral potency; furthermore, amino acid residues in the beta-hairpin structural motif of ECL2 were critical for HIV-1-elicited fusion and binding of these spirodiketopiperazine-based inhibitors to CCR5. The direct ECL2-engaging property of the inhibitors likely produces an ECL2 conformation, which HIV-1 gp120 cannot bind to, but it also prohibits the virus from utilizing the "inhibitor-bound" CCR5 for cellular entry - a mechanism of HIV-1's resistance to CCR5 inhibitors, as discussed in the next section.

5. Generation of resistance to small molecule CCR5 inhibitors

The most parsimonious escape pathway from the selection pressure of a CCR5 inhibitor would be coreceptor switching to CXCR4 use, with its well documented devastating consequences on the rate of $CD4^+$ T cell depletion and disease progression of patients [22, 53, 67]. Both *in vitro* and *in vivo* studies have nevertheless shown that this is not the preferred escape pathway by HIV-1 despite the short distance in sequence space (few mutations) that separate R5 from X4 variants. The reduced replication fitness or the suboptimal coreceptor use, as indicated by the increased sensitivity to the selecting CCR5 antagonist of viral intermediates in the R5 to X4 evolution process compared to baseline virus, may account for this apparently paradoxical phenomenon; the requirements of inserting charged amino acids at specific locations and the strong bias in favor of G-to-A substitutions rather than random mutations are thought to impose additional constraints on the transition [115, 116]. Whatever the reasons may be, when R5 viruses escape from the selection pressure of CCR5 inhibitors they tend to retain the R5 phenotype.

Several factors diversify the pathways of resistance development to CCR5 inhibitors compared to those to conventional antiretroviral drugs [22]. The seemingly facile, for HIV, escape pathway of mutating the active site of a viral enzyme in order to prevent the binding of an antiviral would simply not work in the case of CCR5 antagonists that target a host- rather than a virus-encoded gene. Instead, the virus must devise a strategy to recognize and use the coreceptor to gain access into its target cells despite the presence of the inhibitor. The highly variable nature of the *env* gene certainly facilitates the escape process; however, *env* is also under the constant selection pressure from neutralizing antibodies [34]. Thus, during the development of resistance to CCR5 inhibitors the HIV-1 Env complex must accommodate sequence changes that enable the virus to escape both from the selection pressure of the inhibitors as well as from the humoral immune response, without violating the structural constraints of the Env protein.

5.1. *In vitro* resistance: No coreceptor switch to CXCR4 and no uniform genotypic signature

To gain insights into what may happen *in vivo* if or when small molecule CCR5 inhibitors are used more extensively, resistance is first studied *in vitro*. To generate resistant variants, primary R5 isolates are cultured with physiological target cells that are permissive for replication of both R5 and X4 viruses in the presence of increasing concentrations of the inhibitor under study. Despite the intrinsic difficulty associated with the selection process in each case that proved to require prolonged periods of culture in the presence of these compounds, several such studies have been published (reviewed in [22, 72, 117]). An alternative *in vitro* system that allows for the selection of escape mutants to CCR5 inhibitors over a relatively short period of time is the construction of V3 loop libraries of R5 infectious clones (reviewed in [118]). The results of these studies collectively show that the escape mutants tend to retain usage of CCR5 despite the availability of CXCR4. The mechanism that allows resistant viruses to continue to use CCR5 in the presence of the inhibitor is discussed in the next section. X4 viruses have been observed in CCR5 inhibitor-selection experiments, either in the control culture alone [119] or in both the selection and the control cultures [110], but their emergence was probably due to adaptation to growth in culture rather than the inhibitor escape process. Conditional recognition of CXCR4 in specific cell lines has also been reported for one VCV-resistant virus [109]. HIV-1 can be "forced" to escape CCR5 drug pressure through coreceptor switch under certain experimental conditions, which may not be very relevant physiologically [120].

To date, no clear signature resistance mutations have been identified for CCR5 antagonists and different genetic pathways can lead to the same resistance phenotype (Table 2).

The determinants of resistance commonly map to the V3 region of gp120, a localization that is consistent with the highly variable nature of this region as well as with its role in coreceptor engagement [22, 45]. Four V3 substitutions (K305R, H308P, A316V and G321E) were, for example, responsible for the resistant phenotype of isolate CC101.19 when the CCR5-using, subtype B virus CC1/85 [62] was cultured with the small molecule CCR5 inhibitor AD101, a preclinical precursor of VCV [107, 108]. A much rarer route to resistance was undertaken by viruses derived from the same CC1/85 lineage in an AD101/VCV selection culture [109]; the resulting D101.12 escape mutants contained at least one substitution in V3 (H308P) as well as either of the following combinations of substitutions within and downstream of the gp41 fusion peptide (FP): G514V+V535M (Pattern I) or M518V+F519L+V535M (Pattern II) [127]. We have also described a unique VCV escape pathway for viruses from the D1/85.16 lineage that involved no V3 changes; instead, resistance mapped to three conservative substitutions in the FP: G516V, M518V and F519I [126]. As shown recently [131], the G516V change is critical to VCV resistance, although it must be accompanied by either M518V or F519I to have a substantial impact phenotypically. Nevertheless, introducing the three FP changes together into a heterologous virus, JR-FL, did not create a VCV-resistant variant [126]. CCR5 inhibitor resistance is usually dependent upon the Env genetic context and it is not transferred when introduced into other viruses [124, 126, 132], but that is not always the case [129].

Drug	Parental virus: Name	Parental virus: Subtype	Resistance mutations: gp120: V3	Resistance mutations: gp120: Elsewhere	Resistance mutations: gp41	References
TAK-779	JR-FLV3Lib	B	I304V, H305N, I306M, F312L, E317D	None	None	[121]
TAK-652	KK	Unknown	ND	ND	ND	[119]
AD101	CC1/85	B	K305R, H308P, A316V, G321E	None	None	[107, 108]
VCV	Clinical isolate	C	K305R, T307I, F316I, T318R, G319E and S306P	None	None	[122]
VCV	Clinical isolate S91	D	Q315E, R321G	E328K, G429R (C4)	None	[123]
VCV	RU570	G	K305R, R315Q, K319T	P437S (C4)	None	[124, 125]
VCV	CC1/85	B	None	None	G516V, M518V, F519I	[109, 126]
VCV	CC101.6 (CC1/85 passage 6 AD101 selection)	B	H308P and one or more of: K305R, A316V, G321E	None	G514V, V535M (Pattern I) or M518V, F519L, V535M (Pattern II)	[109, 127]
AVC	Clinical isolates	Unknown	Several	Several	Several	[128]
MVC	Clinical isolate	B	P/T308H, T320H, I322aV	D407G, ΔN386 (V4)	None	[129]
MVC	CC1/85	B	A316T, I323V	ND	ND	[110]
MVC	RU570	G	ΔQAI (315-317)	ND	ND	[110]
MVC	JR-FLV3Lib	B	I304V, F312W, T314A, E317D, I318V	T199K, T275M (C2)	None	[130]

ND, Not determined; **I322aV** occurs at an amino acid not present in HXB2 located between residues 322 and 323 and is designated 322a.

Table 2. Genetics of HIV-1 escape from the selection pressure of small molecule CCR5 inhibitors

The findings of these studies have important implications for the clinical use of small molecule inhibitors, particularly for the generation of genotypic algorithms and phenotypic assays to predict the emergence of resistant viruses and the likelihood of cross-resistance to other members of this drug class. Cross-resistance to other CCR5 antagonists may or may not arise with these molecules that retain sensitivity to all other drug classes (e.g. nucleoside and non-nucleoside reverse transcriptase inhibitors, protease and integrase inhibitors) as well as to other entry inhibitors acting at different stages of the entry process (e.g. the fusion inhibitor enfuvirtide) [117]. Small molecule CCR5 inhibitors also retain sensitivity to anti-CCR5 MAbs that act by a dissimilar mechanism.

Viral fitness. When HIV-1 develops resistance to conventional antiretroviral drugs such as reverse transcriptase or protease inhibitors, its fitness is often impaired. To investigate whether the *in vitro* development of resistance to small molecule CCR5 inhibitors has an associated fitness cost, we developed a growth-competition assay involving dual infections with molecularly cloned viruses that are essentially isogenic outside the *env* genes under study. Real-time TaqMan quantitative PCR (QPCR) was used to quantify each competing virus individually via probes specific to different, phenotypically silent target sequences engineered within their *vif* genes. Head-to-head competition assays of *env* clones derived from the AD101 and VCV resistant isolate, the inhibitor-sensitive parental virus, and a passage control virus showed that CCR5 inhibitor resistance was not associated with a fitness loss [133]. This observation is consistent with the retention of the resistant phenotype when the escape mutant virus CC101.19 was cultured for a total of 20 passages in the absence of the selecting compound [133]. Amino acid substitutions in the V3 region of gp120 that confer complete resistance cause a fitness loss when introduced into an inhibitor-sensitive, parental clone; however, in the resistant isolate, changes elsewhere in *env* that occurred prior to the substitutions within V3, appear to compensate for the adverse effect of the V3 changes on replicative capacity. Hence, a decrease in fitness resulting from CCR5 inhibitor resistance may not be as common as with the fitness loss observed with resistance to almost all other antiretroviral drugs (reviewed in [72]).

The *in vivo* situation may differ, but further studies are needed to explore the fitness impact of HIV-1 with acquired resistance to CCR5 antagonists. In one case, pre-treatment V3 sequences reemerged in a subtype C-infected patient following VCV discontinuation, implying that VCV resistance has associated fitness costs [122]. Nonetheless, all the VCV-resistant isolates we have studied (CC101.19, D101.12 and D1/85.16) have highly stable phenotypes in peripheral blood mononuclear cells (PBMC), in that they do not rapidly revert to sensitivity when cultured without the inhibitor [108, 126, 127, 133]. During reversion experiments of individual resistant clones in the absence of the inhibitor, we discovered that M518V, which has little or no effect on VCV sensitivity on its own, appears to be under no pressure to revert either [131]. Val-518 is a naturally occurring FP polymorphism that becomes enriched during VCV or AD101 selection [126]. However, a resistant clone D1/85.16 cl.23 (= R) reverted to a sensitive phenotype by five weekly, VCV-free passages in PBMC culture. Interestingly, the complete cluster of the three FP changes persisted within the genetic context of the gp120 derived from the resistant clone R; however, the three FP changes were accompanied by a Thr-to-Ala substitution at position 244 of the second conserved region (C2) of gp120 that appears to counter the VCV-resistance phenotype created by the FP substitutions. This residue is located in strand β7, part of a β-sandwich structure in the inner domain that is involved in CD4-induced conformational changes within gp120 and the interaction with gp41 [134-137]. Examining the interplay of these changes will enhance our understanding of Env complex interactions that influence both HIV-1 entry and resistance to CCR5 inhibitors.

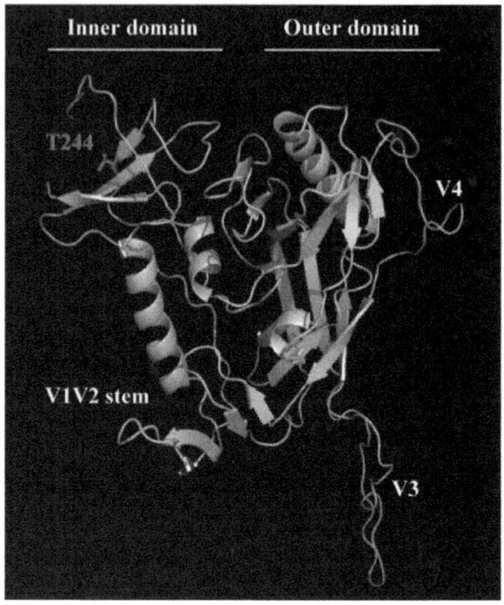

Figure 3. Mapping residue 244 on the structure of the gp120 of the representative clone, CC1/85 cl.7, of the parental, inhibitor-sensitive virus CC1/85. Residue 244 (magenta) is located in strand β7, part of a β-sandwich structure in the inner domain of gp120 that is thought to be involved in interactions with gp41. The CC1/85 cl.7 gp120 core structure was modeled based on the V3-containing structure of gp120 [138] with Swiss-Model [139] using 2B4C.pdb as template and visualized using PyMOL [140].

5.2. Mechanisms of resistance to small molecule CCR5 inhibitors

As portrayed graphically in Figure 4, resistance to small molecule CCR5 inhibitors may likely develop via two, not necessarily exclusive, mechanisms: competitive resistance and noncompetitive or allosteric resistance (reviewed in [22, 72, 117, 118, 141]), not to be confused with the competitive or not, properties of the inhibitors themselves [142]. Either mechanism may be effective at overcoming inhibition for some CCR5 inhibitors, while some HIV-1 escape mutants may undertake a combination of the two mechanisms. Understanding how resistance arises is relevant to how it is detected and quantified.

Competitive resistance. Competitive resistance (Figure 4A) is defined as resistance that results in a shift in the IC_{50} of an inhibitor to a higher concentration; complete inhibition can still be achieved at sufficient inhibitor concentrations [142]. Competitive resistance could arise from more efficient utilization of inhibitor-free CCR5 to gain access into target cells; in turn, this could arise either from a greater affinity of Env for the coreceptor, or from an increase in the kinetics of Env-mediated fusion after CCR5 engagement. Either scenario would allow the virus to better compete with the inhibitor for the coreceptor, reflecting its adaptation to scavenge low levels of inhibitor-free CCR5 [142]. A partially (~5-fold) AD101-resistant isolate had this ability [108]; however, this mechanism alone cannot count for complete resistance to CCR5 antagonists [117].

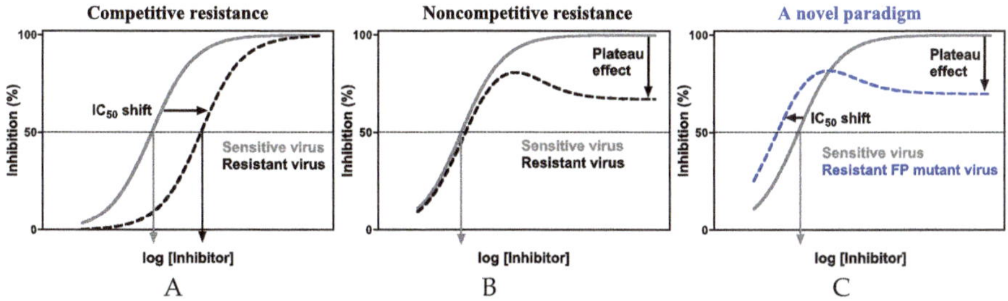

Figure 4. Resistance mechanisms for viral escape from CCR5 inhibitors. Model inhibition curves are displayed for sensitive and resistant viruses (solid grey and dashed black curves, respectively). The atypical dose-response curves of resistant viruses with gp41 fusion peptide (FP) mutations are shown in blue. **A.** Competitive resistance results in a shift in the IC_{50} of an inhibitor to a higher concentration, with complete inhibition potentially achievable at a high enough inhibitor concentration. **B.** In noncompetitive resistance, the IC_{50} values are typically equivalent to those for the sensitive virus, but the extent of inhibition is incomplete for the resistant virus. The maximum percent inhibition (MPI) value, at a saturating inhibitor concentration, reflects the efficiency with which the inhibitor-CCR5 complex is used relative to free CCR5, thereby providing a measure of the degree of resistance of the HIV-1 variant under study. MPI values vary by cell type for inhibition by VCV and related compounds. **C.** In the novel paradigm of noncompetitive resistance, resistant FP mutant viruses display reduced MPI and IC_{50} values. Adapted from [143].

Noncompetitive or "allosteric" resistance. Noncompetitive resistance (Figure 4B) is defined as resistance that results in saturable inhibition, such that increasing concentrations of the inhibitor have no effect on the virus; the EC_{50} required to reach this saturation level is the same as the IC_{50} for the fully sensitive virus [142]. Phenotypically, resistance manifests as a plateau in the maximum achievable suppression of viral replication. The implication of this mechanism is that the resistant Env has adapted to use the inhibitor bound form of CCR5 as a coreceptor as well as, but not instead of, the free coreceptor [110, 142]. The level of residual inhibition, termed the "plateau" or the maximum percent inhibition (MPI), once inhibition has reached saturation reflects the efficiency with which the inhibitor-CCR5 complex is used relative to free CCR5; the higher the MPI value, the less efficiently a resistant virus uses the inhibitor-CCR5 complex [110, 142]. This mechanism is consistent with the allosteric mode of action of small molecule CCR5 inhibitors; these compounds lock the extracellular domains of CCR5 in a conformation that can be recognized only by resistant variants -in addition to the natural coreceptor-, but not by wild-type HIV-1 [117]. In a few instances, the preferred use of the inhibitor-bound CCR5 over the unbound receptor by some CCR5 antagonist-resistant viruses leads to modestly increased replication of resistant viruses in the presence of the inhibitor *in vitro* [142]. The cell type influences the mode in which resistance to small molecule CCR5 inhibitors is manifested, particularly MPI values [110, 124, 126, 127, 131, 142]. Moreover, the differences between the MPI values of VCV-resistant and sensitive viruses we have studied are generally much smaller in cell lines engineered to express CCR5, such as TZM-bl or U87.CD4.CCR5 (that serves as the basis of the PhenoSense and Trofile tropism assays), than in PBMC [126, 127, 131].

Resistant FP mutants: A novel paradigm of noncompetitive resistance. The VCV-resistant viruses carrying FP changes represent a novel paradigm of noncompetitive resistance (Figure 4C); apart from the plateau effect, these FP mutants paradoxically have lower IC_{50} values than wild-type viruses, particularly in certain cell types (e.g. TZM-bl cells). Hence, although by one measure (MPI) the FP-mutant viruses display a modest level of resistance, by another (IC_{50}) they appear to be hypersensitive [126, 127, 131]. To explain this paradox, we created a theoretical model of resistance [126]. The mathematical formulation of the model is presented in detail in the Supporting Information (SI) section of [126]. The model is based on the assumption that distinct forms of CCR5, with varying affinities (ranging from low to high) for small molecule CCR5 inhibitors, are present in different proportions on disparate cell types; these coreceptor forms, which could be conformers (conformational isomers) or differentially Tyr-sulfated forms, are used selectively by resistant HIV-1 variants when ligated with an inhibitor. According to the model, wild-type virus can use both forms of unligated CCR5 for entry, possibly with a preference between them, but it cannot enter via the inhibitor-coreceptor complexes. The resistant virus, on the other hand, uses preferentially the unoccupied high-affinity coreceptor and the occupied low-affinity coreceptor. Applying this model led to the generation of theoretical inhibition curves that closely mimic the experimental data for resistant viruses in each case [126, 127, 131]. Using the model, we have recently identified the third FP mutation, F519I, (of the V3-independent or FP only- genetic pathway to resistance) as an independent determinant of preference for the unoccupied, high-VCV affinity form of CCR5 [131]. Modeling the inhibition data from two cell types, PBMC and TZM-bl cells, suggested that D101.12, which harbors both V3 and gp41 substitutions, discriminates between high- and low-affinity forms of CCR5 less than D1/85.16, the resistant virus with three FP substitutions [127].

Although derived from a common parent, CC1/85, two resistant viruses that we have described, CC101.19 and D1/85.16, followed different genetic pathways to reach the same phenotypic endpoint: CC101.19 acquired four substitutions (K305R, H308P, A316V and G321E) in the V3 region [107], while the key determinants of resistance in D1/85.16 were three changes in the gp41 FP (G516V, M518V and F519I) [126] (Table 2). Both resistant variants acquired the ability to use the VCV–CCR5 complex for entry [107, 108, 126, 142]. However, unlike a clone derived from CC101.19 (V3 mutations), the D1/85.16 cl.23 virus (FP mutations) did not have an increased dependency on the CCR5 Nt, and its CCR5 binding site was not obviously more exposed [144]. The FP-mutant was, however, atypically sensitive to a CCR5 MAb that stains discrete cell surface clusters of CCR5 that might correspond to lipid rafts [145]. The precise molecular mechanism by which the FP changes confer resistance remains to be determined.

The V3 changes that confer resistance to CCR5 inhibitors have been suggested to render the virus more dependent on the CCR5 Nt, to compensate for impaired interactions between the V3-crown and ECL2 [144]. Accordingly, substantial deletions in V3 from both HIV-1 and HIV-2 confer complete resistance to coreceptor antagonists, presumably by disrupting the interaction between V3 and ECL2 [146-150]. Any adverse effect the V3 sequence changes have at the CCR5-binding stage may be compensated for by increases in the affinity of resistant viruses for CD4 and/or in the kinetics of virus entry [147, 151]. The altered virus–

CCR5 interactions are nonetheless characterized by considerable complexity. Thus, a subtype D, VCV-resistant patient isolate recognizes the drug-bound form of CCR5 more efficiently but still uses both the Nt and ECL2 [123]. A recently proposed model suggests that broad cross-resistance to multiple inhibitors is associated with an increased dependence on the N-terminus, while a more specific pattern of resistance to individual compounds involves more subtle changes in how the virus interacts with both the Nt and ECL2 [129].

5.3. *In vivo* resistance: Potential expansion of pre-existing, CXCR4-using viruses

The limited information currently available from published results of clinical studies suggests that the escape process from small molecule CCR5 inhibitors *in vivo* bears similarities to that observed *in vitro*; clinical resistance is also likely to map to the V3 region of gp120, but the lack of consistency of observed mutations renders impossible the prediction of *in vivo* resistance by sequence analysis at present (reviewed in [72, 77, 117, 141]). As mentioned above, two pathways of virological escape from the selection pressure of CCR5 antagonists have been identified: continued use of CCR5 via selection of R5 virus that can use drug-bound CCR5 for entry in addition to free coreceptor and expansion of pre-existing minority populations of dual-tropic or X4 virus (collectively called "CXCR4-using" viruses). The first pathway of R5 virological failure with reduced susceptibility to CCR5 antagonists is not the most common mechanism of failure. Virologic failure most commonly involves expansion of pre-existing, CXCR4-using viruses that are insensitive to CCR5 inhibitors. This outcome underscores the importance of developing tropism assays with improved ability to detect minor or archived virus populations capable of using the CXCR4 coreceptor.

The Trofile assay has been the assay of choice for clinical trials of CCR5 inhibitors. However, the sensitivity of the original commercially available assay was compromised with respect to the detection of low abundance (minority) CXCR4-using variants. As a result, a number of subjects were misjudged to have R5 virus at screening, whereas they actually harbored Dual/Mixed (D/M) virus populations when they entered clinical trials of CCR5 inhibitors; these patients appeared to have a blunted virologic response and high rates of early virologic failure [152-154]. Application of an enhanced-sensitivity Trofile assay or "deep sequencing" and re-analysis of the data showed that virologic failure in a significant proportion of these patients stemmed from the expansion of pre-existing minority CXCR4-using variants that went undetected during the first round of testing [155-157]. Accurate determination of coreceptor usage is therefore necessary to optimize treatment strategies before the initiation of and during therapy with CCR5 inhibitors. Techniques such as deep V3 sequencing may be useful for identifying treatment-experienced individuals who could benefit from CCR5-antagonist-containing regimens [158]. Ongoing improvements in genotypic methodologies and algorithms may eventually render them a viable alternative to phenotypic assays, much like the genotypic resistance methods.

6. Conclusions and future directions

The identification of CCR5 as the principal HIV coreceptor for cellular entry over a decade ago combined with the observed effects of the CCR5Δ32 polymorphism (natural resistance to HIV infection in homozygotes and delayed disease progression in heterozygotes) in the absence of any overt pathology, sparked great interest in its pharmaceutical blockade. The orally bioavailable small molecule CCR5 inhibitors are perhaps the most promising drugs that have been developed to block CCR5. In 2007, Maraviroc (MVC) became the first member of this new class of antiretrovirals, which target host- rather than virus-encoded structures, to receive regulatory approval for clinical use in the treatment of HIV infection. The theoretical virological concern that use of CCR5 antagonists in therapy may accelerate the evolution towards the more pathogenic CXCR4-using viruses has not been observed in clinical studies to date. MVC and other CCR5 antagonists have the potential for use in a variety of other clinical situations, such as the prevention of HIV transmission, intensification of HIV treatment and prevention of rejection in organ transplantation (reviewed in [159]). Moreover, CCR5 antagonists may be used in combination with other entry inhibitors or with agents such as rapamycin which downregulates CCR5 receptors thus decreasing CCR5 density [159]. New drugs that promote CCR5 and CXCR4 internalization, independent of cellular signaling, might also provide clinical benefits with minimum side effects [13].

Abbreviations

AIDS	Acquired immunodeficiency syndrome
ART	Antiretroviral therapy
CCR5	C-C chemokine receptor type 5
CNS	Central nervous system
CXCR4	C-X-C chemokine receptor type 4
ECL2	Second extracellular loop
Env	Envelope glycoprotein
FP	Fusion peptide
GALT	Gut-associated lymphoid tissue
GPCRs	G protein-coupled receptors
HIV	Human immunodeficiency virus
MAb	Monoclonal antibody
MVC	Maraviroc
MIP-1α	Macrophage inflammatory protein-1-alpha
MIP-1β	Macrophage inflammatory protein-1-beta
Nt	Amino terminus
PBMC	Peripheral blood mononuclear cells
RANTES	Regulated on activation, normal T cell expressed and secreted
R5 HIV	CCR5-tropic HIV
R5X4 HIV	Dual-tropic HIV
RNAi	RNA interference
SDF-1	Stromal derived factor-1
SIV	Simian immunodeficiency virus
7-TM	Seven-transmembrane

VCV	Vicriviroc
V3	Variable loop 3
X4 HIV	CXCR4-tropic HIV
ZFNs	Zinc-finger nucleases

Author details

Cleo G. Anastassopoulou
Division of Genetics, Cell and Developmental Biology, Department of Biology, University of Patras, Patras, Greece

Acknowledgement

I thank Dr. Rogier Sanders for assistance with the preparation of Figure 3.

7. References

[1] Centers for Disease Control (CDC). Kaposi's sarcoma and Pneumocystis pneumonia among homosexual men--New York City and California. Morbidity and Mortality Weekly Report (MMWR) 1981; 30(25): 305-308.
[2] Barre-Sinoussi F, Chermann JC, Rey F, et al. Isolation of a T-lymphotropic retrovirus from a patient at risk for acquired immune deficiency syndrome (AIDS). Science 1983; 220(4599): 868-871.
[3] Gallo RC, Sarin PS, Gelmann EP, et al. Isolation of human T-cell leukemia virus in acquired immune deficiency syndrome (AIDS). Science 1983; 220(4599): 865-867.
[4] Anastassopoulou CG, Kostrikis LG. Global genetic variation of HIV-1 infection. Current HIV Research 2006; 4(3): 365-373.
[5] UNAIDS. UNAIDS World AIDS Day Report I 2011. 2011.
[6] Dieffenbach CW, Fauci AS. Thirty years of HIV and AIDS: future challenges and opportunities. Annals of Internal Medicine 2011; 154(11): 766-771.
[7] Dalgleish AG, Beverley PC, Clapham PR, Crawford DH, Greaves MF, Weiss RA. The CD4 (T4) antigen is an essential component of the receptor for the AIDS retrovirus. Nature 1984; 312(5996): 763-767.
[8] Klatzmann D, Champagne E, Chamaret S, et al. T-lymphocyte T4 molecule behaves as the receptor for human retrovirus LAV. Nature 1984; 312(5996): 767-768.
[9] Broder CC, Berger EA. Fusogenic selectivity of the envelope glycoprotein is a major determinant of human immunodeficiency virus type 1 tropism for CD4+ T-cell lines vs. primary macrophages. Proceedings of the National Academy of Sciences of the United States of America 1995; 92(19): 9004-9008.
[10] Feng Y, Broder CC, Kennedy PE, Berger EA. HIV-1 entry cofactor: functional cDNA cloning of a seven-transmembrane, G protein-coupled receptor. Science 1996; 272(5263): 872-877.

[11] Bleul CC, Farzan M, Choe H, et al. The lymphocyte chemoattractant SDF-1 is a ligand for LESTR/fusin and blocks HIV-1 entry. Nature 1996; 382(6594): 829-833.
[12] Oberlin E, Amara A, Bachelerie F, et al. The CXC chemokine SDF-1 is the ligand for LESTR/fusin and prevents infection by T-cell-line-adapted HIV-1. Nature 1996; 382(6594): 833-835.
[13] Alkhatib G. The biology of CCR5 and CXCR4. Current Opinion in HIV and AIDS 2009; 4(2): 96-103.
[14] Cocchi F, DeVico AL, Garzino-Demo A, Arya SK, Gallo RC, Lusso P. Identification of RANTES, MIP-1 alpha, and MIP-1 beta as the major HIV-suppressive factors produced by CD8+ T cells. Science 1995; 270(5243): 1811-1815.
[15] Alkhatib G, Combadiere C, Broder CC, et al. CC CKR5: a RANTES, MIP-1alpha, MIP-1beta receptor as a fusion cofactor for macrophage-tropic HIV-1. Science 1996; 272(5270): 1955-1958.
[16] Choe H, Farzan M, Sun Y, et al. The beta-chemokine receptors CCR3 and CCR5 facilitate infection by primary HIV-1 isolates. Cell 1996; 85(7): 1135-1148.
[17] Deng H, Liu R, Ellmeier W, et al. Identification of a major co-receptor for primary isolates of HIV-1. Nature 1996; 381(6584): 661-666.
[18] Doranz BJ, Rucker J, Yi Y, et al. A dual-tropic primary HIV-1 isolate that uses fusin and the beta-chemokine receptors CKR-5, CKR-3, and CKR-2b as fusion cofactors. Cell 1996; 85(7): 1149-1158.
[19] Dragic T, Litwin V, Allaway GP, et al. HIV-1 entry into CD4+ cells is mediated by the chemokine receptor CC-CKR-5. Nature 1996; 381(6584): 667-673.
[20] Moore JP, Kitchen SG, Pugach P, Zack JA. The CCR5 and CXCR4 coreceptors--central to understanding the transmission and pathogenesis of human immunodeficiency virus type 1 infection. AIDS Research and Human Retroviruses 2004; 20(1): 111-126.
[21] Berger EA, Murphy PM, Farber JM. Chemokine receptors as HIV-1 coreceptors: roles in viral entry, tropism, and disease. Annual Review of Immunology 1999; 17: 657-700.
[22] Kuhmann SE, Hartley O. Targeting chemokine receptors in HIV: a status report. Annual Review of Pharmacology and Toxicology 2008; 48: 425-461.
[23] Allen SJ, Crown SE, Handel TM. Chemokine: receptor structure, interactions, and antagonism. Annual Review of Immunology 2007; 25: 787-820.
[24] Choi WT, An J. Biology and clinical relevance of chemokines and chemokine receptors CXCR4 and CCR5 in human diseases. Experimental Biology and Medicine 2011; 236(6): 637-647.
[25] Pollakis G, Paxton WA. HIV-1 (co)receptors: implications for vaccine and therapy design. Current Pharmaceutical Design 2010; 16(33): 3701-3715.
[26] Schlyer S, Horuk R. I want a new drug: G-protein-coupled receptors in drug development. Drug Discovery Today 2006; 11(11-12): 481-493.
[27] Marchese A, Paing MM, Temple BR, Trejo J. G protein-coupled receptor sorting to endosomes and lysosomes. Annual Review of Pharmacology and Toxicology 2008; 48: 601-629.

[28] Viola A, Luster AD. Chemokines and their receptors: drug targets in immunity and inflammation. Annual Review of Pharmacology and Toxicology 2008; 48: 171-197.

[29] Lederman MM, Penn-Nicholson A, Cho M, Mosier D. Biology of CCR5 and its role in HIV infection and treatment. Journal of the American Medical Association 2006; 296(7): 815-826.

[30] Oppermann M. Chemokine receptor CCR5: insights into structure, function, and regulation. Cellular Signalling 2004; 16(11): 1201-1210.

[31] Anastassopoulou CG, Kostrikis LG. The impact of human allelic variation on HIV-1 disease. Current HIV Research 2003; 1(2): 185-203.

[32] Steen A, Schwartz TW, Rosenkilde MM. Targeting CXCR4 in HIV cell-entry inhibition. Mini Reviews in Medicinal Chemistry 2009; 9(14): 1605-1621.

[33] McCandless EE, Zhang B, Diamond MS, Klein RS. CXCR4 antagonism increases T cell trafficking in the central nervous system and improves survival from West Nile virus encephalitis. Proceedings of the National Academy of Sciences of the United States of America 2008; 105(32): 11270-11275.

[34] Wilen CB, Tilton JC, Doms RW. Molecular mechanisms of HIV entry. Advances in Experimental Medicine and Biology 2012; 726: 223-242.

[35] Wyatt R, Sodroski J. The HIV-1 envelope glycoproteins: fusogens, antigens, and immunogens. Science 1998; 280(5371): 1884-1888.

[36] Stein BS, Gowda SD, Lifson JD, Penhallow RC, Bensch KG, Engleman EG. pH-independent HIV entry into CD4-positive T cells via virus envelope fusion to the plasma membrane. Cell 1987; 49(5): 659-668.

[37] Miyauchi K, Kim Y, Latinovic O, Morozov V, Melikyan GB. HIV enters cells via endocytosis and dynamin-dependent fusion with endosomes. Cell 2009; 137(3): 433-444.

[38] Daecke J, Fackler OT, Dittmar MT, Krausslich HG. Involvement of clathrin-mediated endocytosis in human immunodeficiency virus type 1 entry. Journal of Virology 2005; 79(3): 1581-1594.

[39] Gorry PR, Ancuta P. Coreceptors and HIV-1 pathogenesis. Current HIV/AIDS reports 2011; 8(1): 45-53.

[40] Cormier EG, Dragic T. The crown and stem of the V3 loop play distinct roles in human immunodeficiency virus type 1 envelope glycoprotein interactions with the CCR5 coreceptor. Journal of Virology 2002; 76(17): 8953-8957.

[41] Dragic T. An overview of the determinants of CCR5 and CXCR4 co-receptor function. The Journal of General Virology 2001; 82(Pt 8): 1807-1814.

[42] Huang CC, Lam SN, Acharya P, et al. Structures of the CCR5 N terminus and of a tyrosine-sulfated antibody with HIV-1 gp120 and CD4. Science 2007; 317(5846): 1930-1934.

[43] Anastassopoulou CG, Kostrikis LG. Viral correlates of HIV-1 disease. Current HIV Research 2005; 3(2): 113-132.

[44] Berger EA, Doms RW, Fenyo EM, et al. A new classification for HIV-1. Nature 1998; 391(6664): 240.

[45] Hartley O, Klasse PJ, Sattentau QJ, Moore JP. V3: HIV's switch-hitter. AIDS Research and Human Retroviruses 2005; 21(2): 171-189.
[46] De Jong JJ, De Ronde A, Keulen W, Tersmette M, Goudsmit J. Minimal requirements for the human immunodeficiency virus type 1 V3 domain to support the syncytium-inducing phenotype: analysis by single amino acid substitution. Journal of Virology 1992; 66(11): 6777-6780.
[47] Fouchier RA, Groenink M, Kootstra NA, et al. Phenotype-associated sequence variation in the third variable domain of the human immunodeficiency virus type 1 gp120 molecule. Journal of Virology 1992; 66(5): 3183-3187.
[48] Schuitemaker H, van 't Wout AB, Lusso P. Clinical significance of HIV-1 coreceptor usage. Journal of Translational Medicine 2011; 9 Suppl 1: S5.
[49] Rose JD, Rhea AM, Weber J, Quinones-Mateu ME. Current tests to evaluate HIV-1 coreceptor tropism. Current Opinion in HIV and AIDS 2009; 4(2): 136-142.
[50] Lin NH, Kuritzkes DR. Tropism testing in the clinical management of HIV-1 infection. Current Opinion in HIV and AIDS 2009; 4(6): 481-487.
[51] Low AJ, Swenson LC, Harrigan PR. HIV coreceptor phenotyping in the clinical setting. AIDS Reviews 2008; 10(3): 143-151.
[52] Braun P, Wiesmann F. Phenotypic assays for the determination of coreceptor tropism in HIV-1 infected individuals. European Journal of Medical Research 2007; 12(9): 463-472.
[53] Kuhmann S, Moore JP. The HIV-1 Phenotypic Variants: Deadly and Deadlier. Journal of Viral Entry 2005; 1(1): 4-16.
[54] Keele BF, Derdeyn CA. Genetic and antigenic features of the transmitted virus. Current Opinion in HIV and AIDS 2009; 4(5): 352-357.
[55] Salazar-Gonzalez JF, Salazar MG, Keele BF, et al. Genetic identity, biological phenotype, and evolutionary pathways of transmitted/founder viruses in acute and early HIV-1 infection. The Journal of Experimental Medicine 2009; 206(6): 1273-1289.
[56] Grivel JC, Shattock RJ, Margolis LB. Selective transmission of R5 HIV-1 variants: where is the gatekeeper? Journal of Translational Medicine 2011; 9 Suppl 1: S6.
[57] Gorry PR, Churchill M, Crowe SM, Cunningham AL, Gabuzda D. Pathogenesis of macrophage tropic HIV-1. Current HIV Research 2005; 3(1): 53-60.
[58] Repits J, Sterjovski J, Badia-Martinez D, et al. Primary HIV-1 R5 isolates from end-stage disease display enhanced viral fitness in parallel with increased gp120 net charge. Virology 2008; 379(1): 125-134.
[59] Moir S, Chun TW, Fauci AS. Pathogenic mechanisms of HIV disease. Annual Review of Pathology 2011; 6: 223-248.
[60] Cicala C, Arthos J, Fauci AS. HIV-1 envelope, integrins and co-receptor use in mucosal transmission of HIV. Journal of Translational Medicine 2011; 9 Suppl 1: S2.
[61] Shankarappa R, Margolick JB, Gange SJ, et al. Consistent viral evolutionary changes associated with the progression of human immunodeficiency virus type 1 infection. Journal of Virology 1999; 73(12): 10489-10502.

[62] Connor RI, Sheridan KE, Ceradini D, Choe S, Landau NR. Change in coreceptor use correlates with disease progression in HIV-1--infected individuals. The Journal of Experimental Medicine 1997; 185(4): 621-628.
[63] Hutter G, Nowak D, Mossner M, et al. Long-term control of HIV by CCR5 Delta32/Delta32 stem-cell transplantation. The New England Journal of Medicine 2009; 360(7): 692-698.
[64] Allers K, Hutter G, Hofmann J, et al. Evidence for the cure of HIV infection by CCR5Delta32/Delta32 stem cell transplantation. Blood 2011; 117(10): 2791-2799.
[65] Telenti A. Safety concerns about CCR5 as an antiviral target. Current Opinion in HIV and AIDS 2009; 4(2): 131-135.
[66] de Silva E, Stumpf MP. HIV and the CCR5-Delta32 resistance allele. FEMS Microbiology Letters 2004; 241(1): 1-12.
[67] Tsibris AM, Kuritzkes DR. Chemokine antagonists as therapeutics: focus on HIV-1. Annual Review of Medicine 2007; 58: 445-459.
[68] Glass WG, McDermott DH, Lim JK, et al. CCR5 deficiency increases risk of symptomatic West Nile virus infection. The Journal of Experimental Medicine 2006; 203(1): 35-40.
[69] Lim JK, Louie CY, Glaser C, et al. Genetic deficiency of chemokine receptor CCR5 is a strong risk factor for symptomatic West Nile virus infection: a meta-analysis of 4 cohorts in the US epidemic. The Journal of Infectious Diseases 2008; 197(2): 262-265.
[70] Kindberg E, Mickiene A, Ax C, et al. A deletion in the chemokine receptor 5 (CCR5) gene is associated with tickborne encephalitis. The Journal of Infectious Diseases 2008; 197(2): 266-269.
[71] Hartley O, Offord RE. Engineering chemokines to develop optimized HIV inhibitors. Current Protein & Peptide Science 2005; 6(3): 207-219.
[72] Lobritz MA, Ratcliff AN, Arts EJ. HIV-1 Entry, Inhibitors, and Resistance. Viruses 2010; 2(5): 1069-1105.
[73] Simmons G, Clapham PR, Picard L, et al. Potent inhibition of HIV-1 infectivity in macrophages and lymphocytes by a novel CCR5 antagonist. Science 1997; 276(5310): 276-279.
[74] Hartley O, Gaertner H, Wilken J, et al. Medicinal chemistry applied to a synthetic protein: development of highly potent HIV entry inhibitors. Proceedings of the National Academy of Sciences of the United States of America 2004; 101(47): 16460-16465.
[75] Khatib N, Das S. PRO 140--a novel CCR5 co-receptor inhibitor. Recent Patents on Anti-Infective Drug Discovery 2010; 5(1): 18-22.
[76] Pugach P, Ketas TJ, Michael E, Moore JP. Neutralizing antibody and anti-retroviral drug sensitivities of HIV-1 isolates resistant to small molecule CCR5 inhibitors. Virology 2008; 377(2): 401-407.
[77] Westby M, van der Ryst E. CCR5 antagonists: host-targeted antiviral agents for the treatment of HIV infection, 4 years on. Antiviral Chemistry & Chemotherapy 2010; 20(5): 179-192.

[78] Hannon GJ. RNA interference. Nature 2002; 418(6894): 244-251.
[79] Dykxhoorn DM, Lieberman J. The silent revolution: RNA interference as basic biology, research tool, and therapeutic. Annual Review of Medicine 2005; 56: 401-423.
[80] Boden D, Pusch O, Ramratnam B. HIV-1-specific RNA interference. Current Opinion in Molecular Therapeutics 2004; 6(4): 373-380.
[81] Zhou J, Rossi JJ. Current progress in the development of RNAi-based therapeutics for HIV-1. Gene Therapy 2011; 18(12): 1134-1138.
[82] Urnov FD, Rebar EJ, Holmes MC, Zhang HS, Gregory PD. Genome editing with engineered zinc finger nucleases. Nature Reviews 2010; 11(9): 636-646.
[83] Cannon P, June C. Chemokine receptor 5 knockout strategies. Current Opinion in HIV and AIDS 2011; 6(1): 74-79.
[84] Baba M, Nishimura O, Kanzaki N, et al. A small-molecule, nonpeptide CCR5 antagonist with highly potent and selective anti-HIV-1 activity. Proceedings of the National Academy of Sciences of the United States of America 1999; 96(10): 5698-5703.
[85] Baba M, Takashima K, Miyake H, et al. TAK-652 inhibits CCR5-mediated human immunodeficiency virus type 1 infection in vitro and has favorable pharmacokinetics in humans. Antimicrobial Agents and Chemotherapy 2005; 49(11): 4584-4591.
[86] Klibanov OM, Williams SH, Iler CA. Cenicriviroc, an orally active CCR5 antagonist for the potential treatment of HIV infection. Current Opinion in Investigational Drugs 2010; 11(8): 940-950.
[87] Tagat JR, McCombie SW, Steensma RW, et al. Piperazine-based CCR5 antagonists as HIV-1 inhibitors. I: 2(S)-methyl piperazine as a key pharmacophore element. Bioorganic & Medicinal Chemistry Letters 2001; 11(16): 2143-2146.
[88] Tagat JR, Steensma RW, McCombie SW, et al. Piperazine-based CCR5 antagonists as HIV-1 inhibitors. II. Discovery of 1-[(2,4-dimethyl-3-pyridinyl)carbonyl]-4- methyl-4-[3(S)-methyl-4-[1(S)-[4-(trifluoromethyl)phenyl]ethyl]-1-piperazinyl]-piperidine N1-oxide (Sch-350634), an orally bioavailable, potent CCR5 antagonist. Journal of Medicinal Chemistry 2001; 44(21): 3343-3346.
[89] Billick E, Seibert C, Pugach P, et al. The differential sensitivity of human and rhesus macaque CCR5 to small-molecule inhibitors of human immunodeficiency virus type 1 entry is explained by a single amino acid difference and suggests a mechanism of action for these inhibitors. Journal of Virology 2004; 78(8): 4134-4144.
[90] Palani A, Shapiro S, Clader JW, et al. Discovery of 4-[(Z)-(4-bromophenyl)-(ethoxyimino)methyl]-1'-[(2,4-dimethyl-3- pyridinyl)carbonyl]-4'-methyl-1,4'-bipiperidine N-oxide (SCH 351125): an orally bioavailable human CCR5 antagonist for the treatment of HIV infection. Journal of Medicinal Chemistry 2001; 44(21): 3339-3342.
[91] Strizki JM, Xu S, Wagner NE, et al. SCH-C (SCH 351125), an orally bioavailable, small molecule antagonist of the chemokine receptor CCR5, is a potent inhibitor of HIV-1 infection in vitro and in vivo. Proceedings of the National Academy of Sciences of the United States of America 2001; 98(22): 12718-12723.

[92] Palani A, Shapiro S, Josien H, et al. Synthesis, SAR, and biological evaluation of oximino-piperidino-piperidine amides. 1. Orally bioavailable CCR5 receptor antagonists with potent anti-HIV activity. Journal of Medicinal Chemistry 2002; 45(14): 3143-3160.

[93] Strizki JM, Tremblay C, Xu S, et al. Discovery and characterization of vicriviroc (SCH 417690), a CCR5 antagonist with potent activity against human immunodeficiency virus type 1. Antimicrobial Agents and Chemotherapy 2005; 49(12): 4911-4919.

[94] Tagat JR, McCombie SW, Nazareno D, et al. Piperazine-based CCR5 antagonists as HIV-1 inhibitors. IV. Discovery of 1-[(4,6-dimethyl-5-pyrimidinyl)carbonyl]-4-[4-[2-methoxy-1(R)-4-(trifluoromethyl)phenyl]ethyl-3(S)-methyl-1-piperazinyl]-4-methylpiperidine (Sch-417690/Sch-D), a potent, highly selective, and orally bioavailable CCR5 antagonist. Journal of Medicinal Chemistry 2004; 47(10): 2405-2408.

[95] Maeda K, Nakata H, Koh Y, et al. Spirodiketopiperazine-based CCR5 inhibitor which preserves CC-chemokine/CCR5 interactions and exerts potent activity against R5 human immunodeficiency virus type 1 in vitro. Journal of Virology 2004; 78(16): 8654-8662.

[96] Dorr P, Westby M, Dobbs S, et al. Maraviroc (UK-427,857), a potent, orally bioavailable, and selective small-molecule inhibitor of chemokine receptor CCR5 with broad-spectrum anti-human immunodeficiency virus type 1 activity. Antimicrobial Agents and Chemotherapy 2005; 49(11): 4721-4732.

[97] Fatkenheuer G, Pozniak AL, Johnson MA, et al. Efficacy of short-term monotherapy with maraviroc, a new CCR5 antagonist, in patients infected with HIV-1. Nature Medicine 2005; 11(11): 1170-1172.

[98] Veazey RS, Springer MS, Marx PA, Dufour J, Klasse PJ, Moore JP. Protection of macaques from vaginal SHIV challenge by an orally delivered CCR5 inhibitor. Nature Medicine 2005; 11(12): 1293-1294.

[99] MacArthur RD, Novak RM. Reviews of anti-infective agents: maraviroc: the first of a new class of antiretroviral agents. Clinical Infectious Diseases 2008; 47(2): 236-241.

[100] Castonguay LA, Weng Y, Adolfsen W, et al. Binding of 2-aryl-4-(piperidin-1-yl)butanamines and 1,3,4-trisubstituted pyrrolidines to human CCR5: a molecular modeling-guided mutagenesis study of the binding pocket. Biochemistry 2003; 42(6): 1544-1550.

[101] Maeda K, Das D, Ogata-Aoki H, et al. Structural and molecular interactions of CCR5 inhibitors with CCR5. The Journal of Biological Chemistry 2006; 281(18): 12688-12698.

[102] Dragic T, Trkola A, Thompson DA, et al. A binding pocket for a small molecule inhibitor of HIV-1 entry within the transmembrane helices of CCR5. Proceedings of the National Academy of Sciences of the United States of America 2000; 97(10): 5639-5644.

[103] Tsamis F, Gavrilov S, Kajumo F, et al. Analysis of the mechanism by which the small-molecule CCR5 antagonists SCH-351125 and SCH-350581 inhibit human immunodeficiency virus type 1 entry. Journal of Virology 2003; 77(9): 5201-5208.

[104] Watson C, Jenkinson S, Kazmierski W, Kenakin T. The CCR5 receptor-based mechanism of action of 873140, a potent allosteric noncompetitive HIV entry inhibitor. Molecular Pharmacology 2005; 67(4): 1268-1282.

[105] Seibert C, Ying W, Gavrilov S, et al. Interaction of small molecule inhibitors of HIV-1 entry with CCR5. Virology 2006; 349(1): 41-54.

[106] Kondru R, Zhang J, Ji C, et al. Molecular interactions of CCR5 with major classes of small-molecule anti-HIV CCR5 antagonists. Molecular Pharmacology 2008; 73(3): 789-800.

[107] Kuhmann SE, Pugach P, Kunstman KJ, et al. Genetic and phenotypic analyses of human immunodeficiency virus type 1 escape from a small-molecule CCR5 inhibitor. Journal of Virology 2004; 78(6): 2790-2807.

[108] Trkola A, Kuhmann SE, Strizki JM, et al. HIV-1 escape from a small molecule, CCR5-specific entry inhibitor does not involve CXCR4 use. Proceedings of the National Academy of Sciences of the United States of America 2002; 99(1): 395-400.

[109] Marozsan AJ, Kuhmann SE, Morgan T, et al. Generation and properties of a human immunodeficiency virus type 1 isolate resistant to the small molecule CCR5 inhibitor, SCH-417690 (SCH-D). Virology 2005; 338(1): 182-199.

[110] Westby M, Smith-Burchnell C, Mori J, et al. Reduced maximal inhibition in phenotypic susceptibility assays indicates that viral strains resistant to the CCR5 antagonist maraviroc utilize inhibitor-bound receptor for entry. Journal of Virology 2007; 81(5): 2359-2371.

[111] Ray N, Harrison JE, Blackburn LA, Martin JN, Deeks SG, Doms RW. Clinical resistance to enfuvirtide does not affect susceptibility of human immunodeficiency virus type 1 to other classes of entry inhibitors. Journal of Virology 2007; 81(7): 3240-3250.

[112] Garcia-Perez J, Rueda P, Staropoli I, et al. New insights into the mechanisms whereby low molecular weight CCR5 ligands inhibit HIV-1 infection. The Journal of Biological Chemistry 2011; 286(7): 4978-4990.

[113] Garcia-Perez J, Rueda P, Alcami J, et al. Allosteric model of maraviroc binding to CC chemokine receptor 5 (CCR5). The Journal of Biological Chemistry 2011; 286(38): 33409-33421.

[114] Maeda K, Das D, Yin PD, et al. Involvement of the second extracellular loop and transmembrane residues of CCR5 in inhibitor binding and HIV-1 fusion: insights into the mechanism of allosteric inhibition. Journal of Molecular Biology 2008; 381(4): 956-974.

[115] Pastore C, Ramos A, Mosier DE. Intrinsic obstacles to human immunodeficiency virus type 1 coreceptor switching. Journal of Virology 2004; 78(14): 7565-7574.

[116] Pastore C, Nedellec R, Ramos A, et al. Conserved changes in envelope function during human immunodeficiency virus type 1 coreceptor switching. Journal of Virology 2007; 81(15): 8165-8179.

[117] Moore JP, Kuritzkes DR. A piece de resistance: how HIV-1 escapes small molecule CCR5 inhibitors. Current Opinion in HIV and AIDS 2009; 4(2): 118-124.

[118] Maeda Y, Yoshimura K, Miyamoto F, et al. In vitro and In vivo Resistance to Human Immunodeficiency Virus Type 1 Entry Inhibitors. Journal of AIDS & Clinical Research 2011; S2: 004.

[119] Baba M, Miyake H, Wang X, Okamoto M, Takashima K. Isolation and characterization of human immunodeficiency virus type 1 resistant to the small-molecule CCR5 antagonist TAK-652. Antimicrobial Agents and Chemotherapy 2007; 51(2): 707-715.

[120] Moncunill G, Armand-Ugon M, Pauls E, Clotet B, Este JA. HIV-1 escape to CCR5 coreceptor antagonism through selection of CXCR4-using variants in vitro. AIDS 2008; 22(1): 23-31.

[121] Yusa K, Maeda Y, Fujioka A, Monde K, Harada S. Isolation of TAK-779-resistant HIV-1 from an R5 HIV-1 GP120 V3 loop library. The Journal of Biological Chemistry 2005; 280(34): 30083-30090.

[122] Tsibris AM, Sagar M, Gulick RM, et al. In vivo emergence of vicriviroc resistance in a human immunodeficiency virus type 1 subtype C-infected subject. Journal of Virology 2008; 82(16): 8210-8214.

[123] Ogert RA, Hou Y, Ba L, et al. Clinical resistance to vicriviroc through adaptive V3 loop mutations in HIV-1 subtype D gp120 that alter interactions with the N-terminus and ECL2 of CCR5. Virology 2010; 400(1): 145-155.

[124] Ogert RA, Wojcik L, Buontempo C, et al. Mapping resistance to the CCR5 co-receptor antagonist vicriviroc using heterologous chimeric HIV-1 envelope genes reveals key determinants in the C2-V5 domain of gp120. Virology 2008; 373(2): 387-399.

[125] Ogert RA, Ba L, Hou Y, et al. Structure-function analysis of human immunodeficiency virus type 1 gp120 amino acid mutations associated with resistance to the CCR5 coreceptor antagonist vicriviroc. Journal of Virology 2009; 83(23): 12151-12163.

[126] Anastassopoulou CG, Ketas TJ, Klasse PJ, Moore JP. Resistance to CCR5 inhibitors caused by sequence changes in the fusion peptide of HIV-1 gp41. Proceedings of the National Academy of Sciences of the United States of America 2009; 106(13): 5318-5323.

[127] Anastassopoulou CG, Ketas TJ, Depetris RS, Thomas AM, Klasse PJ, Moore JP. Resistance of a human immunodeficiency virus type 1 isolate to a small molecule CCR5 inhibitor can involve sequence changes in both gp120 and gp41. Virology 2011; 413(1): 47-59.

[128] Kitrinos KM, Amrine-Madsen H, Irlbeck DM, Word JM, Demarest JF. Virologic failure in therapy-naive subjects on aplaviroc plus lopinavir-ritonavir: detection of aplaviroc resistance requires clonal analysis of envelope. Antimicrobial Agents and Chemotherapy 2009; 53(3): 1124-1131.

[129] Tilton JC, Wilen CB, Didigu CA, et al. A maraviroc-resistant HIV-1 with narrow cross-resistance to other CCR5 antagonists depends on both N-terminal and extracellular loop domains of drug-bound CCR5. Journal of Virology 2010; 84(20): 10863-10876.

[130] Yuan Y, Maeda Y, Terasawa H, Monde K, Harada S, Yusa K. A combination of polymorphic mutations in V3 loop of HIV-1 gp120 can confer noncompetitive resistance to maraviroc. Virology 2011; 413(2): 293-299.
[131] Anastassopoulou CG, Ketas TJ, Sanders RW, Klasse PJ, Moore JP. Effects of sequence changes in the HIV-1 gp41 fusion peptide on CCR5 inhibitor resistance. Virology 2012; 428(2): 86-97.
[132] Pfaff JM, Wilen CB, Harrison JE, et al. HIV-1 resistance to CCR5 antagonists associated with highly efficient use of CCR5 and altered tropism on primary CD4+ T cells. Journal of Virology 2010; 84(13): 6505-6514.
[133] Anastassopoulou CG, Marozsan AJ, Matet A, et al. Escape of HIV-1 from a small molecule CCR5 inhibitor is not associated with a fitness loss. PLoS Pathogens 2007; 3(6): e79.
[134] Finzi A, Xiang SH, Pacheco B, et al. Topological layers in the HIV-1 gp120 inner domain regulate gp41 interaction and CD4-triggered conformational transitions. Molecular Cell 2010; 37(5): 656-667.
[135] Helseth E, Olshevsky U, Furman C, Sodroski J. Human immunodeficiency virus type 1 gp120 envelope glycoprotein regions important for association with the gp41 transmembrane glycoprotein. Journal of Virology 1991; 65(4): 2119-2123.
[136] Pancera M, Majeed S, Ban YE, et al. Structure of HIV-1 gp120 with gp41-interactive region reveals layered envelope architecture and basis of conformational mobility. Proceedings of the National Academy of Sciences of the United States of America 2010; 107(3): 1166-1171.
[137] Yang X, Mahony E, Holm GH, Kassa A, Sodroski J. Role of the gp120 inner domain beta-sandwich in the interaction between the human immunodeficiency virus envelope glycoprotein subunits. Virology 2003; 313(1): 117-125.
[138] Huang CC, Tang M, Zhang MY, et al. Structure of a V3-containing HIV-1 gp120 core. Science 2005; 310(5750): 1025-1028.
[139] Swiss-Model. http://swissmodel.expasy.org/ (accessed 1 July 2009).
[140] PyMOL. http://www.pymol.org/ (accessed 1 July 2009).
[141] Westby M. Resistance to CCR5 antagonists. Current Opinion in HIV and AIDS 2007; 2(2): 137-144.
[142] Pugach P, Marozsan AJ, Ketas TJ, Landes EL, Moore JP, Kuhmann SE. HIV-1 clones resistant to a small molecule CCR5 inhibitor use the inhibitor-bound form of CCR5 for entry. Virology 2007; 361(1): 212-228.
[143] Hirsch MS, Gunthard HF, Schapiro JM, et al. Antiretroviral drug resistance testing in adult HIV-1 infection: 2008 recommendations of an International AIDS Society-USA panel. Clinical Infectious Diseases 2008; 47(2): 266-285.
[144] Berro R, Sanders RW, Lu M, Klasse PJ, Moore JP. Two HIV-1 variants resistant to small molecule CCR5 inhibitors differ in how they use CCR5 for entry. PLoS Pathogens 2009; 5(8): e1000548.

[145] Berro R, Klasse PJ, Lascano D, et al. Multiple CCR5 conformations on the cell surface are used differentially by human immunodeficiency viruses resistant or sensitive to CCR5 inhibitors. Journal of Virology 2011; 85(16): 8227-8240.
[146] Laakso MM, Lee FH, Haggarty B, et al. V3 loop truncations in HIV-1 envelope impart resistance to coreceptor inhibitors and enhanced sensitivity to neutralizing antibodies. PLoS Pathogens 2007; 3(8): e117.
[147] Agrawal-Gamse C, Lee FH, Haggarty B, et al. Adaptive mutations in a human immunodeficiency virus type 1 envelope protein with a truncated V3 loop restore function by improving interactions with CD4. Journal of Virology 2009; 83(21): 11005-11015.
[148] Lin G, Bertolotti-Ciarlet A, Haggarty B, et al. Replication-competent variants of human immunodeficiency virus type 2 lacking the V3 loop exhibit resistance to chemokine receptor antagonists. Journal of Virology 2007; 81(18): 9956-9966.
[149] Nolan KM, Jordan AP, Hoxie JA. Effects of partial deletions within the human immunodeficiency virus type 1 V3 loop on coreceptor tropism and sensitivity to entry inhibitors. Journal of Virology 2008; 82(2): 664-673.
[150] Nolan KM, Del Prete GQ, Jordan AP, et al. Characterization of a human immunodeficiency virus type 1 V3 deletion mutation that confers resistance to CCR5 inhibitors and the ability to use aplaviroc-bound receptor. Journal of Virology 2009; 83(8): 3798-3809.
[151] Platt EJ, Kozak SL, Durnin JP, Hope TJ, Kabat D. Rapid dissociation of HIV-1 from cultured cells severely limits infectivity assays, causes the inactivation ascribed to entry inhibitors, and masks the inherently high level of infectivity of virions. Journal of Virology 2010; 84(6): 3106-3110.
[152] Fatkenheuer G, Nelson M, Lazzarin A, et al. Subgroup analyses of maraviroc in previously treated R5 HIV-1 infection. The New England Journal of Medicine 2008; 359(14): 1442-1455.
[153] Gulick RM, Su Z, Flexner C, et al. Phase 2 study of the safety and efficacy of vicriviroc, a CCR5 inhibitor, in HIV-1-Infected, treatment-experienced patients: AIDS clinical trials group 5211. The Journal of Infectious Diseases 2007; 196(2): 304-312.
[154] Gulick RM, Lalezari J, Goodrich J, et al. Maraviroc for previously treated patients with R5 HIV-1 infection. The New England Journal of Medicine 2008; 359(14): 1429-1441.
[155] Whitcomb JM, Huang W, Fransen S, et al. Development and characterization of a novel single-cycle recombinant-virus assay to determine human immunodeficiency virus type 1 coreceptor tropism. Antimicrobial Agents and Chemotherapy 2007; 51(2): 566-575.
[156] Su Z, Gulick RM, Krambrink A, et al. Response to vicriviroc in treatment-experienced subjects, as determined by an enhanced-sensitivity coreceptor tropism assay: reanalysis of AIDS clinical trials group A5211. The Journal of Infectious Diseases 2009; 200(11): 1724-1728.

[157] Swenson LC, Mo T, Dong WW, et al. Deep V3 sequencing for HIV type 1 tropism in treatment-naive patients: a reanalysis of the MERIT trial of maraviroc. Clinical Infectious Diseases 2011; 53(7): 732-742.

[158] Swenson LC, Mo T, Dong WW, et al. Deep sequencing to infer HIV-1 co-receptor usage: application to three clinical trials of maraviroc in treatment-experienced patients. The Journal of Infectious Diseases 2011; 203(2): 237-245.

[159] Gilliam BL, Riedel DJ, Redfield RR. Clinical use of CCR5 inhibitors in HIV and beyond. Journal of Translational Medicine 2011; 9 Suppl 1: S9.

Chapter 8

Selective Antibody Deficiency with Normal Immunoglobulins

Ricardo U. Sorensen, Tammy Harvey and Lily E. Leiva

Additional information is available at the end of the chapter

1. Introduction

Specific antibody deficiency (SAD) is a common antibody immunodeficiency defined as a poor antibody response to unconjugated pneumococcal polysccharides present in the 23-valent pneumococcal vaccine (PPV23). Clinical manifestations of specific antibody deficiency include recurrent sinopulmonary infections, such as sinusitis, otitis media, bronchitis, and pneumonia. All immunoglobulin concentrations, including IgG subclasses, are normal, and antibody response to protein antigens (eg, tetanus toxoid, diphtheria toxoid) and the conjugate H influenzae b vaccine are also normal in most patients. [11, 44, 56] In some patients with SAD, the response to the pneumococcal conjugate vaccines (PCV7, PCV10, and PCV13) is also normal.

SAD was first reported in a small group of patients in the early 1980s. [6, 46] The widespread use of pneumococcal immunization to assess antibody responses has revealed that specific unresponsiveness to polysaccharide antigens is not unusual. [21, 25]

The vast majority of SAD patients have a deficiency of specific antibodies to polysaccharides but normal antibodies to protein antigens, resembling the developing immunologic status of human newborns and infants. Infants readily produce antibodies against vaccine proteins but fail to respond to most vaccine polysaccharides until approximately two years of age. In some patient with early onset SAD, this condition may represent a delayed maturation of the immune response to polysaccharides.

SAD is also found in association with many primary and secondary immunodeficiencies. An association of SAD with IgG subclass deficiencies, particulary IgG2 deficiencies, has been described. [9] IgG2 subclass deficient patients have antibody responses to a restricted number of polysaccharides in the PPV vaccine. Frequently, these patients also have poor immunological memory, with IgG antibody titers decreasing to pre-immunization levels within 6 to 12 months. [51]

Other primary immunodeficiency disorders with an immunologic phenotype associated with specific antibody deficiency include Wiskott-Aldrich syndrome, partial DiGeorge syndrome, asplenia, hyper-IgE syndrome, and selective IgA deficiency (without IgG subclass deficiency). [30] In addition, specific antibody deficiency can be identified in some patients with congenital dysmorphic syndromes or chromosomal abnormalities associated with recurrent sinopulmonary infections. Acquired or secondary immunodeficiencies associated with specific antibody deficiency include splenectomy, immunosuppression, chronic lung disease, protein-calorie malnutrition, and human immunodeficiency virus infection.

There is not a single pathogenic mechanism for specific anti-polysaccharide antibody deficiencies. The variable conditions in which an inability to respond to polysaccharides is found suggest that many different immunologic phenotypes may lead to the same clinical phenotypic antibody deficiency. Further defining different SAD phenotypes and relating these phenotypes to associated conditions may shed further insight into possible pathogenic mechanisms.

2. Assessment of specific antibodies

The assessment of specific antibodies always needs to take into account:

1. Evidence of exposure to vaccines or infections. In the case of vaccines, this includes an exact record of immunizations;
2. Time since last exposure or vaccination to the time of obtaining the blood sample to be tested ;
3. Method of antibody measurement, including the method, the antigen used, the standards used to normalize values and normal values for different age groups obtained with the same method used to test the patient sample.

All this information is essential to determine if the antibody response is normal or abnormal and also to determine if further immunization is likely to increase antibody titers and protection.

Pneumococcal vaccines are an ideal tool to evaluate the ability to produce specific antibodies in response to a known stimulus. All pneumococcal vaccines contain antigens from several serotypes so the immunologic evaluation is not based on a single antibody response. More recently, research has also revealed that these serotypes allow for clear differentiation between antibody responses to conjugate and pure polysaccharide vaccines, a difference that is clinically relevant.

Current recommendations for the use of pneumococcal vaccines are based on the age at which immunization began. Pneumococcal conjugate vaccines (PCV) are recommended for all infants at 2, 4, 6 and 12 months of age. PCV has also been used in children 24 to 59 months of age who are unimmunized, had incomplete vaccination prior to age 24 months, or are at high risk of acquired invasive pneumococcal disease [2].

The pneumococcal polysaccharide vaccine (PPV23) is not recommended for children under 24 months since the responses to polysaccharide antigens is considered absent or ineffective in the first 2 years of life. Pneumococcal polysaccharide vaccines (PPV23) are recommended for in high risk patients over age 5 and for individuals over age 65. [1]

Serotypes	Vaccines		
	23-PPV	7-PCV	13-PCV
1	X		X
2	X		
3	X		X
4	X	X	X
5	X		X
6A			X
6B	X	X	X
7F	X		X
8	X		
9N	X		
9V	X	X	X
10A	X		
11A	X		
12F	X		
14	X	X	X
15B	X		
17F	X		
18C	X	X	X
19A	X		X
19F	X	X	X
20	X		
22F	X		
23F	X	X	X
33F	X		

23-PPV: 23-valent polysaccharide vaccine; 7-PCV: heptavalent conjugate vaccine; 13-PCV: 13-valent conjugate vaccine PCV: 13-valent conjugate vaccine. *Courtesy of RU Sorensen, MD.*

Table 1. Pneumococcal vaccines and antibody testing for conjugate and pure pneumococcal polysaccharides

	Vaccine	
	Conjugate (CV)*	Polysaccharide (PV)
Normal infants	2, 4, 6, 12-15 months	Not given to patients this age
7 to 11 months	3 doses•	Not given to patients this age
12 to 23 months	2 doses	Not given to patients this age Δ
2 to 5 years	1 dose◊	1 dose
>5 years		1 dose §

The measurement of pre-immunization immunoglobulin and serotype-specific antibody concentrations, as well as 4 - to-6-week post immunization serotype-specific antibody concentrations are recommended.

* Recommendations for the use of CV are based upon the recommendations of the CDC Advisory Committee (press release 10/22/99), FDA (HHS News release 2/17/00) and of the American Council on Immunization Practices [4].

• Intervals between doses of any vaccine combination should be ≥ 2 months.

Δ One study showed excellent serological responses to 22 of the 23 serotypes in the PV vaccine in 56 12-month old children. [7] These results support personal observations (Sorensen RU) of good responses to PV in younger children. The use of PV in patients 12-24 months of age could be considered when CVs are not available.

◊ Patients with IgG2 deficiency may require 2 doses at any age [62].

§ If there is no antibody response to PV, give CV; repeating PV is not effective [55].

Adapted from: Sorensen RU, Moore C. Peds Clin N A 2000;42:1225.

Table 2. Pneumococcal immunization in patients with recurrent infections

Severity of deficiency	IgG anti-pneumococcal antibodies	
	Post-immunization	
	2-5 years of age	≥6 years of age
Severe	No protective antibody levels for any serotype	No protective antibody levels for any serotype
Moderate	Protective antibody levels for <50% of serotypes administered	Protective antibody levels for <70% of serotypes administered

A protective antibody concentration is defined as ≥1.3 micrograms/mL, based on response to polysaccharide vaccine serotypes in patients >2 years of age.

If a patient previously received the conjugate pneumococcal vaccine and had protective titers to those serotypes, then an adequate response would be expected to the age-appropriate percentage (50% or 70%) of those serotypes exclusive to the polysaccharide vaccine.

%: percent of polysaccharide vaccine serotypes administered and tested.

Adapted from Sorensen, RU, Moore, C. Peds Clin N A 2000;43:1225.

Table 3. Classification of deficient response to pneumococcal vaccination

3. Measurement of specific antibody responses

Various methods for the measurement of antigen-specific antibodies include nephelometry, turbidimetry, chemiluminescence and enzyme-linked assay (ELISA) .

Although infections and immunizations elicit IgM, IgA, and IgG antibody responses, only IgG titers are relevant to the assessment of vaccine responses. IgG antibodies confer long-term protection and are considered indicative of immunity. The specific IgG titer represents the total of all IgG subclass concentrations, since most antibody tests do not differentiate among Ig subclasses.

For IgG anti-pneumococcal antibody assessment, the standard method is the third generation WHO ELISA, which incorporates double absorption of samples with capsular polysaccharide (CPS) and serotype 22F and correlates closely with OPA measurements [Concepcion 2001]. Multiplex technologies allow simultaneous quantitation of multiple serotype-specific antibodies. There has been limited validation against the established gold standard ELISA and assay performance in the clinical setting has not been carefully examined.

Measurements of antibodies to all 23 pneumococcal serotypes in a single test, without differentiating specific antibodies to single serotypes, is not useful. The correlation of this test with the standard ELISA test is poor. For instance, the presence of a high concentration antibody to a single serotype may give a falsely high antibody concentration, though the antibody response to other serotypes may be deficient.

Ideally, evaluation of antibody-mediated immunity includes the measurement of immunoglobulin and pre-immunization anti-pneumococcal antibody concentrations, with follow-up assessment of post immunization antibodies four to six weeks later. In practice today, most patients needing evaluation for recurrent infections have already received one or more pneumococcal vaccines and pre-immunization antibody concentrations cannot be measured. So, an exact immunization history becomes essential for the adequate interpretation of results [43].

When there is a good initial clinical and serological response to vaccination but clinical infections recur after a period of time, usually 6 to 12 months, the antibody evaluation is repeated to rule out a rapid loss of antibody concentration down to non-protective concentrations.

In most cases, evaluation of specific antibody deficiency is based on the response to pneumococcal polysaccharides. In some circumstances, it is also important to consider the response to other vaccines or infections. In patients with hypogammaglobulinemia in the first year of life, the response to protein antigens such as tetanus and diphtheria toxoids may help to predict whether the patients has transient hypogammaglobulinemia of infancy, and whether the low IgG concentrations will spontaneously increase into the normal range. The present role of the response to the conjugate *Hemophilus influenzae* type b vaccine has not been well defined.

The measurement of anti-A and B isoagglutinins is not useful in the diagnosis of specific antibody deficiency. Blood groups A and B are galactosamines on red blood cells that cross-react with galactosamines on the capsule of gut E coli bacteria. The method currently in use does not differentiate between IgM and IgG responses so is not clinical useful except for in rare instances, such as suspected Wiskott-Aldrich syndrome that needs evaluation in the first year of life. A normal child should have detectable isogglutinin titers after age 6 months.

In patients with persistent or recurrent infections with a single pathogen, such as varicella, shingles, or a specific hepatitis, assessing the specific antibody response to a causative pathogen may be clinically relevant. However, such evaluations are usually not part of the evaluation for SAD.

4. Diagnostic criteria

The interpretation of anti-pneumococcal antibody concentration results is based on increased post-immunization antibody concentrations over pre-immunization concentrations (immune response) and on the final post-immunization antibody concentrations, regardless of increase from pre-immunization concentrations (antibody concentration). Patients who already have high baseline antibody concentrations of specific antibodies to a pneumococcal serotype are less likely to have a significant increase in antibody concentrations after immunization.

The definition of adequate response to individual pneumococcal polysaccharides is not well defined. Protection against invasive disease, as assessed in clinical vaccine trials, may require lower antibody concentrations that protection against mucosal diseases like sinusitis and otitis [10]. Immunocompetence, as a reflection of the ability of producing a response for clinical protection against mucosal infections and pneumonia, has been arbitrarily defined as a post-immunization antibody concentration ≥1.3 mcg/mL. This antibody concentration can be used as a marker of immunocompetence, regardless of degree of response over pre-immunization baseline antibody concentrations [56]. For instance, a patient with a pre-immunization titer of 0.15 mcg/mL may have a 4-fold increase to 0.6 mcg/ml, still significantly below the level needed to show immunocompetence.

The number of individual polysaccharide responses required in the immunologic evaluation for a reliable assessment of the antibody response to polysaccharides has not been established. Response to a single serotype-specific polysaccharide does not predict the ability or inability to respond to most or all other serotypes. Therefore, measuring response of at least **six** different antibodies to vaccine serotypes is recommended to obtain a reliable estimate of the spectrum of responses of a given patient. For patients who received one or more doses of the conjugate pneumococcal vaccine, at least six or more non-conjugate vaccine serotypes (present only in polysaccharide vaccine) need to be measured. A patient that responds to the conjugate vaccine may still be unresponsive to pure polysaccharides, which is an immunologic abnormality that may be clinically relevant.

The age of the patient significantly affects the intensity of the antibody response to individual serotypes and the number of serotypes inducing an adequate response [56].

Normal children between two and five years of age are expected to have an adequate response to >50 percent of serotypes evaluated. Older patients are expected to respond to >70 percent of serotypes evaluated. These criteria have not been tested critically; however, they have allowed us to predict a clinical course and decide upon treatment options in over 1000 patients of all ages tested since 1995 (Sorensen et al, unpublished observations).

Other factors that affect pneumococcal antibody concentrations in the evaluation of SAD include treatment with intravenous or subcutaneous gammaglobulin within the previous 6 months and underlying diseases and/or treatments possibly affecting immune response. Examples include long-term steroid therapy, malignancy, and chemotherapy.

In addition to immunization, responses to natural, often subclinical, infection influence the antibody concentrations in patients. In fact, absent protective antibodies in unimmunized patients above 2 years of age are unusual. However, upon vaccination, older patients who never developed protective antibodies to pneumococcal serotypes often have adequate response to most serotypes. Low antibody concentrations in an unimmunized individual do not define an immunodeficiency syndrome unless there is inadequate response to immunization.

5. Clinical manifestations

The clinical manifestations of patients with selective anti-polysaccharide antibody deficiency are similar to those of all antibody deficiency syndromes. The majority of patients have recurrent upper and/or lower respiratory infections such as sinusitis, otitis, bronchitis or pneumonia due to *Streptococcus pneumoniae, Haemophilus influenzae, Branhamella catarrhalis, or Staphylococcus aureus.*

The sinopulmonary infections must be more frequent or severe that normally expected for the age group of the patient. Most of these infections require antibiotic treatment for clinical improvement, and an evaluation is warranted when multiple antibiotic treatments are needed, even when antibiotics effectively resolve each infection.

For a common infection such as otitis media, characteristics frequently found in patients with SAD include:

- Early onset of infections, as early as 3-4 months of age
- Recurrence of infection after antibiotic treatment
- Infectious complications such as mastoiditis
- Association with invasive infections
- Recurrence after ear tubes
- Repeated ear tube placement
- Clinical change to sinusitis after ear tubes

Very few patients with specific antibody deficiency also present with atopic diseases, including atopic dermatitis and asthma, complicated by recurrent infections requiring frequent antibiotic treatments for improvement. Patients with asthma and selective antibody deficiency may also have chronic sinusitis or other recurrent sinopulmonary infections.

6. Sad phenotypes

There are many different forms of SAD based on the immunologic and clinical phenotypes, the transient or permanent nature of the defect, and the maintenance or loss of antibody concentrations after an initial normal response.

The classic SAD with absent or poor responses to pneumococcal polysaccharides is well defined and is based on the response to polysaccharides from serotypes present in PPV23. When patients have received one or more conjugate pneumococcal vaccines, differentiating antibody responses to serotypes present in the conjugate vaccines from responses to serotypes present only in the polysaccharide vaccines is important. In specific antibody deficiency, antibody response to the conjugate serotypes may be normal with poor responses to polysaccharide serotypes.

The intensity of antibody responses to polysaccharides and the number of polysaccharides eliciting antibody responses vary considerably from one individual to another, even in the same age group. This variability makes it difficult to clearly define immunologic phenotypes of polysaccharide antibody unresponsiveness.

The severe immunologic phenotype of SAD is the easiest phenotype to define. These patients have little or no antibody response and no protective antibody concentrations to any pneumococcal serotype evaluated . Some patients with a severe immunologic phenotype have protective titers to one serotype, and the titer tends to be low (1.3 to 2.0 ug/ml) [45, 51].

A moderate immunologic SAD phenotype is characterized by partial antibody responses, with less than the expected arbitrarily defined adequate response to serotypes for their age group. Some of these patients can have a severe clinical phenotype despite their relatively mild or moderate immunological abnormality.

Since the introduction of conjugate pneumococcal vaccines in the USA in 2000, patients with recurrent respiratory infections who are fully immunized with 4 doses of PCV may be clearly unresponsive to conjugate polysaccharides. These patients usually are able to develop protective antibody concentrations against protein antigens such as diphtheria and tetanus toxoids and to the single antigen conjugate *Haempphilus influenza* vaccine. The immunologic and clinical severity of these patients is similar to the phenotypes of patients unresponsive to PPV. There is a large subgroup of PCV-SAD patients that respond only to serotype 14, revealing that the immunologic properties of the polysaccharide in serotype 14 is different from other penumococccal polysaccharides.

A different clinical phenotype of SAD occurs in patients who have an initial adequate response to a pneumococcal vaccine, followed by a rapid loss of antibody concentrations over time. This form of SAD, based on poor persistence of IgG antibodies against pneumococci, is usually suspected when a patient who had a significant improvement with decreased infections after immunization begins again to have recurrent infections, typically six or more months post-immunization.

Some unimmunized patients in all age groups fail to develop protective antibody concentrations to any pneumococcal serotype tested. This lack of antibody response is unusual in individuals above two years of age who typically develop antibodies in response to natural infections. Most unimmunized adults have protective antibodies to at least 80 percent of serotypes tested. The lack of pre-immunization protective antibodies does not define an immunodeficiency, and most of these patients have a normal response to immunization. Those patients that completely fail to respond to natural infection and immunization have a severe form of selective antibody deficiency. Responders to immunization cannot be differentiated from non-responders without evaluation with immunization and retesting after immunization.

7. Management of SAD

The management of SAD, including prevention and treatment of recurrent infections, can be classified into the following broad categories: additional immunization, antibiotic prophylaxis and treatment, and immune serum globulin therapy.

8. Immunization

Immunization beyond the suggested regular immunization schedule should be the first step in a newly diagnosed SAD patient. Patients who fail to respond to a complete series of PCV vaccinations, PCV-SAD patients, should be immunized with one dose of PPV. This vaccine should increase the patient's protection against bacterial polysaccharide infections, and this immunization allows for assessment of the patient's immunologic response to polysaccharides. Clinical experience shows that these patients typically have good immunologic response to most or all 23 PPV serotypes (Sorensen, unpublished observations).

Patients with recurrent infections despite good response to PCV may benefit from immunization with PPV. PPV contains serotypes common to PCV and serotypes no present in PCV, so this vaccine may increase antibody response to PCV and nonPCV serotypes. For less severe mucosal infections not requiring multiple antibiotic treatments, it may be possible to immunize the patient first, with a subsequent complete immunological evaluation only if infections persist.

After immunizing with one dose of PPV initially, repeated immunization with PPV should not be considered a routine therapeutic option in patients with recurrent infections that fail to respond to PPV. If patients do not respond to one dose of PPV-23, our experience suggests that these patients likely do not have an appropriate immunologic response to polysaccharide antigens. So, a second dose of PPV-23 generally has little benefit. An exception may be re-immunization of otherwise immunologically normal patients who partially responded to PPV initially, with resulting titers slightly below protective levels.. Reimmunization of partial responders to PPV may result in protective antibody levels.

In contrast to the ineffectiveness of repeated PPV immunization, 80 to 90 percent of patients with classic PPV-SAD do have a serological response to the serotypes present in the conjugate vaccine that can be used to overcome the unresponsiveness to pure polysaccharides [56]. Conjugate vaccines were developed to immunize children younger than 2 years of age, as children below age 2 years typically demonstrate poor responses to polysaccharide antigens alone. Conjugation helps direct the immune response toward the immunogenic protein complexed to the polysaccharide antigen, thereby stimulating protective immune responses in those individuals. Therefore, it is not surprising that PPV-nonresponders typically have a good serological response to PCV serotypes.

Although most patients benefit from immunization with the conjugate vaccine by improving protection against common pneumococcal serotypes, none of the conjugate vaccines has all 23 serotypes present in the polysaccharide vaccine. This clinical improvement after a PCV immunization is notable because recurrent respiratory infections are caused by a much larger variety of pathogens than just the vaccine pneumococcal serotypes.

If there is a serological response to the conjugate vaccine without clinical improvement, then the PPV-SAD persists and further treatment options need to be considered. In PPV-SAD patients who are clinically unresponsive to immunization with additional PCV, reimmunizing with PPV is generally ineffective if repeated within one year of the initial PPV vaccine. After a period of IgG therapy, many patients respond to an additional PPV dose with or without clinical improvement, so a second PPV dose should be given after completion of 1-2 years of IgG replacement therapy.

For patients with poor immunological memory (loss of antibody concentrations after an adequate initial response), immunization with a second dose of polysaccharide vaccine generally triggers a vigorous IgG antibody response. Further study is needed since this phenotype may not be attributable only to poor immunological memory.

9. Antibiotics

If the frequency and severity of infections persists after additional immunization, antibiotic prophylaxis should be considered, especially in younger patients who will likely outgrow their selective antibody deficiency. When an oral antibiotic is considered for prophylaxis, treatment doses of trimetroprim-sulfa can be very effective. Prolonged daily use of topical mupirocin intranasally, for several months to a year, is a safe alternative treatment plan.

Appropriate antibiotic selection and duration for any febrile and/or purulent respiratory infection is important. Treatment with high doses of antibiotics for periods of at least 2 to 3 weeks is necessary. When antibiotic use alone improves the patient's quality of life and prevents infectious complications, no additional treatment is needed.

10. IgG replacement therapy

IgG replacement by the intravenous or the subcutaneous route is appropriate when the infection history is well documented, when immunizations have been utilized, and most of all, when proper antibiotic prophylaxis and treatment has been optimized. Patients with any form of SAD need decreased infections to improve quality of life and to prevent complications such hearing loss, sinus damage or bronchiectasis.

The recommended IgG dose is 400 to 600 mg/kg calculated on a monthly basis. ItgG can be given intravenously every four weeks or subcutaneously in divided doses one or twice weekly. Occasional patients require either higher doses if they have breakthrough infections or complications such as bronchiectasis.

When the severity of infections warrants the use of IgG replacement treatment, patients should be advised that treatment will be discontinued after a period of one to two years and the immune response will be reevaluated four to six months after discontinuation of IgG replacement. Whenever possible, the discontinuation of IVIG should be scheduled for during the spring or summer time when the incidence of infections typically decreases.

Four to six months after the IgG dose, a complete immunological evaluation of antibody mediated immunity should be performed. This evaluation includes an additional dose of PPV and measurement of antibodies 3 to 6 weeks after immunizations. Many children do not require further IgG replacement therapy, but some continue to have persistent infections and need continue replacement IgG therapy. These patients are likely to have additional immunological abnormalities that presently under evaluation. Patient management, IgG replacement therapy, and post treatment evaluation is best done by experts in the management of patients with all forms of primary immunodeficiency diseases.

11. Prognosis

The immunologic phenotypes of specific antibody deficiency may be transient or permanent. Transient forms are common in children two to five years of age. Even in permanent phenotypes, the natural history of specific antibody deficiency is usually benign with proper management of these patients.

Reassessment of antibody-mediated immunity should always be performed after discontinuation of IVIG therapy and in patients with recurrent infections. In particular, older patients with selective antibody deficiencies with normal immunoglobulin concentrations should be monitored closely, as they may eventually develop common variable immunodeficiency.

Further insights into the pathogenesis of this immunodeficiency by studying larger numbers of patients will allow further understanding of the correlation between immunologic and clinical phenotypes of specific antibody deficiency. Further study will result in a more reliable assessment of the risk for persistent immune abnormalities and recurrent sinopulmonary infections in subgroups of these patients.

Author details

Ricardo U. Sorensen, and
Department of Pediatrics, New Orleans, Louisiana, USA

Tammy Harvey
Jeffrey Modell Center for Immunodeficiencies, New Orleans, Louisiana, USA

Lily E. Leiva
Louisiana State University Health Science Center, New Orleans, Louisiana, USA

12. References

[1] Centers of Disease Control and Prevention. Prevention of pneumococcal disease: Recommendations of the Advisory Committee on Immunization Practices (ACIP). MMWR Morb Mortal Wkly Rep 1997;46:1-24.

[2] American Academy of Pediatrics: Pneumococcal infections. In: In: Pickering LK BC, Long SS, Kimberlin DW, Long SS, editor. Red Book: 2009 Report of the Committee on Infectious Diseases. 28 ed. Elk Grove Village,.IL; 2009. p. 524-535.

[3] Recommendations for the prevention of Streptococcus pneumoniae infections in infants and children: use of 13-valent pneumococcal conjugate vaccine (PCV13) and pneumococcal polysaccharide vaccine (PPSV23). Pediatrics 2010;126(1):186-90.

[4] Recommended childhood immunization schedule--United States. MMWR Morb Mortal Wkly Rep 2002;51:31.

[5] Ambrosino D, Umetsu D, Siber G, Howie G, Goularte T, Michaels R, et al. Selective defect in the antibody response to Haemophilus influenzae type b in children with recurrent infections and normal serum IgG subclass levels. . J Allergy Clin Immunol 1988;81:1175.

[6] Ambrosino DM, Siber GR, Chilmonczyk BA, Jernberg JB, Finberg RW. An immunodeficiency characterized by impaired antibody responses to polysaccharides. N Engl J Med 1987;316(13):790-3.

[7] Balloch A, Licciardi P, Russell F, et al. Infants aged 12 months can mount adequate serotype-specific IgG responses to pneumococcal polysaccharide vaccine. J Allergy Clin Immunol 2010;126:395.

[8] Barrett D, Ayoub E. IgG2 subclass restriction of antibody to pneumococcal polysaccharides. Clin Exp Immunol 1986;63:127.

[9] Bernatowska-Matuszkiewicz E, Pac M, Pum M, Liszka K, Leibl H, Eibl MM. IgG subclasses and antibody response to pneumococcal capsular polysaccharides in children with severe sinopulmonary infections and asthma. Immunol Invest 1991;20(2):173-85.

[10] Black S, Eskola J, Whitney C, Shinefield H. Pneumococcal conjugate vaccine and pneumococcal common protein vaccines,. In: Plotkin SA OW, Offit, PA,, editor. Vaccines. 5 ed. Philadelphia: Elsevier; 2006. p. 521-567.

[11] Bonilla FA, Bernstein IL, Khan DA, Ballas ZK, Chinen J, Frank MM, et al. Practice parameter for the diagnosis and management of primary immunodeficiency. Ann Allergy Asthma Immunol 2005;94(5 Suppl 1):S1-63.

[12] Bossuyt X, Borgers H, Moens L, et al. Age- and serotype-dependent antibody response to pneumococcal polysaccharides. J Allergy Clin Immunol 2011;127:1079.

[13] Boyle R, Le C, Balloch A, et al. The clinical syndrome of specific antibody deficiency in children. Clin Exper Immunol 2006;146:486-92.

[14] Burton R, Nahm M. Development and validation of a fourfold multiplexed opsonization assay (MOPA4) for pneumococcal antibodies. Clin Vaccine Immunol 2006;13:1004-9.

[15] Concepcion N, Frasch C. Pneumococcal type 22f polysaccharide absorption improves the specificity of a pneumococcal-polysaccharide enzyme-linked immunosorbent assay. Clin Diagn Lab Immunol 2001;8:266-72.

[16] Epstein M, Gruskay F. Selective deficiency in pneumococcal antibody response in children with recurrent infections. Ann Allergy Asthma Immunol 1995;75:125.

[17] Eskola J. Polysaccharide-based pneumococcal vaccines in the prevention of acute otitis media. Vaccine 2001;19:S78-S82.

[18] Fong S, Qaqundah B, Taylor W. Developmental patterns of ABO isoagglutinins in normal children correlated with the effects of age, sex, and maternal isoagglutinins. Transfusion 1974;14(14):551.

[19] French M, Harrison G. Systemic antibody deficiency in patients without serum immunoglobulin deficiency or with selective IgA deficiency. Clin Exp Immunol 1984;56:18.

[20] Go E, Ballas Z. Anti-pneumococcal antibody response in normal subjects: A meta-analysis. J Allergy Clin Immunol 1996;98:205-15.

[21] Gross S, Blaiss M, Herrod H. Role of immunoglobulin subclasses and specific antibody determinations in the evaluation of recurrent infection in children. J Pediatr 1992;121:516.

[22] Hare N, Smith B, Ballas Z. Antibody response to pneumococcal vaccination as a function of preimmunization titer. J Allergy Clin Immunol 2009;123:195.

[23] Herer B, Labrousse F, Mordelet-Dambrine M, et al. Selective IgG subclass deficiencies and antibody responses to pneumococcal polysaccharide antigen in adult community-acquired pneumonia. Am Rev Respir Dis 1990;142:854.

[24] Hidalgo H, Inostroza J, Leiva L, Sorensen RU. [immunization and immune response to pneumococcal vaccination]. Rev Med Chil 1996;124(3):287-92.

[25] Hidalgo H, Moore C, Leiva LE, Sorensen RU. Preimmunization and postimmunization pneumococcal antibody titers in children with recurrent infections. Ann Allergy Asthma Immunol 1996;76(4):341-6.

[26] Jackson L, Neuzil K. Pneumococcal vaccines. In: Plotkin S, Orenstein W, Offit P, editors. Vaccines. 5 ed. Philadelphia, PA: Elsevier; 2006. p. 569-604.

[27] Jackson LA, Baxter R, Naleway AL, Belongia EA, Baggs J. Patterns of pneumococcal vaccination and revaccination in elderly and non-elderly adults: a Vaccine Safety Datalink study. BMC Infect Dis 2009;9:37.

[28] Javier F, Moore C, Sorensen R. Distribution of primary immunodeficiency diseases diagnosed in a pediatric tertiary hospital. Ann Allergy Asthma Immunol 2000;84:25.
[29] Kamchaisatian W, Wamwatsuntikul W, Sleasman J, et al. Validation of current joint AAAAI and ACAAI guidelines for antibody response to the 23-valent pneumococcal vaccine using a population of HIV-infected children. J Allergy Clin Immunol 2006;118:1336-41.
[30] Knutsen A. Patients with IgG subclass and/or selective antibody deficiency to polysaccharide antigens: initiation of a controlled clinical trial of intravenous immune globulin. J Allergy Clin Immunol 1989;84:640.
[31] Landesman S, Schiffman G. Assessment of the antibody response to pneumococcal vaccine in high-risk populations. Rev Infect Dis 1981;3 Suppl:S184.
[32] Lawrence E, Edwards K, Schiffmann G, et al. Pneumococcal vaccine in normal children. Am J Dis Child 1983;137:846.
[33] Lim P, Lau Y. Occurrence of IgG subclass antibodies to ovalbumin, avidin, and pneumococcal polysaccharide in children. Int Arch Allergy Immunol 1994;104:137.
[34] Lortan J, Kaniuk A, Monteil M. Relationship of in vitro phagocytosis of serotype 14 Streptococcus pneumoniae to specific class and IgG subclass antibody levels in healthy adults. Clin Exp Immunol 1993;91:54.
[35] Makela P, Herva E, Sibakov M, et al. Pneumococcal vaccine and otitis media. Lancet 1980;2:547-51.
[36] McQuillan G, Kruszon-Moran D, Deforest A, et al. Serologic immunity to diphtheria and tetanus in the United States. Ann Intern Med 2002;136:660.
[37] Ochs H, Buckley R, Kobayashi R, et al. Antibody responses to bacteriophage phi X174 in patients with adenosine deaminase deficiency. Blood 1992;80:1163.
[38] Ortigas A, Leiva L, Moore C, et al. Natural history of specific antibody deficiency after IgG replacement therapy. Ann Allergy Asthma Immunol 1999;82:71.
[39] Paris K, Sorensen R. Assessment and clinical interpretation of polysaccharide antibody responses. Ann Allergy Asthm Immunol 2007;99:462-4.
[40] Ridda I, Macintyre C, Lindley R, et al. Immunological responses to pneumococcal vaccine in frail older people. Vaccine 2009;27:1628.
[41] Rijkers G, Sanders L, Zegers B. Anti-Capsular polysaccharide antibody deficiency states. Immunodeficiency 1993;5:1.
[42] Romero-Steiner S, Frasch C, Carlone G, Fleck R, Goldblatt D, Nahm M. Use of opsonophagocytosis for the serologic evaluation of pneumococcal vaccines. Clin Vaccine Immunol 2006;13:165-9.
[43] Rose MA, Schubert R, Strnad N, Zielen S. Priming of immunological memory by pneumococcal conjugate vaccine in children unresponsive to 23-valent polysaccharide pneumococcal vaccine. Clin Diagn Lab Immunol 2005;12(10):1216-22.
[44] Sanders LA, Rijkers GT, Kuis W, Tenbergen-Meekes AJ, de Graeff-Meeder BR, Hiemstra I, et al. Defective antipneumococcal polysaccharide antibody response in children with recurrent respiratory tract infections. J Allergy Clin Immunol 1993;91(1 Pt 1):110-9.
[45] Sanders LA, Rijkers GT, Tenbergen-Meekes AM, Voorhorst-Ogink MM, Zegers BJ. Immunoglobulin isotype-specific antibody responses to pneumococcal polysaccharide

vaccine in patients with recurrent bacterial respiratory tract infections. Pediatr Res 1995;37(6):812-9.
[46] Saxon A, Kobayashi RH, Stevens RH, Singer AD, Stiehm ER, Siegel SC. In vitro analysis of humoral immunity in antibody deficiency with normal immunoglobulins. Clin Immunol Immunopathol 1980;17(2):235-44.
[47] Schenkein J, Park S, Nahm M. Pneumococcal vaccination in older adults induces antibodies with low opsonic capacity and reduced antibody potency. Vaccine 2008;26:5521.
[48] Shrimpton A, Duddridge M, Ziegler-Heitbrock L. Vaccination with polysaccharide-conjugate-vaccines in adult patients with specific antibody deficiency. Vaccine 2006;24:3574.
[49] Siber G, Schur P, Aisenberg A, et al. Correlation between serum IgG-2 concentrations and the antibody response to bacterial polysaccharide antigens. N Engl J Med 1980;303:178.
[50] Simell B, Kilpi T, Kayhry H. Pneumococcal carriage and otitis media induce salivary antibodies to pneumococcal capsular polysaccharides in children. J Infect Dis 2002;186:1106-14.
[51] Sorensen R, Hidalgo H, Moore C, Leiva L. Anti-pneumococcal antibody titers and IgG subclasses in children with recurrent respiratory infections. Pediatr Pulmonol 1996;22:167.
[52] Sorensen R, Moore C. Immunology in the pediatrician's office. Pediatr Clin North Am 1994;41:691.
[53] Sorensen R, Moore C. Antibody deficiency syndromes. Pediatr Clin North Am 2000;47:1225.
[54] Sorensen RU, Hidalgo H, Moore C, Leiva LE. Post-immunization pneumococcal antibody titers and IgG subclasses. Pediatr Pulmonol 1996;22(3):167-73.
[55] Sorensen RU, Leiva LE, Giangrosso PA, Butler B, Javier FC, 3rd, Sacerdote DM, et al. Response to a heptavalent conjugate Streptococcus pneumoniae vaccine in children with recurrent infections who are unresponsive to the polysaccharide vaccine. Pediatr Infect Dis J 1998;17(8):685-91.
[56] Sorensen RU, Leiva LE, Javier FC, 3rd, Sacerdote DM, Bradford N, Butler B, et al. Influence of age on the response to Streptococcus pneumoniae vaccine in patients with recurrent infections and normal immunoglobulin concentrations. J Allergy Clin Immunol 1998;102(2):215-21.
[57] Straetemans M, Sanders E, Veenhoven R, et al. Review of randomized controlled trials on pneumococcal vaccination for prevention of otitis media. Pediatr Infect Dis J 2003;22:515-24.
[58] Uddin S, Borrow R, Haeneuy M, et al. Total and serotype specific pneumococcal antibody titres in children with normal and abnormal humoral immunity. Vaccine 2006;24:5637-44.
[59] Wasserman R, Sorensen R. Evaluating children with respiratory tract infections: the role of immunization with bacterial polysaccharide vaccine. Pediatr Infect Dis J 1999;18:157.

[60] Wood P, Mayne A, Joyce H, et al. A mutation in Bruton's tyrosine kinase as a cause of selective anti-polysaccharide antibody deficiency. J Pediatr 2001;139:148.
[61] Zhang Q, Finn A. Mucosal immunology of vaccines against pathogenic nasopharyngeal bacteria. J Clin Pathol 2004;57:1015-21.
[62] Zielen S, Buhring I, Strnad N, et al. Immunogenicity and tolerance of a 7-valent pneumococcal conjugate vaccine in nonresponders to the 23-valent pneumococcal vaccine. Infect Immun 2000;68:1435.
[63] Zora J, Silk H, Tinkelman D. Evaluation of postimmunization pneumococcal titers in children with recurrent infections and normal levels of immunoglobulin. Ann Allergy 1993;70:283.

Chapter 9

Emerging Role of MicroRNAs in the Pathophysiology of Immune System

Marco Rossi, Pierosandro Tagliaferri and
Pierfrancesco Tassone

Additional information is available at the end of the chapter

1. Introduction

1.1. Overview of MiRNA biology

MicroRNAs are small (22 nucleotides), noncoding, double-stranded RNA molecules, that can regulate gene expression primarily by reducing the abilities of specific mRNAs to be transduced to their encoded proteins. The first recognized miRNA found in 1993 is lin-4, that controls the cell fate at larval stages in Caenorhabditis elegans [1, 2]. Bioinformatic approaches suggested that the mammalian miRNA repertoire is involved in regulation of 30% of all protein-encoding genes [3].

Human miRNAs are encoded within introns of coding genes and introns and exons of noncoding transcripts [4]. Generation of mature miRNAs is due to a series of endonucleolytic steps starting from long primary transcripts (pri-miRNAs). The pri-miRNAs are cleaved in the nucleus to a_70 nt intermediate with the typical stem-loop hairpin structure, precursor miRNAs (pre-miRNAs) by the Drosha- DGCR8 microprocessor complex [5, 6]. The pre-miRNAs are further processed into_22 nt double-stranded miRNA duplex by the cytoplasmic RNase III enzyme Dicer [7]. One strand of this miRNA duplex (the guide strand) incorporates into a large protein complex, RNA-induced silencing complex (RISC), formed by Dicer, TRBP (a dsRNA-binding domain protein) and Ago2 (the Argonaute protein 2), and finally becomes the mature miRNA. The other strand, the so-called passenger strand, is degraded.

Each mature miRNA interacts with a specific mRNA in the mRNA's 3′-untranslated region (3′UTR), leading to translational repression or mRNA degradation. Besides, some evidences have shown that miRNA can increase translation [8].

2. The role of MiRNAs in hematopoietic cell development

The development of hematopoietic and immune system requires an integrated network of survival, proliferation and apoptotic signals that are finely tuned along differentiation. miRNAs represent efficient modulators of such a system as they can affect the expression of multiple genes at different stages. The identification of putative miRNA involved in hematopoietic ontogeny has been one of primary topic of miRNA studies since their discovery. To clarify the role of specific miRNAs, Chen et al. [9] first cloned about 100 previously identified miRNAs and analyzed only those expressed in hematopoietic cells (miR181, 142 and 223). miR181 was found in lineage negative (Lin -) mouse bone marrow undifferentiated cells and strongly upregulated in mature B cells and within the thymus; miR142 was more ubiquitously expressed, while 223 was mostly confined to myeloid lineage. miR181 was then cloned into a GFP gene carrying retroviral vector and ectopically expressed in Lin- bone marrow cells. Infected cells were then followed in vitro to check their lineage commitment. A preferential development of B cells was observed. When Lin- miR181+ cells were transplanted in irradiated mice, lymphoid repopulation showed a prevalence of B cell population as compared to control (80% vs 32%, respectively). This study was of primary relevance as it has shown the effects of a single miRNA in lymphopoiesis and addressed a method to study next candidate miRNAs. De Yebenes and colleagues [10] observed that miR181b is involved also in immunoglobulin class switch at activated B cell level. Hence, miR 181 family is involved in early (switch from pro B cell to pre B cell) and late (from centroblasts to activated B cells) stages of B cell development.

The expression of miR181 in mouse thymus prompted investigators to evaluate their role in T cell selection. Interestingly, miR181 is expressed at higher levels in early T cell differentiation as its expression drops from double negative/double positive cells to single positive CD4/CD8 cells [11] MiR17-92 cluster (miR17, 18a, 19a, 20a, 19b and 92) has been implicated in B cell lymphopoiesis (transition pro B to pre B cells) by Ventura et al. [12]. Interestingly, in mice this cluster is homologous to the miR-106a-63 (except miR18 and 19), although only mice lacking miR17-92 show a relevant phenotype, including B cell differentation arrest. It is likely that miR17-92 cluster controls apoptotic signals through suppression of Bim and PTEN [13] miR-150 has been involved in the transition pro B to pre B cells through suppression of c-Myb [14-16], a transcription factor that leads this phase. miR-150 is strongly upregulated along T cell development beginning from double positive stage and modulates expression of NOTCH3 [17]. NOTCH3 gene is known to be involved in T cell differentiation and leukemogenesis.

Overall, these data indicate that miR181/miR17-92/miR150 are among the main regulators of early T and B lymphopoiesis from the common lymphoid precursor.

An analogue role is played by miR 223 in myeloid lineage. Chen et al [9] observed that miR223 is highly expressed in mouse bone marrow. Indeed, miR223 tunes granulocytic differentation both at an early and late phase [18]. MiR223 knock out mice show expansion of granulocyte precursors and hyper mature circulating granulocytes. miR223 targets ELF-1-like factor (mef) 2c, a transcription factor that promotes myeloid differentiation and IGFR1, thus affecting expansion of myeloid precursors committed to granulocytic differentiation [18].

Granulocytic differentiation is further regulated through a critical transcription factor, GFI1 (growth factor independent-1). GFI1 expression depends upon miR21 as demonstrated in a knockout model [19].

3. MiRNAs at the cross-roads between innate and adaptive immune responses

3.1. Innate immune responses

Innate responses imply the final differentiation and interaction of intervening cells to the site where inflammatory stimuli were generated. Several miRNAs have been described as implicated in a complex network, that controls the on and off phases of the response.

miR146a is upregulated upon LPS stimulation in monocytes and is likely to be responsible of the phenomenon known as hyporesponsiveness to prolonged LPS exposure. Indeed, miR146a acts as a negative regulator of LPS induced responses. LPS-induced NF Kb promotes miR146a upregulation, which in turns suppresses TRAF6 (TNF receptor associated factor 6), IRAK1/2 (Interleukin 1 receptor associated kinase 1). These genes encode key adaptor molecules along TLR related pathways and are involved in innate responses through TNF activation and production of IL-1 dependent molecules such as IL-8 and RANTES [20-22]. Therefore, monocytes become hyporesponsive to further stimulation with LPS and relevant pro inflammatory molecules are reduced in the microenvironment.

miR155 seems to act on the same pathways but with opposite effects to miR146a. Indeed, engagement of several TLRs (3,4 and 9) promotes miR155 transcription through AP1 and NFkb. miR155 main targets are SOCS1 (suppressor of cytokine signaling 1) and SHIP1(Src Homology-2 domain-containing inositol-5′-phosphatase 1) that lead to release of proinflammatory cytokines in the microenvironment such as TNF alpha and IFN gamma [23-26].

miR223 can regulate also monocyte-macrophage differentiation by targeting IKK-alpha (IKb kinase) and leaving NFKb to promote inflammatory genes transcription. The final result is the transition of monocyte to macrophage [27].

The emerging data suggest that miRNA regulation of inflammatory and innate responses is timely tuned according to microenviromental stimuli. Indeed, TLR stimulation evokes miR155 upregulation within 2hr , while other miRNAs, such as miR21 are produced according to a delayed time frame. These observations are likely related to a differential role of miRNAs in turning on and off the inflammatory/innate responses. In this setting, miR21 should turn off the response, by increasing IL-10 levels [28].

3.2. Adaptive responses

Immune responses require an integration between the innate/inflammatory and adaptive arm. According to their specific functions, miRNAs represent a perfect set of molecules to finely regulate and coordinate also adaptive responses. miRNAs that are involved in developmental stages of hematopoiesis can show additional functions in differentiated immune cells. Indeed, miR181a, which is implicated in thymic selection, is able to strengthen TCR signaling and reinforce T cell activation upon antigen engagement [11]. This effect likely relies on phosphatase suppression and increase in ERK phosphorylation. A member of the same family, miR181b has been proposed as regulating CSR (class switch recombination) of B cells. CSR is induced by activation induced cytidine deaminase (AID) and is likely targeted by miR181b. Indeed, IgG switch promoted by LPS and IL-4 stimulation is impaired when levels of endogenous miR181b are increased [10].

The role of miRNAs in T cell responses can be also variable according to its endogenous levels and/or contemporary expression in antigen presenting cells (APCs). This might be the case of miR155. miR155 is encoded within the BIC region (B cell integration cluster), which is often involved in lymphomas. BIC deficient mice, which lacked miR155 production, did not show significant impairment in hematopoiesis. When immunization with different bacterial strains and subsequent challenge with the same pathogens were administered to BIC deficient mice, the animals died of infection. Indeed, immunizations did not translate into protective immunity as compared with wild type mice. The authors have shown that T cell activity was compromised because there was a shift towards Th2 phenotype due to downregulation of c-Maf, which is a transcription factor that drives Th2 cytokine secretion [29]. Furthermore, BIC deficient DCs failed to adequately activate T cell responses. In this model, B cells were not able to differentiate to plasmablasts and showed alterations in CSR (class switch recombination). This phenomenon may be due to miR155, that targets AID [30].

Overall, these data indicate that miR155 has a pivotal role in sustaining adaptive immune responses.

However, these data are partly in contrast with the study from Mao et al. [31], who showed that miR155 is upregulated upon TLR stimulation in murine bone marrow derived dendritic cells. Furthermore, transfection of murine epidermal DCs with miR155 coding plasmid increased its endogenous levels and attenuated T cells responses driven by DCs. These effects were reverted when a miR155 antisense sequence was co-transfected into epidermal DCs. The authors try to reconcile these conflicting data, explaining that endogenous levels may induce different effects of the same miRNA in different cell types. However, since epidermal DC population is heterogeneous and not pure, it is possible that high levels of miR155 promote attenuation of T cell responses through APCs different from differentiated DCs.

The plasticity of miRNAs in controlling overall immune responses is further demonstrated by the miR29 activity. Interestingly, recent findings of Ma et al. [32], who have shown that miR29 suppresses IFN-γ secretion in NK and T cells, thereby linking together innate and adaptive responses. Indeed, responses to pathogen are mainly regulated through this mechanism as for the case of L. Monocytogenes and M. Tuberculosis.

4. MiRNAs and autoimmune diseases

The emerging picture of a central role played by miRNAs in the onset, development and turning off of immune responses is strictly related to the findings of their involvement in autoimmune diseases. In some cases, the functions of specific miRNAs have been first elucidated in the disease and then in immune system physiology. The possibility to use murine models of autoimmunity allows investigators to study the selected miRNAs *in vivo* in order to understand how they facilitate or attenuate the disease. However, the identification of a specific miRNA in the mouse model does not mean a direct translation into human disease. Overall, disregulation of miRNAs observed in autoimmunity promote either activation of immune effectors and/or suppression of immune regulatory cells, thus contributing to disease development. In the following section, the contribution of miRNAs will be discussed according to the specific autoimmune disorder.

5. Systemic Lupus Erythematosus (SLE)

SLE is a chronic autoimmune disease with a complex pathogenesis, involving different organs [33]. Since systemic inflammation is the hallmark of the disease, deregulation of critical pro inflammatory pathways have been described [34]. Indeed, miRNAs deregulated in SLE target genes involved in the inflammatory responses

5.1. miR146a

Type I IFN pathway is widely recognized as a primary deregulation of inflammatory responses in SLE pathogenesis [34]. IFN I pathway is elicited by TLR engagement. Among TLRs, TLR-7 contributes the most to this phenomenon. In 2009, Tang et al. [35] have shown that underexpression of miR146a is tightly related to the upregulation of type I IFN pathway. They analyzed 52 patients with SLE, 6 with Behcet'disease and 29 normal subjects and evaluated miR146a levels from PBMCs. Interestingly, miR146a was proportionally decreased according to disease state (no disease, inactive SLE and active SLE, with active SLE having the lowest levels). miR146a levels were inversely related to IFN score, which was calculated considering the expression of three representative inducible genes. Finally, IFN pathway could be downregulated when overexpression of miR146a was attained in PBMCs taken from normal donors and SLE patients. The same group [36] has identified a genetic variant of the miR146a promoter region, that confers reduced binding affinity to the transcription factor ETS1, thus leading to reduced levels of miR146a and increased susceptibility to SLE. These data have been further confirmed by a genomic analysis, where a SLE associated polymorphic SNP variant, rs2431697, was found to be related to low expression levels of miR146a gene [37]. Overall, these findings suggest a pivotal role of miR146a in SLE susceptibility and development.

5.2. miR125a, 126, 21 and 148a

Autoimmune disorders are often characterized by disregulated expression of pro-inflammatory chemokines and its receptor that drive and sustain unchecked immune responses, favoring autoimmunity. This is the case for RANTES (Regulated upon Activation, Normal T-cell Expressed, and Secreted), also known as CCL5, whose elevated levels are observed in the context of chronic systemic inflammations such as arthritis and nephritis. Renal damage is initiated by RANTES over-expression in mouse models of SLE [38].

Zhao et al. [39] have shown that miR125a levels are underexpressed in T cells of SLE patients, while its predicted target KLF13 (Kruppel like factor 13) was upregulated. KLF13 directly controls the expression of RANTES in T cells. Interestingly, prolonged mitogenic stimuli evoke miR125a upregulation in normal T cells, providing a negative feedback loop that controls chemokine expression and helps to turn off inflammatory responses. The deficiency of this mechanism in SLE patients provide further insights on the onset and progression of the disease.

DNA methylation is a relevant mechanism to regulate gene transcription in eukaryotic cells [40] and any perturbation of these pathways can have crucial impact in health and disease. T cells from SLE patients suffer of a global hypomethylation [41], which is related to disease activity. The reduction of DNA methylation depends upon the reduced levels of Dnmt1 (Dna methyl transferase-1), the key enzyme that transfers methyl groups to CpG islands. The paired analysis of CD4 T cells from normal donors and SLE patients revealed the presence of an upregulated miRNA in SLE-T cells, miR126, that was independent from costimulatory signals [42]. miR126 targets Dnmt1 and reduces its levels in SLE- CD4 T cells. miR126 downstream effects include hypomethylation of critical genes in autoimmune pathogenesis such as TNSFS7 and ITGAL, that encode CD70 and CD11a [43], respectively. Indeed, CD70 [44] is the cellular ligand for the tumor necrosis factor receptor family member CD27,and is required on activated T cells and B cells to stimulate the synthesis of IgG. CD11a, also known as lymphocyte function–associated antigen 1, belongs to the integrin family of cell surface receptors and can strengthen the adhesion of T lymphocytes to other immune cells. These events could be reverted by miR126 inhibition. A similar activity of Dnmt1 suppression in CD4 T cells from SLE has been ascribed to miR21 and 148a [45]

6. Rheumathoid Arthritis (RA)

RA is a systemic inflammatory disorder, primary involving synovial joints. The inflammatory milieu is the base for disease onset and progression. Several groups reported an increase of miR155 and 146a in synovial fibroblasts and PBMCs from RA patients [46, 47]. Interestingly, these miRNAs can be stimulated by inflammatory stimuli, though promoting opposite effects. miR155 sustains inflammation, while miR146a attenuates through TNFα suppression. In this setting, miR146a seems not able to promote its action. A possible explanation is that both miRNAs are elicited by the pro-inflammatory environment of RA, with miR155 enforcing inflammation, while miR146a should shut off it, but it is unable to exert its activity.

7. Multiple Sclerosis (MS)

MS is an autoimmune disease of the central nervous system characterized by chronic inflammation, demyelination, and axonal damage. Demyelination is due to pro inflammatory T cells. Mireia Guerau-de-Arellano et al. [48] identified increased levels of miR128 and 27b in naive and miR340 in memory CD4 T cells from MS patients, favoring switch to Th1 phenotype. Gain-of-function experiments with these micro-RNAs enhanced the encephalitogenic potential of myelin-specific T cells in experimental autoimmune encephalomyelitis, while treatment with specific oligonucleotide miRNA inhibitors reverted to normal Th2 shift. These data further clarified the role of these miRNAs in MS pathogenesis and suggested a therapeutic strategy based on miR suppression by selected inhibitors.

8. Conclusions

The increasing evidences on the role of miRNAs in pathophysiology are radically changing the established paradigms of disease onset and development. However, we can assert that our undestanding of miRNA functions is still preliminary and further work is awaited to better define how these molecules integrate with known intracellular pathways. Indeed, we know that miRNAs exert a very finely tuned regulation of intracellular pathways. This effect is attained through a modulation of miR levels, that is very complex to study in simplified models both in vitro and in vivo. Indeed, the best method to study miRNAs is to over express or completely inhibit its expression, but it is unlikely that this method can perfectly mirror the real intracellular conditions. Immune responses represent an attracting system to explore miR functions, since they have to be tightly regulated. The data have shown that miRNA modulation is an efficient way to rapidly turn on and off immune responses, both preceding and integrating with the classical gene mastered pathways. Therefore, we believe that the study of miRNAs within immune system may represent an excellent model to understand miRNA pathophysiology, providing critical insights to be extended to the other branches of biopathology.

Author details

Marco Rossi and Pierosandro Tagliaferri
Translational Medical Oncology Unit, Department of Experimental and Clinical Medicine, Magna Græcia University and Tommaso Campanella Cancer Center, Catanzaro, Italy

Pierfrancesco Tassone
Translational Medical Oncology Unit, Department of Experimental and Clinical Medicine, Magna Græcia University and Tommaso Campanella Cancer Center, Catanzaro, Italy
Temple University's College of Science & Technology, Philadelphia, PA, USA

9. References

[1] Lee, R. C., Feinbaum, R. L., Ambros V. The C. elegans heterochronic gene lin-4 encodes small RNAs with antisense complementarity to lin-14. *Cell*, 1993, *75*, 843–854

[2] Wightman, B, Ha, I, Ruvkun, G. Posttranscriptional regulation of the heterochronic gene lin- 14 by lin-4 mediates temporal pattern formation in C. elegans. *Cell*, 1993, *75*, 855–862

[3] Bartel, D. P. MicroRNAs: Genomics, biogenesis, mechanism, and function. *Cell*, 2004, *116*, 281–297

[4] Rodriguez, A, Griffiths-Jones, S, Ashurst, J. L., Bradley A. Identification of mammalian microRNA host genes and transcription units. *Genome Res*, 2004, *14*, 1902–1910

[5] Denli, A. M., Tops, B. B., Plasterk, R. H., Ketting, R.F., Hannon, G. J. Processing of primary microRNAs by the Microprocessor complex. *Nature*, 2004, *432*, 231–235

[6] Han, J, Lee, Y, Yeom, K. H., Kim, Y. K., Jin, H, Kim, V. N. The Drosha-DGCR8 complex in primary microRNA processing. *Genes Dev*, 2004, *18*, 3016–3027.

[7] Ketting, R. F., Fischer, S. E., Bernstein, E, Sijen, T, Hannon, G. J., Plasterk, R.H. Dicer functions in RNA interference and in synthesis of small RNA involved in developmental timing in C. Elegans. *Genes Dev*, 2001, *15*, 2654–2659

[8] Vasudevan, S, Tong, Y, Steitz, J. A. Switching from repression to activation: microRNAs can up-regulate translation. *Science*, 2007, *318*, 1931–1934

[9] Chen, C.Z., Li, L, Lodish, H.F., Bartel, D.P. MicroRNAs modulate hematopoietic lineage differentiation. *Science*, 2004, *303*, 83-86

[10] de Yébenes, V.G., Belver, L, Pisano, D. G., González, S, Villasante, A, Croce, C, He L, Ramiro, A.R. miR-181b negatively regulates activation-induced cytidine deaminase in B cells. *J.Exp. Med.* 2008, *205*, 2199–2206

[11] Li, Q. J., Chau, J, Ebert, P. J. R., Sylvester, G, Min, H, Liu, G, Braich, R, Manoharan, M Soutschek, J, Skare, P, Klein, L. O., Davis, M. M., and Chen, C. Z. miR-181a is an intrinsic modulatorof T Cell sensitivity and selection *Cell*, 2007, *129*, 147–161.

[12] Ventura, A, Young, A. G, Winslow, M. M, Lintault, L, Meissner, A, Erkeland, S. J, Newman, J, Bronson, R. T., Crowley, D, Stone, J. R., Jaenisch, R, Sharp, P. A., Jacks, T. Targeted deletion reveals essential and overlapping functions of the miR-17 through 92 family of miRNA clusters. *Cell*, 2008, *132*, 875–886

[13] Xiao, C, Rajewsky, K. MicroRNA control in the immune system: basic principles. *Cell*, 2009, *136*, 26-36

[14] Lin, Y. C., Kuo, M. W., Yu, J, Kuo, H. H., Lin, R. J., Lo, W. L., Yu, A. L. c-Myb is an evolutionary conserved miR-150 target and miR-150/c-Myb interaction is important for embryonic development. *Mol. Biol. Evol.* 2008, *25*, 2189–2198

[15] Thomas, M. D., Kremer, C. S., Ravichandran, K. S., rajewsky, K, Bender, T. P. c-Myb is critical for B cell development and maintenance of follicular B cells. *Immunity*, 2005, *23*, 275–286

[16] Xiao, C., Calado, D. P., Galler, G, Thai, T.H., Patterson, H. C., Wang, J, Rajewsky, N, Bender, T. P., Rajewsky, K. MiR-150 controls B cell differentiation by targeting the transcription factor c-Myb. Cell, 2007, *131*, 146–159

[17] Ghisi, M, Corradin, A, Basso, K, Frasson, C, Serafin, V, Mukherjee, S, Mussolin, L, Ruggero, K, Bonanno, L, Guffanti, A, De Bellis, G, Gerosa, G, Stellin, G, D'agostino, D. M., Basso, G, Bronte, V, Indraccolo, S, Amadori, A, Zanovello, P. Modulation of microRNA expression in human T-cell development: targeting of NOTCH3 by miR-150. *Blood*, 2011, *117*, 7053-7062

[18] Johnnidis, J. B., Harris, M. H., Wheeler, R. T., Stehling-Sun, S, Lam M. H., Kirak, O, Brummelkamp, T. R., Fleming, M. D., Camargo, F. D. Regulation of progenitor cell proliferation and granulocyte function by microRNA-223. *Nature*, 2008, *451*, 1125-1129

[19] Velu, C. S., Baktula, A. M., Grimes, H. L. Gfi1 regulates miR-21 and miR-196b to control myelopoiesis. *Blood*, 2009, *113*, 4720–4728

[20] Taganov, K. D., Boldin, M. P., Chang, K. J., Baltimore, D. NF-kappaB-dependent induction of microRNA miR-146, an inhibitor targeted to signaling proteins of innate immune responses. *Proc Natl Acad Sci USA*, 2006, *103*, 12481–12486

[21] Hou, J, Wang, P, Liu, L, Liu, X, Ma, F, An, H, Wang, Z, Cao, X. MicroRNA-146a feedback inhibits RIG-1-dependent type I IFN production in macrophage by targeting TRAF6, IRAK1 and IRAK2. *J Immunol*, 2009, *183*, 2150–2158

[22] Rom, S, Rom, I, Passiatore, G, Pacifici M, Radhakrishnan, S, Del Valle, L, Pina-Oveido, S, Khalili, K, Eletto D, Peruzzi F. CCL8/MCP-2 is a target for miR-146a in HIV1-infected human microglial cells. *FASEB J*, 2010, *24*, 2292–2300

[23] Androulidaki, A, Iliopoulos, D, Arranz, A, Doxaki, C, Schworer, S, Zacharioudaki, V, Margioris, A. N., Tsichlis, P. N., Tsatsanis, C. The kinase Akt1 controls

macrophage response to lipopolysaccharide by regulating microRNAs. *Immunity* 2009, *31*, 220–231

[24] O'Connell, R. M., Kahn, D, Gibson, W. S., Round, J. L., Scholz, R. L., Chaudhuri, A. A., Kahn, M. E., Rao, D. S., Baltimore, D. MicroRNA-155 promotes autoimmune inflammation by enhancing inflammatory T cell development. *Immunity*, 2010, *33*, 607–619

[25] O'Connell, R. M., Taganov, K. D., Boldin, M. P., Cheng, G, Baltimore, D. MicroRNA-155 is induced during the macrophage inflammatory response. *Proc. Natl. Acad. Sci. U. S. A.* 2007, *104*, 1604–1609

[26] Tili, E., Michaille, J. J., Cimino, A, Costinean, S, Dumitru, C. D., Adair, B, fabbri, M, Alder, H, Liu, C. G., Croce, C. M. Modulation of miR-155 and miR-125b Levels following Lipopolysaccharide/TNF-alpha stimulation and their possible roles in regulating the response to endotoxin shock. *J. Immunol*, 2007, *179*, 5082–5089

[27] Li, T, Morgan, M. J., Choksi, S, Zhang, Y, Kim, Y. S., Liu, Z. G. MicroRNAs modulate the non canonical transcription factor NF-kappaB pathway by regulating expression of the kinase IKK alpha during macrophage differentiation. *Nat Immunol*, 2010, *11*, 799–805

[28] Sheedy, F. J., Palsson-McDermott, E, Hennessy, E. J., Martin, C, O'Leary, J. J., Ruan, Q, Johnson, D. S., Chen, Y, O'neill, L. A. Negative regulation of TLR4 via targeting of the proinflammatory tumor suppressor PDCD4 by the microRNA miR-21. *Nat Immunol*, 2010, *11*, 141– 147

[29] Rodriguez, A, Vigorito, E, Clare, S, Warren, M. V., Couttet, P, Soond, D. R., Van Dongen , S, Grocock, R. J., Das, P. P., Miska, E. A., Vetrie, D, Okkenhaug, K, Enright, A. J., Dougan, G, Turner, M, Bradley, A. Requirement of bic/microRNA-155 for normal immune function. *Science*, 2007, *316*, 608–611

[30] Teng, G, Hakimpour, P, Landgraf, P, Rice, A, Tuschl, T, Casellas, R, Papavasiliou, F. N. MicroRNA-155 is a negative regulator of activation-induced cytidine deaminase. *Immunity*, 2008, *28*, 621–629

[31] Mao, C. H., Liangmei He, Tsai, Y. C., Peng, S, Kang, T. H., Pang, X, Monie, A, Hung, C. F., Wu, T-C. In vivo microRNA-155 expression influences antigen-specific T cell-mediated immune responses generated by DNA vaccination. *Cell Biosci*, 2011, *1*, 1-11

[32] Ma, F, Xu, S, Liu, X, Zhang, Q, Xu, X, Liu, M, Hua, M, Li, N, Yao, H, Cao, X. The microRNA miR-29 controls innate and adaptive immune responses to intracellular bacterial infection by targeting interferon-γ. *Nat Immunol*, 2011, *12*, 861-869

[33] Crow MK. Collaboration, genetic associations, and lupus erythematosus. *N Engl J Med* 2008, *358*, 956–61

[34] Ohl, K, Tenbrock, K. Inflammatory cytokines in systemic lupus erythematosus. *J Biomed Biotechnol*. 2011, 432595

[35] Tang, Y, Luo, X, Cui, H, Ni, X Yuan, M, Guo, Y, Huang, X, Zhou, H, De Vries, N, Tak, P. P., Chen, S, Shen, N. MicroRNA-146a Contributes to Abnormal Activation of the Type I Interferon Pathway in Human Lupus by Targeting the Key Signaling Proteins *Arthritis and Reumathisms* 2009, *60*, 1065–1075

[36] Luo, X., Yang, W, Ye, D-Q, Cui, H, Zhang, H, Hirankarn, N, Qian, X, Tang, Y, Lau, Y. L., De Vries, N, Tak, P. P., Tsao, B. P., Shen, N. A Functional Variant in MicroRNA-146a Promoter Modulates Its Expression and Confers Disease Risk for Systemic Lupus Erythematosus. *Plos Genet*, 2011, *7*, e1002128

[37] Lofgren, S. E., Frostegard, J., Truedsson, L., Pons-Estel, B. A., D'Alfonso, S., Witte, T, Lauwerys, B. A., Endreffy, E, Kovacs, L, Vasconcelos, C, Martins da Silva, B, Kozyrev, S. V., Alarcon-Riquelme, M. E. Genetic association of miRNA-146a with systemic lupus erythematosus in Europeans through decreased expression of the gene. *Genes and Immunity*, 2012 *13*, 268 – 274

[38] Moore, K. J., Wada, T, Barbee, S. D., Kelley, V. R. Gene transfer of RANTES elicits autoimmune renal injury in MRL-Faslpr mice. Kidney Int 1998, *53*, 1631–41

[39] Zhao, X, Tang, Y, Qu, B, Cui, H, Wang, S, Wang, L, Luo, X, Huang, X, Li, J, Chen, S, Shen, N. MicroRNA-125a Contributes to Elevated Inflammatory Chemokine RANTES Levels via Targeting KLF13 in Systemic Lupus Erythematosus. *Arthritis Rheum*, 2010, *62*, 3425–3435

[40] Weber M, Schubeler D. Genomic patterns of DNA methylation: targets and function of an epigenetic mark. *Curr Opin Cell Biol*, 2007, *19*, 273–80

[41] Richardson B, Scheinbart L, Strahler J, Gross L, Hanash S, Johnson M. Evidence for impaired T cell DNA methylation in systemic lupus erythematosus and rheumatoid arthritis. Arthritis Rheum 1990, *33*, 1665–73

[42] Zhao, S, Wang, Y, Liang, Y, Zhao, M, Long, H, Ding, S, Yin, H, Lu, Q. MicroRNA-126 Regulates DNA Methylation in CD4-T Cells and Contributes to Systemic Lupus Erythematosus by Targeting DNA Methyltransferase 1. *Arthritis Rheum*, 2011, 63, 1376–1386

[43] Lu Q, Kaplan M, Ray D, Zacharek S, Gutsch D, Richardson B. Demethylation of ITGAL (CD11a) regulatory sequences in systemic lupus erythematosus. *Arthritis Rheum* 2002, *46*, 1282–91

[44] Hogg N, Laschinger M, Giles K, McDowall A. T-cell integrins: more than just sticking points. *J Cell Sci*, 2003, *116*, 4695–705

[45] Pan, W, Zhu, S, Yuan, M, Cui, H, Wang, L, Luo, X, Li, J, Zhou, H, Tang, Y, Shen, N. MicroRNA-21 and microRNA-148a contribute to DNA hypomethylation in lupus CD4+ T cells by directly and indirectly targeting DNA methyltransferase 1. *J Immunol*, 2010, *184*, 6773-6781

[46] Stanczyk, J, Pedrioli, D. M., Brentano, F, Sanchez-Pernaute, O, Kolling, C, Gay, R. E., Detmar, M, Gay, S, Kyburz, D. Altered expression of MicroRNA in synovial fibroblasts and synovial tissue in rheumatoid arthritis. *Arthritis Rheum*, 2008, *58*, 1001-1009

[47] Li, J, Wan, Y, Guo, Q, Zou , L, Zhang, J, Fang, Y, Fu, X, Liu, H, Lu, L, Wu, Y. Altered microRNA expression profi le with miR-146a upregulation in CD4+ T cells from patients with rheumatoid arthritis. *Arthritis Res Ther*, 2010, *12*, R81

[48] Guerau-de-Arellano, M, Smith, K. M., Godlewski, J, Liu, Y, Winger, Lawler, R. S. E., Whitacre, C. C., Racke, M. K., Lovett-Racke, A. E. Micro-RNA dysregulation in multiple sclerosis favours pro-inflammatory T-cell-mediated autoimmunity. *Brain*, 2011, *134*, 3578-3589

Section 3

Immunodeficiency – HIV, Human Model

Chapter 10

Coreceptor Usage in HIV Infection

Kerina Duri

Additional information is available at the end of the chapter

1. Introduction

Chemokines are small low molecular weight proteins or cytokines secreted by cells that function as chemical messengers. They were originally found to attract leukocytes to site(s) of inflammation. As ligands they activate and signal through their respective chemokine receptors triggering an influx of intracellular calcium (Ca^{2+}) ions causing a process known as chemotaxis. Chemokine receptors are integral membrane proteins that specifically bind and respond to chemokines. They are members of the class A subfamily of G-protein coupled receptor (GPCRs) superfamily, a name derived from the characteristic cysteine motif of the group of chemokines they interact with. Despite their pivotal roles in the immune system and angiogenesis, chemokines as well as their receptors have been associated with a number of pathologies including autoimmune disorders, pulmonary diseases, transplant rejection, cancers, vascular diseases and human immunodeficiency virus (HIV) infection. Scientists have noted that while the CD4 receptor is necessary for the successful infection of host immune cells by all naturally occurring HIV-1 strains it is not sufficient. Thus, another specific cell surface molecule called chemokine receptor is required. The recent introduction of entry inhibitors in the clinic as components of antiretroviral treatment has increased the research interest of coreceptor usage in HIV infection. Chemokine receptors are subjects of significant medical importance which not only provide new insights into the mechanisms of viral entry, tropism and pathogenesis, but have also culminated into new control strategies from the host's perspective influencing HIV transmission along with disease progression. Identification of the different phenotypes of HIV-1 strains with different prevalence during various stages of disease progression and the role of these phenotypes in treatment outcome has further revolutionalised research in this field. This chapter seeks to depict a simple and clear understanding of the basics of HIV phenotypes or genotypes and the respective current as well as prospective diagnostic tools. Milestones and challenges in this relatively new class of antiretroviral therapy of coreceptor antagonists will also be highlighted.

2. Structure of chemokine receptors

Chemokine receptors consist of about 350 amino acids that are divided into a short and acidic N-terminal end, seven helical transmembrane domains since they span the cell membrane seven times with three intracellular and three extracellular hydrophilic loops, and an intracellular C-terminus containing serine and threonine residues that act as phosphorylation sites during receptor regulation as shown in **Figure 1** below. Chemokine receptors are usually linked to a G-protein through which they signal. The N-terminus of the chemokine receptor is an extracellular domain that binds the chemokine(s) and has been shown to influence infection tropism. The first two extracellular loops of chemokine receptors are linked together by disulphide bonding between two conserved cysteine residues. The disulfide bonds keep the extracellular loops in place thereby maintaining the structural integrity necessary for ligand binding and signal transduction. In spite of the high amino acid similarity of their primary sequences, chemokine receptors bind a limited number of ligands.

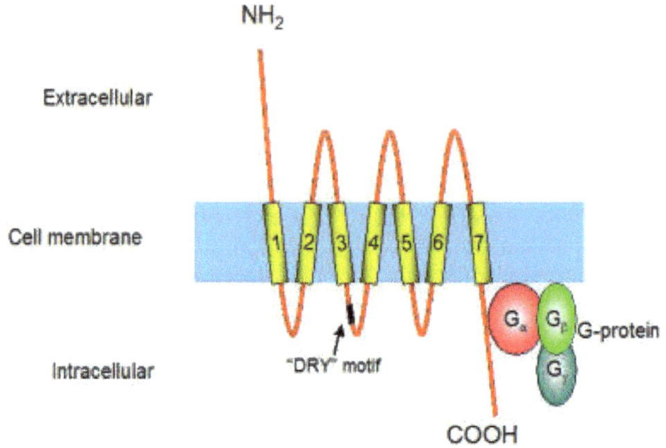

Figure 1. Typical structure of a chemokine receptor

3. Classification of chemokine receptors

To date, approximately 50 human chemokines and 20 receptors have been discovered. Basically chemokines and their receptors are divided into four subfamilies; CXC, CC, CX3C and XC depending on the position of the two pairs of the highly conserved cysteine residues on the ligands, where C denotes the cysteine amino acid residue whilst X represents non-cysteine amino acids. For the main subfamilies, the first two cysteines are either contiguous (CC) or intercalated by one non cysteine amino acid residue (CXC). A system of nomenclature has been introduced where each ligand and receptor is identified by its subfamily and an identifying number. For example, CCL2 refers to a chemokine ligand of the CC subfamily, number 2. Similarly, the receptors are referred to by subfamily **R** and similarly an identifying number. Thus, for instance one of the receptors of CCL5 is called CCR5. Despite the numerous chemokine receptors that are prospective coreceptors for HIV *in vitro*, only CCR5 and CXCR4 have attracted substantial interest because they form portals of cellular entry for both HIV-1 and HIV-2 inclusive of other related simian or feline retroviruses. The lack of crystallography for these two highly hydrophobic coreceptors makes them difficult to isolate.

4. CXC chemokine receptors

The first HIV coreceptor to be identified was CXCR4 which was originally an orphan receptor called leukocyte-derived seven-transmembrane domain receptor (LESTR). By then it did not receive much attention until it was recognized as a coreceptor for HIV-1. Thus, in the mid 1990s the second receptor, CXCR4, needed for successful entry of HIV into cells was discovered. At that time this coreceptor was termed "fusin" as it facilitated certain HIV strains to fuse with and enter immune cells called T cells. A detailed analysis of the structure of fusin revealed that it was a receptor for chemokines which were previously shown to suppress HIV activity. CXCR4 has a wide cellular distribution. It is commonly expressed on most immature and mature hematopoietic cell types, cells of the central nervous system, neutrophils, monocytes, T and B cells, dendritic cells (DCs), Langerhans cells and macrophages. To date there are seven CXC chemokine receptors in mammals, named CXCR1 through CXCR7. The CXC chemokines include stromal cell-derived factor-1 alpha and beta now officially designated CXCL12a and CXCL12b respectively. CXCL12 is often induced by pro-inflammatory stimuli such as lipopolysaccharide, interleukin-1 (IL-1) or tumour necrosis factor-alpha (TNF-α) and has been shown to be strongly chemotactic for lymphocytes. Its high level of expression in the genital mucosa may help to explain the inefficient transmission of CXCR4-tropic HIV isolates.

5. CC chemokine receptors

Another chemokine receptor necessary for the entry of HIV into macrophages called CCR5 that was subsequently identified. CCR5 receptors have been shown to be involved in leukocyte activation and mobilization. CCR5 is expressed on several cell types including peripheral blood-derived DCs, CD34+ hematopoietic progenitor cells and some activated/memory Th1 lymphocyte. Chemokines that bind these receptors are RANTES (regulated-upon-activation normal T expressed and secreted); MIP-1α and MIP-1β (macrophage inflammatory protein-1 alpha and beta) previously observed to suppress HIV infection but now officially called CCL5, CCL3 and CCL4 respectively. *In vitro* studies have demonstrated several CC chemokines bind CCR5. However, CCL3, CCL4, CCL5, and CCL8 have shown the most suppressive effects in HIV-1 infection assays. To date ten members of the CC chemokine receptor subfamily have been described, namely CCR1 through to CCR10 according to the IUIS/WHO Subcommittee on Chemokine Nomenclature. CCR5 is one of the major coreceptor implicated in susceptibility to HIV-1 infection and disease progression. The lack of CCR5 gene expression has been associated with resistant to HIV-1 infection as will be discussed later on.

6. CX3CR1

CX3C chemokine receptor 1 (CX3CR1) also known as the fractalkine receptor or G-protein coupled receptor 13 (GPR13) has been shown to bind chemokine CX3CL1, also called fractalkine. Fractalkine is a transmembrane chemokine involved in the adhesion and migration of leukocytes. CX3CR1 is expressed on monocytes and plays a major role in the survival of monocytes. It has been shown to interact with human respiratory syncytial virus protein G consequently, modulating the host immune response. It also interacts with HIV-1 envelope (env) polyprotein glycoprotein (gp) 160. Thus CX3CR1 is also a minor coreceptor for HIV-1. Certain variations in the expression this gene has been associated with increased susceptibility to HIV-1 infection and rapid progression to AIDS.

7. XCR1

The "C" sub-family of chemokine receptors contains only one member: XCR1, also known as GPR5. It is the receptor for chemokines XCL1 and XCL2 formerly, lymphotactin-1 and-2, respectively. This receptor is closely related to the MIP-1 α and RANTES yet to date its expression and the function of its ligand XCL1 remain elusive. However, at least in murine models, XCR1 has been shown to be expressed on $CD8^+$ DCs and that its ligand XCL1 has shown to be a potent and highly specific chemo-attractant for this subset of DCs.

8. Tropism

HIV-1 was initially isolated from peripheral blood cells and consequently characterised as a virus that infects the CD4+ T-lymphocyte population, T tropic isolates. However, subsequent isolation of HIV-1 from non-lymphoid organs demonstrated that HIV-1 could also infect cells of the monocyte-macrophage lineage; macrophage tropic isolates. Studies have shown that T-cell and macrophage isolates display significant different biological properties with respect to cellular tropism, genetic diversity and relative replication rates including their inherent ability to induce syncytia.

9. MT-2 cell tropism

Biological differences of HIV-1 isolates and depletion of CD4 positive lymphocytes have been shown to correlate with the pathogenesis of AIDS. Direct cytopathic effects of HIV can be studied *in vitro* in T cell lines. An MT-2 tumour cell line assay is generally used for the phenotypic characterisation of HIV-1 isolates. The ability of HIV-1 isolates to replicate in MT-2 cell lines is a prototype where viruses that do not infect MT-2 cells are designated non-syncytium inducing (NSI), while those that infect cells are termed syncytium inducing (SI). Studies have shown that HIV-1 isolates from patients with low CD4 counts have been shown to replicate rapidly to high titres in peripheral blood mononuclear cells (PBMCs) with the infected cells forming syncytia and such isolates are called rapid/high replicating or syncytium inducing (SI). HIV-1 isolates from asymptomatic individuals replicate much slowly with low titres and such isolates are termed slow/low or NSI. Consequently, HIV-1 isolates can be classified into two main groups; those that replicate in T–cell lines, grow rapidly in cultures forming syncytia in target cells and the other group that replicate in macrophages, grow relatively slowly in culture but are not able to induce syncytia, SI and NSI, respectively. The formation of syncytia does not always happen in HIV infected people. However, autopsies have found syncytia in the spleens of some patients. More frequently CD4 syncytia have been observed in the brains of patients who would have died from serious AIDS related neurological complications.

10. HIV strains classification based on tropism

Following the identification of the coreceptors, HIV-1 isolates have also been characterized based on their ability to infect and induce syncytia in $CD4^+$ T-cell lines that express CXCR4 but not CCR5.While all the HIV-1 strains require CD4 to enter and infect cells, some isolates utilize the chemokine receptors X4 or R5 while other variants use both receptors, dual tropic (R5X4) strains for binding and entry. Coreceptor usages correspond to the phenotypes previously defined by the MT-2 assay with SI and NSI viruses using CXCR4 and CCR5, respectively. Dual tropic isolates exhibit both the M and T tropic characteristics. They are further classified as dual-R; R5X4 variants with more efficient use of CCR5 than of CXCR4 or dual-X; R5X4 with more efficient use of CXCR4 than of CCR5. *In vitro* studies have shown that some HIV-1 strains can use a variety of other chemokine receptors. Interestingly, this does not appear to have major relevance to HIV infection nor pathogenesis *in vivo*. MT-2 positive variants are defined as either X4 or R5X4. Absence of viral growth in this assay may be either due to the exclusive presence of R5 variants or failure to isolate HIV.

Frequencies of R5 HIV-1 variants vary among different populations, being 80% and 50% in drug naïve individuals and patients receiving antiretroviral therapy, respectively. Tropism shifts have been associated with long term use of antiretroviral therapy. Some studies have shown that drug selection pressure may gradually select for pre-existing X4 virus from cellular reservoirs during sustained highly active antiretroviral therapy. Thus, the use of CCR5 coreceptor antagonists is associated with a selective pressure that promotes the emergence of CXCR4-using variants.

11. Evolution of X4 viruses

There are different theories regarding the origin of X4 viruses. One theory postulates that X4 viruses emerge directly from the pre-existing R5 pool as a result of mutations within the HIV V3 loop *env* gene. At least for HIV-1 subtype C, X4 variants have been associated with an amino acid substitution mutation from the conserved GPGQ crown motif to a GPGR. Still some authors argue that X4 viruses are already in the existing pool of viruses but somehow the X4 viruses and R5/X4 viruses remain suppressed by varied host mechanisms and only to be detected in the late phases of infection suggestive that the immune system exerts a selective pressure that hinders the emergence of CXCR4-using variants. However, when the host immune competence begins to deteriorate during the HIV disease progression, it paves way for the emergence of CXCR4-using variants. Another hypothesis proposes that chemokines and the C2-V3-C3 region of HIV gp120 have a common origin such that the HIV ancestor incorporated a chemokine gene into its *env* gene such that this captured chemokine gene rapidly diverge by frequent mutations thereby attaining the ability to effectively interact with various chemokine receptors in a short period of time. Another possible explanation is based on cell division rate where it has been observed that X4 and R5 viruses show preferential tropism for naive and memory T cells, respectively. Since memory T cells divide 10 times more frequently than naive cells, it would be an advantage to have a tropism for CCR5 coreceptor during the first stages of infection.

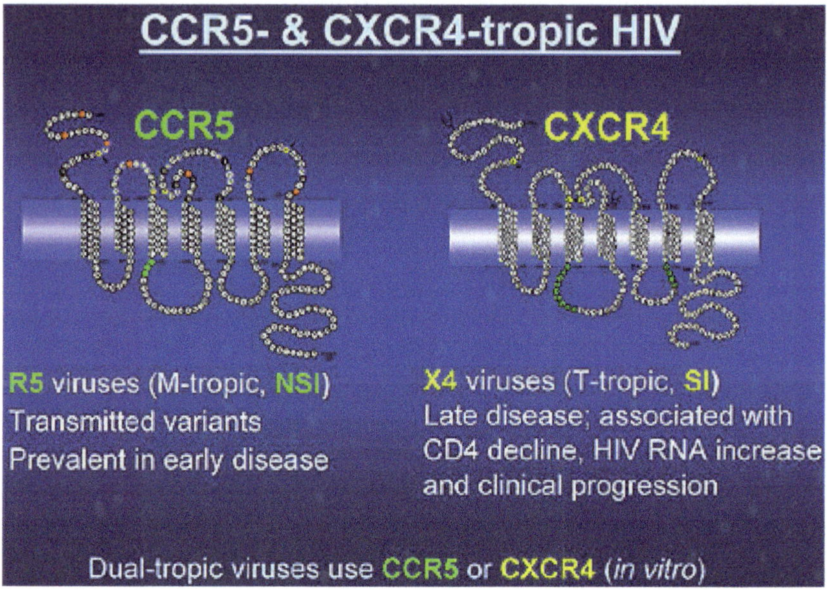

Figure 2. HIV classification adopted from Moyle G, 2008.

12. Coreceptor usage in HIV-2

Studies have shown that the use of coreceptors is much broader in HIV-2 infections relative to HIV-1. In addition to CCR5 and CXCR4 HIV-2 is able to utilise alternative coreceptors such as GPR15, or CXCR6 and to a lesser extent CCR1, CCR2b or CCR3 in aviremic patients whilst CXCR4 is only used in viremic individuals. It still needs to be explored whether this wide use of coreceptors is the underlying reason behind the less virulent phenotype associated with HIV-2, compared to HIV-1.

13. Clinical application of tropism

One property that has been closely correlated with clinical prognosis is the ability to induce syncytia formation in susceptible cells with clinical course of AIDS being associated with a shift from NSI to SI. HIV isolates obtained during early acute infection are generally M-tropic/NSI whilst T-tropic/ SI are associated with disease progression. The emergence of CXCR4-using HIV-1 variants in a patient is almost invariably associated with a subsequent increase in the rate of decline of circulating $CD4^+$ T cells, an accelerated disease progression and a poor prognosis for survival. While CXCR4-using variants can emerge at any stage of infection, untreated individuals who develop such variants progress to AIDS within an average of two years after their first detection. However, the presence of CXCR4-using variants is not an obligatory prerequisite for disease progression as a significant proportion of individuals' progress to AIDS whilst harbouring exclusive R5 HIV-1 variants. The emergence of SI HIV-1 in a sero-positive individual is now generally regarded as a negative prognostic indicator and thus considerable interest has been focused on the HIV-1 genetic determinants of the SI phenotype. Tropism assays are important for determining HIV phenotype before administering coreceptor antagonists in combination antiretroviral therapy. In view of this, tropism assays must taken by HIV infected people with drug resistance who are considering taking coreceptor antagonists. This new class of anti-retroviral targets CCR5-specific HIV during entry into the cell. Thus, knowing the patient's viral tropism can assist and guide the clinician make an informed and effective HIV treatment plan. Consequently, the importance of tropism screening to detect the presence of R5-using HIV may not be over emphasized.

14. Methods for determination of coreceptor usage

With the recent introduction of HIV-1 chemokine receptor antagonists on the market as components of antiretroviral therapy, it is increasingly important to screen HIV patients' coreceptor phenotype or genotype prior to therapy. Hence simple and efficient methods for routinely characterising and monitoring HIV-1 coreceptor phenotypes or genotypes are of paramount importance. Studies have demonstrated that the ability to induce syncytia is determined by regions of env outside the V3 loop that encompass residues that contribute to the binding of CD4 by gp120. Such observations suggest that areas of the HIV-1 *env* gene contributing to the CD4 binding site may also contribute to the determination of SI and NSI genotypes. HIV-1 tropism can be determined by phenotypic or genotypic based methods.

15. Phenotypic methods

HIV-1 tropism can be assessed using phenotypic assays which are currently the most accurate method based on recombinant viruses. Determination of coreceptor use of HIV-1 isolates is done in cell lines such as U87 and GHOST transfected with CCR5 or CXCR4. Patients' plasma is used to generate pseudoviruses or infectious recombinant viruses of full-length or partial viral envelopes derived from the patient's viral population. The recombinants are subsequently tested on indicator cell lines expressing CD4 and either CCR5 or CXCR4. The first commercially available tropism assay became available on the market almost at the same time of approval of the CCR5 antagonist, maraviroc. Its brand name of phenotypic assay is Trofile® manufactured by Monogram Biosciences South San

Francisco, USA. The test can detect 10% of X4 variants with 100% sensitivity. More recently, an enhanced Trofile® assay with better sensitivity to improve detection of low level X4-using variants has been developed that can detect 0.3% of these variants with 100% sensitivity. Trofile® phenotypic assay continues to be the only clinically validated assay to identify coreceptor tropism and is considered the gold standard for tropism testing capable of distinguishing pure R5, D/M and pure X4 populations.

Another phenotypic tropism assay, Phenoscript-tropism; Eurofins is also on the market. It was specifically developed to cater for phenotypic test for the evaluation of viral tropism in HIV-1 non-B subtypes. It is worthwhile to appreciate that the HIV-1 env V3 loop is implicated in the determination of phenotypic tropisms

16. Challenges of phenotypic methods

Despite having high sensitivity phenotypic assays are laborious, expensive, and time-consuming and can only be done in sophisticated laboratories by highly qualified personnel. More so the presence of CXCR4 viruses, which frequently constitute less than 5% of viral population is a challenge as phenotypic assays' sensitivity does not seem to permit this range of detection threshold. Consequently, individuals may be misdiagnosed as harboring only CCR5 coreceptor using virus, when in actual fact they may also be harbouring R4 virus in very low quantities such that once initiated on CCR5 coreceptor antagonists their CXCR4 tropic viruses may emerge. Due to the foregoing bottlenecks there is need for the development of simple, more sensitive, accurate and less expensive tests with a shorter turnaround time to replace slow and resource intensive phenotypic assays.

17. Genotypic coreceptor analysis methods

HIV env gp120 is composed of about 400 amino acids which consists five relatively conserved constant (C1-C5) and five hyper-variable regions (V1-V5). The genetic determinants of HIV-1 coreceptor usage are localized in the V3 loop of gp120 which has a highly conserved crown motif and glycosylation sites. The third variable region also called the V3 loop is composed of 31-39 amino acids. . The V3 loop is closed by a disulfide bridge formed by two cysteines. Functionally it is critical in maintaining the right conformation to facilitate coreceptor interaction with the virus. This region has been shown to be the major determinant of viral tropism and accordingly, prediction of coreceptor usage based on the interpretation of V3 sequences using bioinformatics tools could be a good alternative to infer tropism in the clinical routine Sequences in the N-terminus of V3 loop have been shown to modulate the levels of infection through CCR5 coreceptor. Minor or a few sequence alterations or mutations in V3 are sufficient to switch coreceptor use from CCR5 to CXCR4 or from dual-tropic to X4-tropic virus. Additional mutations within the V1/V2 have also been observed during coreceptor switching. Studies have shown that such mutations seem to compensate for the harmful V3 mutations. Functional studies have demonstrated that the V3 loop interacts with the N-terminal extra-cellular domain of CCR5 and the extracellular loop 2. Bioinformatics tools based on V3 sequences can be used to predict HIV-1 tropism. The identification of viral genotypic changes associated with different coreceptor usage has led to the development of sequence-based algorithms to predict coreceptor usage. Different rules have been published based on the amino acid sequence of the env V3 region of HIV-gp120, which is known to be the major determinant of coreceptor usage.

18. Predictive algorithms of HIV-1 coreceptor usage

At least eight different bioinformatics tools have been used to predict viral tropism in different HIV-1 subtypes which uses phenotypic data to predict the corresponding viral genotype. Studies of genotypic predictors have been retrospective with patient samples selected based on availability of phenotypic tropism determinations. Three of the interpretation systems namely, WetCat, WebPSSM, geno2pheno [coreceptor] are freely available on internet. All three focus on the env-V3 region and only take the amino acid sequence into account. Such genotypic systems provide the possibility for rapid screening of patients who may be administered with CCR5 blockers like maraviroc. On cloned viruses belonging to genetic subtype B, the specificity and sensitivity of most predictive methods exceed 90% and 80%, respectively. While genotypic assays may have lower specificity and sensitivity, retrospective analyses have found that they are comparable to phenotypic tropism assays for prediction of response to treatment with CCR5 antagonists in populations pre-screened with a phenotypic assay. The first genotypic algorithm designed to predict HIV-1 tropism takes into account only the net charge of amino acids at two key residues located within the V3 loop, amino acids at positions 11 and 25. The most widely used is the 11/25 rule which focuses on identifying sequence patterns within the V3 loop. Predictions using the "11/25 charge rule" are relatively satisfactory.

19. Correlation between phenotypic and bioinformatics tools in determining HIV coreceptor use

Evaluation of the performances of genotypic tools to predict HIV-1 tropism has been investigated. Paired genotypic and phenotypic determination of HIV-1 coreceptor usage has been performed to assess several genotypic approaches for detecting CXCR4-using and CCR5-using viruses in a clinical setting. Excellent correlations between HIV-1 V3 genotype and phenotype have been observed. Overall, the accuracy of the bioinformatics tools to detect CXCR4-using virus was similar for ES Trofile and Trofile. However, the negative predictive values for genotypic tools with ES Trofile were slightly higher than they were with Trofile. The accuracy of genotypic algorithms for detecting CXCR4-using viruses is high when using Trofile as the reference. The concordance with ES Trofile is better with higher CD4 cell counts and non-exposure to antiretroviral therapy. The global concordance between genotypic and phenotypic data is 91% with the rule combining the amino-acid residues at positions 11/25 and V3 net charge. Gaining a better understanding of the output of these assays and correlating them with clinical progression and therapy response will provide some indication on how both genotype-based and phenotypic assays for determining HIV coreceptor usage can be improved. Deep V3 sequencing is a promising tool for identifying treatment-experienced individuals who could benefit from CCR5-antagonist-containing regimens.

20. Challenges of genotypic methods

Genotypic predictions are relatively satisfactory but because not all determinants of coreceptor usage lie within the V3 loop, the region employed by most current predictors, causing occasional disagreements. Accurate prediction is also complicated by the fact that the V3-C4 region of the *env* gene, which has the greatest influence on tropism, also has a relatively high rate of diversity such that the sensitivity drops with uncloned sequences and HIV-1 non-B subtypes. Since non-B subtypes show a wide genetic variability in the V3 region and taking cognisance that X4 viruses might be more prevalent in some subtypes than others, there is an urgent need to know the reliability of genotypic tools for inferring HIV-1 tropism in non-B subtypes, especially in regions where these HIV-1 variants are quite prevalent and may soon have access to CCR5 antagonists. Moreover, technical limitations to the generation of unambiguous DNA sequences from the HIV-1 env region that has insertions and deletions may interfere with the generation of clean and clear electropherograms thereby interfering with a predictive determination of tropism in a significant portion of patients' samples. Prospective studies are needed to firmly establish the clinical usefulness of genotypic tropism determination. Further research is also warranted regarding the need for specific genetic characteristics of dual/mixed-tropic HIV-1 strains which also exist in a significant proportion of patients.

21. HIV-1 coreceptor usage and genetic subtypes

There are remarkable differences in the prevalence of CXCR4-using variants among different HIV-1 genetic subtypes and circulating recombinant forms (CRFs). Since CXCR4-using variants emerge after an accumulation of mutations, the different prevalence observed may reflect the same phenomenon at the population level. Infection with subtype-C accounts for over half of the worldwide HIV-1 epidemics and is rapidly expanding in Southern Africa, South East Asia and India. Studies have shown this rapidly expanding subtype C isolates almost exclusively use the CCR5 coreceptor, with CXCR4 usage being rarely observed. Some authors argue that the predominant usage of CCR5 by HIV-1 subtype C isolates is more due to sampling artifacts rather than any fundamental biological properties of these viruses. Unique to subtype C is the determinant of coreceptor usage, the V3 regions which has been shown to be highly conserved and have a low overall positive charge, which is consistent with the NSI phenotypes compared to other subtypes. Moreover, this atypical property of the subtype C envelope glycoproteins might be the reason behind the rapid expansion of the virus being currently observed. In view of this, there is need for intervention strategies that are subtype specific to curb this pandemic tailor designed for use in areas where subtype C viruses predominate. R5-using viruses have also been found to be more common in subtype A than subtype D HIV-1 infections. The emergence of X4 viruses occurs very early among subtype D-infected individuals. More so, a high proportion of subtype D infections have been shown to display D/M tropism throughout the course of disease. An inverse skewing in coreceptor usage, with an increased presence of CXCR4-using strains, has instead been reported for subtype-D HIV-1. This observation is consistent with the faster pace of disease progression reported for subtype-D infection both in Africa and abroad. An increased rate of CXCR4 usage has also been reported for CRF AE isolates common in South East Asia. There are proposals to the effect that the increase in prevalence of CXCR4-using HIV-1 variants increases with the age of the subtype epidemic. Indeed recent phylogenetic studies suggest that the proportion of patients with detectable CXCR4 using HIV-1 variants varies with subtype D having the highest CXCR4 switch rate being the oldest whilst subtype C with the lowest CXCR4 switch rate being the youngest. Subtype B predominant in North America and Europe has demonstrated that CXCR4 coreceptor usage increases with time following infection with or without concurrent use of R5 in 50% of HIV-1 infected individuals. The HIV-1 subtype-B epidemic has an intermediate pattern, both in terms of age and prevalence of CXCR4-using HIV-1 variants. This assumption is highly speculative and not supported by all the data available at present. However, if confirmed it would imply that all the subtype epidemics are evolving towards a higher prevalence of CXCR4-using HIV-1 variants although it is plausible that each epidemic would reach a point of equilibrium beyond which such prevalence will not further increase.

22. HIV coreceptor usage and compartmentalization

Compartmentalization is the occurrence of distinct yet phylogenetically related HIV-1 phenotypes or genotypes within different anatomic sites, an observation common amongst both treated and untreated individuals. Differences in selective pressures may shape the distinct viral populations in different compartments. Anatomic compartmentalization of HIV coreceptor usage variants has been described in diverse tissues including in blood, lungs, brain, central nervous system, breast milk and genital tract. Studies have shown that the distribution of R5 and CXCR4-using variants differ in different blood compartments. Higher prevalence of predicted CXCR4-using variants in PBMC than in plasma has been reported. The limited compartmentalization and the clonal amplification of evolving functional viruses in milk indicate continual seeding of the mammary gland by blood virus variants, followed by transient local replication of these variants in the breast compartment.

Gender studies have demonstrated different viral variants between genital tract and blood for both women and men. Differences in genetic strains between blood- and semen-derived HIV isolates within the same individual have been documented. Male genital tract tissues such as the prostate, seminal vesicles, and epididymis which serve as sites of viral replication have been found to develop distinct, compartment-specific HIV strains in response to these local selective pressures. Studies seeking to determine chemokine receptor preference for all sequences derived from patients with compartmentalized virus to determine if seminal tropism correlated with altered coreceptor usage have shown a trend towards reduced CXCR4 usage in the male genital tract.

Other environmental factors such as sexually transmitted infections (STIs) have been also shown to exert selective pressures. Genital inflammation can stimulate the expression of R5 receptors dramatically, conferring a selective advantage on R5 virus in the genital tract of women with STIs. A history of intravenous drug use (IDU) among women has been shown to correlate with larger proportions of X4 strains in plasma relative to those without an IDU record. Quantifying the proportion of R5 and X4 viruses in each compartment has been found to vary significantly between them. Thus, the proportion of X4 strains in one compartment does not necessarily reflect coreceptor usage in the other suggesting that measuring coreceptor usage in say the genital tract and blood may aid in effective monitoring of disease progression and response to therapy as efficiencies of antiretroviral drug penetration has also been found to differ with compartments. Hence, there is need for compartment specific treatment outcome monitoring of patients and also the most appropriate choice of patient material for the determination of HIV-1 coreceptor usage remains to be established.

23. Chemokine receptors and viral entry into host cells

The entry of HIV into cells is critically dependent on the sequential interaction of the viral envelope with two cell-surface receptors, the CD4 glycoprotein and CCR5 or CXCR4. The evolutionary choice of HIV of exploiting chemokine receptors as entry gateways has established a tight biological bond between HIV and the chemokine system, making the respective natural ligands of these receptors potent viral inhibitors. Entry into target cells by HIV occurs by a multi-step process that culminates with the fusion of viral and cellular membrane as shown in **figure 3** below. Many enveloped viruses including HIV possess a fusion protein in their envelopes which confers the ability of the virion to fuse with the host cell membrane and thus allowing entry of the infectious genomic material into the cell cytoplasm. Receptor interactions then trigger gp41 to promote membrane fusion. This reaction is thought to involve extension of the gp41 subunit to allow insertion of its N-terminal 'fusion peptide' into the target cell membrane, followed by refolding the prefusion intermediate into an energetically favorable six-helix bundle that brings the two membranes together so that fusion can occur. During replication of the virus, expression of the fusion protein on the cell membrane can result in the fusion of neighbouring cells forming multi-nucleate cells or syncytia.

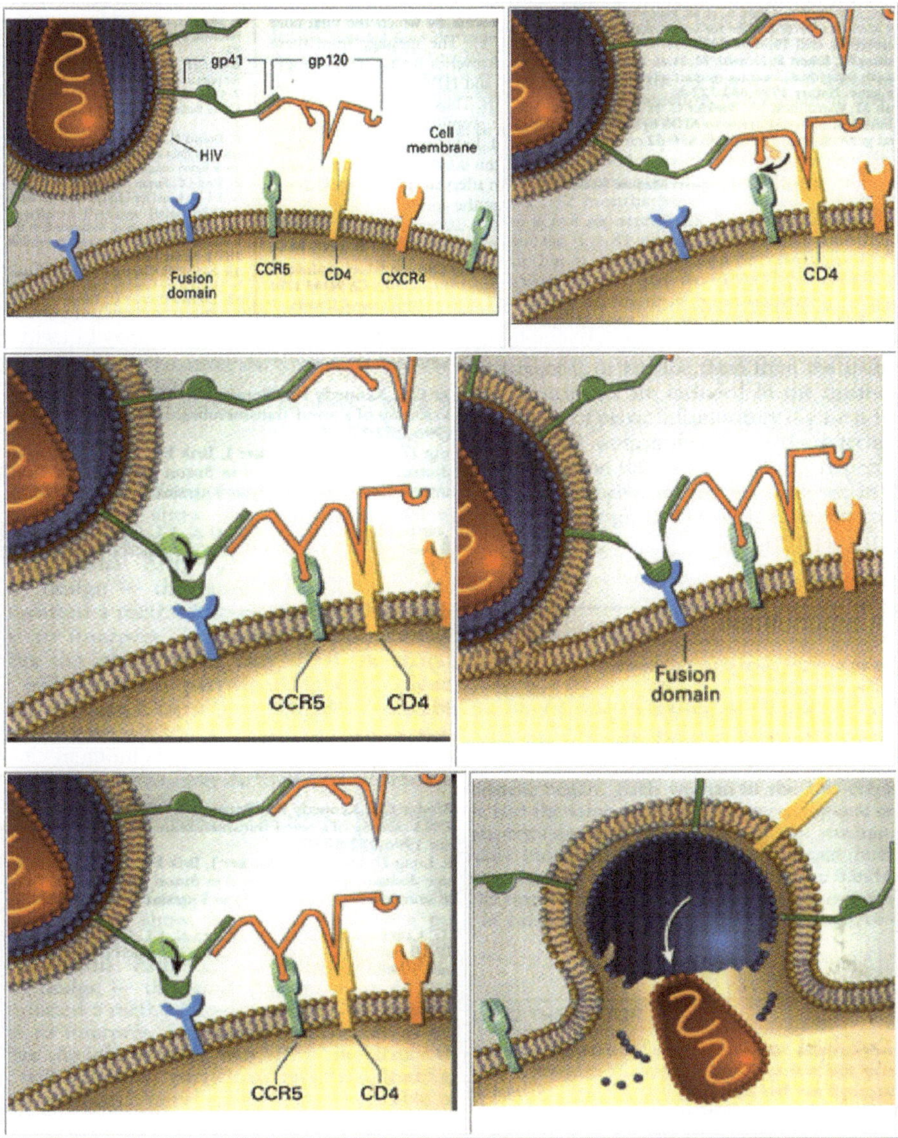

Figure 3. Interaction between HIV-1 and the cell surface Molecules, adopted from Levy J, 1996

24. Coreceptor usage and HIV-1 transmission

Irrespective of the transmission route or HIV-1 subtype, R5 viruses are preferentially transmitted in both horizontal and vertical transmission events except for subtype D. HIV transmission via breastfeeding accounts for a considerable proportion of infant HIV acquisition. However, no conclusive evidence has been provided to indicate that CXCR4-using strains are less able or unable to sustain mucosal transmission. For example simian chimeric immunodeficiency viruses (SHIV) bearing an X4 HIV-1 envelope can be readily transmitted via the mucosal route in macaques, and have widely been used as a reference model. Another important element that is rarely taken into consideration in the HIV-1 transmission equation is the transmitter bias which suggests that individuals with replicating CXCR4- using viruses are more likely to be in a more advanced stage of their disease progression and hence are more likely to be too ill to engage in risky sexual behavior. Majority of transmissions occur from asymptomatic individuals who generally harbor R5 variants. Consequently, the transmission of CXCR4-using variants may in fact be more frequent than it appears, albeit underestimated due to late sampling. Although primary infection with CXCR4-using HIV-1 strains is believed to be a rare event, mixed R5/X4 primary infections have been documented. Vertical transmission of dual tropic HIV-1 has also been demonstrated. Genotypic characteristics of HIV-1 V3 loop that are preferentially vertically transmitted for different subtypes remain unclear yet this information is critical for the development of effective transmission preventive strategies. At least for HIV-1 subtype B maternal viral phenotype can be predictive of the newborn's viral phenotype whilst the dual R5X4 phenotype is predominantly lost during vertical transmission. Antenatal HIV-1 subtype C coreceptor usage is generally preserved in vertical transmission and can be predictive of the newborn's viral genotype.

25. Co receptor usage and HIV Disease progression

Coreceptor usage is a marker for disease progression. There is a continued evolution in viral coreceptor usage in vivo, resulting in a broad range of coreceptor affinities within the HIV-1 quasi-species. Discriminating between these and other alternatives is central to increasing our understanding of the fundamental pathogenic processes involved in HIV-1 infection.

26. CCR5 HIV-1 variants

During the asymptomatic phase of HIV-1 infection a homogeneous R5 virus population is commonly present that can replicate efficiently in both T cells and macrophages. The early stages of HIV infection and the latency phase are characterised by CCR5 coreceptor using viral variants which are less virulent, non-syncytium-inducing and are associated with reduced progression to AIDS. A significant proportion of patients progresses to full-blown AIDS without experiencing an overt switch to CXCR4 usage, indicating that CCR5 usage remains a critical coreceptor throughout the course of HIV infection. This has been supported by the observation that the ability of R5 isolates to replicate in macrophages is progressively reduced during the course of infection, resulting in a predominantly T-cell tropic R5 HIV-1 quasi-species even before the progression to AIDS. However, studies have shown that these late stage homogeneous CCR5 isolates are more pathogenic than the earlier isolates. In line with this observation is the ability of late-stage CCR5-restricted HIV-1 variants to use chimeric coreceptors where some parts of CCR5 would have been replaced with segments of CXCR4 (R5 broad), whilst early CCR5-using HIV-1 variants are restricted to the use of wild-type CCR5 (R5 narrow). This *in vivo* evolution of CCR5-restricted HIV-1 in humans is similar to that observed in non-human primates infected with SIV, which never acquires CXCR4 usage even though its pathogenicity increases during the late disease stages. This evolution is accompanied by improved coreceptor-binding affinity, which in turn is reflected in decreasing sensitivities of R5 variants to inhibition by CCR5-binding chemokines and small- molecule CCR5 antagonists.

27. Co-existence of R5 and CXCR4- HIV-1 variants

Some HIV-1 variants can use either coreceptor hence they are termed dual/mixed (DM)-tropic. These have been detected in all stages of infection although they are more common in infections of longer duration, with lower $CD4^+$ cell counts and higher viral loads. Such strains produce gp120 molecules capable of recognizing the CXCR4 protein on CD4-bearing T-cells. During this phase HIV-1 may infect both macrophages and T-cells. Still later, the bulk of the viral population may switch it's preference to the CXCR4 receptor and become T-tropic. T-tropic viruses readily destroy infected T-cells, contributing to the collapse of the immune system and the onset of AIDS. Evidence suggests that the evolutionary changes in the V3 loop involved in the coreceptor-usage switch are gradual with dual coreceptor usage (R5X4) representing an intermediate transitional phase. Once established the DM–tropic viruses have been shown to develop the optimal fitness to predominate during the transition phase, although they may eventually be outcompeted by HIV-1 variants with a pure X4 phenotype.

28. X4 variants

Following years of chronic HIV infection X4 using strains emerge although this phenomenon is not consistently observed in all patients progressing to AIDS. This switch of coreceptor usage has been shown to be associated with accelerated decrease in CD4 cells and hence it could be an important determinant of HIV pathogenesis and disease progression. The emergence of X4 variants has also been shown to coincide with disease progression and has been associated with longer duration of antiretroviral treatment including higher risk of death. The mechanism by which X4 viruses are associated with accelerated disease progression has never been properly elucidated although one theory proposes that R5-viruses lose their fitness with time, showing an abrupt decline in their ability to use CCR5 coreceptors and to infect cell lines with low CCR5 expression, demonstrating an increased susceptibility to CCR5 inhibitors consequently creating a pro-X4-virus environment. It has also been postulated that the decline of the host immune system associated with clinical AIDS may allow X4 viruses to evolve and replicate freely in late-stage infection. Furthermore, it has also been reported that disease progression among individuals infected with subtypes D and C is faster than in those infected with subtypes A and A/G in Africa and that subtype D infection leads to faster rates of CD4 cell decline and subsequent virological failure compared to infection with subtype B and other non-subtype B HIV strains in England.

29. Host coreceptor genes & insights on resistance to HIV infection

A disproportionate transmission and distribution of HIV epidemic in the world has been observed with alarming rates in Sub Saharan Africa (SSA). Currently there is very little explanation for this observation of differences in susceptibility to HIV infection which could among other factors be attributable to variation in host genetics. Host genetic factors, including some polymorphisms in chemokine receptors and chemokine genes have been identified as having an impact on both HIV-1 infection and disease progression to death. Scientists have observed that despite multiple or repeated unprotected sexual exposures to HIV-1, some individuals remain HIV sero-negative. More so the discovery of long-term non-progressors (LTNP) in HIV infection prompted further investigations to ascertain the role of host genetic factors in the progression of HIV infection to AIDS. Polymorphisms in these human chemokine receptor genes will therefore affect the evolution of HIV-1.

30. CCR5 gene mutation

Analysis of blood samples from infected persons and the repeatedly exposed but somehow uninfected have shown specific molecular differences within the coding and regulatory regions of chemokine receptors and coreceptors genes. There is a deletion of 32 base pairs from the coding region of CCR5 gene in the second ECL. In these individuals the 32-base deletion in the CCR5 gene results in a frame shift and truncation of the normal CCR5 protein which renders them uninfectable after exposure to CCR5 tropic HIV viruses. This aberrant protein has been associated with protection against HIV-1 infection in people who are homozygous for mutant genotypes. Thus individuals resistant to HIV infection inherit two mutated copies of the dysfunctional gene for CCR5 from either parent. Without functional coreceptors, HIV is not able to enter immune cells. Despite the strong protective effect conferred by congenital CCR5 deficiencies, a handful of infected *CCR5-Δ32* homozygotes have been reported, all invariably harboring CXCR4- dependent HIV-1 strains. The rare homozygous individuals that got infected by HIV have been shown to be through CXCR4 coreceptor mediated entry only. Interestingly it has been found that in such homozygous conditions there is no evidence of health/phenotypic impairment caused by the absence of functional CCR5 coreceptors. However, HIV-infected individuals who would have inherited a copy of the defective CCR5 gene from only one parent, heterozygotes for a Δ32 deletion (CCR5-wt/Δ32) are not protected against HIV-1 infection but are associated with a much slow progression to AIDS relative to those with two normal copies of the gene. Heterozygous individuals have lower plasma HIV RNA levels in the early years of infection, which gives them a medical advantage of delaying disease progression. Since these mutations do not account for all cases of resistance to HIV infection, scientists are looking for other possible host factors, including genetic defects involving other coreceptors. It was this protective property of CCR5Δ32 against HIV infection that has prompted pharmaceutical companies to develop a CCR5 antagonist for clinical use in the treatment of HIV/AIDS. Studies have shown that inhibition of CCR5 coreceptor seems not to cause significant clinical harmful consequences yet surprising to date there has not been any description of natural genetic alteration in CXCR4 human gene, suggestive that mutations in this gene are incompatible with life.

31. Epidemiology of CCR5Δ32 gene

A general North to South downhill gradient in CCR5Δ32 gene frequency has been observed. The highest frequency has been found in Northern and North-eastern Europe especially amongst the Finnish and Swedish populations. Data confirm the high frequency of CCR5-Delta 32 among northern European Caucasians, a gene frequency declining across Europe and Asia reflecting recent population admixture. The virtual absence of CCR5-Delta 32 deletion among native Africans, East Asians, and American-Indians is suggestive that the mutation arose in northern Europe in response to selective pressures due to other factors including infection epidemics. The CCR5Δ32 has a prevalence rate of between 20-35% among the Jewish population. In Africa studies indicated that the allelic frequency of CCR5Δ32 mutation is 0.1% in the black South African population.

32. CCR2 –V641 mutation

A CCR2 –V641 mutation from a conservative valine to isoleucine substitution in the transmembrane region has also been associated with some protective effects against HIV infection and reduction in progression of HIV to AIDS. The protective effect of CCR2 –V641 is believed is to be through regulation linkage disequilibrium in the regulatory region or promoter region of this gene. CCR2-V64I is common among Africans, yet this race is one of the most affected populations by the HIV pandemic. Hence, the protective effect of CCR2 –V641 against HIV infection remains controversial. Despite the availability of evidence linking some host genetic factors to protection against HIV infection, very little information is available regarding the role of CCR5-Δ32 and CCR2-V64I polymorphism on HIV transmission.

33. Coreceptor antagonists and antiretroviral therapy

To successfully infect an immune cell HIV env gp 120 has to interact with the host cellular receptor CD4 and either a CCR5 or CXCR4. Both coreceptors are recognized as novel targets for anti-HIV-therapy consequently resulting in the development of a new class of antiretroviral drugs called coreceptor antagonists or blockers. Blocking these coreceptors would protect the host cell from viral entry and would reduce the viral transmission and pathogenesis. Interestingly coreceptor antagonists differ from the other antiretroviral agents that target HIV proteins in the sense that they bind and inhibit receptors encoded by the host itself. Besides blocking replication of the virus in other cells, coreceptor antagonists may reduce the decline of immune system through other ways. It is known that HIV-1 env glycoproteins may trigger autophagy in uninfected CD4 positive T cells, leading to their apoptosis, and consequently increasing immune decline. These cells need to present, among other things, a CXCR4 coreceptor in their surface. The blockage of the interaction between glycoproteins and the coreceptor of uninfected cells could help to avoid immune impairment. CCR5 antagonists design and development are a step ahead relative to their CXCR4 counterparts. This unique new class of drugs not only increases the alternative therapeutic options for HIV treatment but also maximizes potency, minimizes toxicity and reduces the risk of drug resistance development. Range of coreceptor antagonists discovered to date includes modified chemokines monoclonal antibodies, peptides and small organic molecules.

34. Mechanism of action of coreceptor antagonists

Coreceptor antagonists' antiviral properties are related to their ability to internalize the receptor, preventing it from being expressed on the cell surface thereby avoiding viral replication by reducing coreceptors availability to bind to HIV glycoproteins.

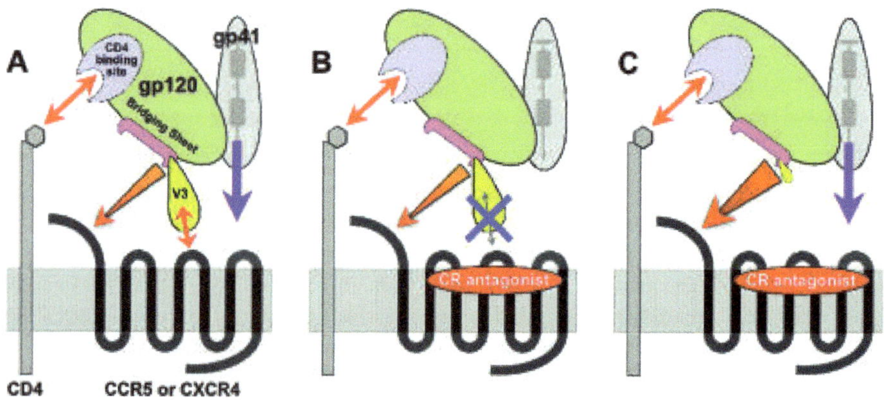

Figure 4. Mode of Action of Coreceptor antagonists

35. Coreceptor antagonists in development

35.1. Modified chemokines

Modified chemokines include RANTES, a natural chemokine ligand for CCR5 manufactured by RANTES engineering technology including other novel agents that have not been very successful and their future remains uncertain. Other possible antagonists are zinc finger nucleases that cause mutagenesis in the CCR5 gene by binding and cleaving the gene, producing abnormal proteins. Zinc fingers, along with RNA interference, ribozymes, intrakines, and intrabodies are HIV-1 vector-delivered genetic disruption mechanisms that target HIV-1 chemokine receptors. Although chemokines or derivative-molecules could be exploited as therapeutic agents against HIV, the risk of inducing inflammatory side-effects or of interfering with the physiology of the homeostatic chemokine system represents a potential limitation.

36. Monoclonal antibodies as coreceptor antagonists

Another type of coreceptor antagonists are monoclonal antibodies. Examples of such agents are CCR5mAb004 of Human Genome Sciences (Rockville, MD, USA) and PRO 140 of Progenics Pharmaceuticals (Tarrytown, NY, USA). They are both mouse-derived but humanized monoclonal antibodies capable of blocking CCR5 without activating the signal transduction pathways. In phase I clinical trials CCR5mAb004 has been shown to be safe and well tolerated.

37. Small molecule CXR4 chemokine receptor antagonists

AMD3100 is a small-molecule CXCR4 antagonist with activity against X4 viruses' in vitro and antiviral activity in vivo, although it is no longer being pursued clinically because of pharmacology and toxicology considerations. More examples of small molecule chemokine receptor antagonists of CXCR4 coreceptor include AMD11070/ AMD070, AMD3465, ALX40-4C, T22, T134 and T140. AMD11070 is known to specifically inhibit CXCR4 in a reversible way. Other CXCR4 selective inhibitor is AMD3100 from AnorMED. AMD3100 is highly specific for CXCR4 that blocks replication of X4 strains. However, clinical trials of AMD3100 have been stopped due to side effects of cardiotoxicity. A relatively safer derivative of AMD3100 known as AMD070 is currently undergoing clinical trials. Previously AMD3100 has proved to be a useful tool to probe interactions between env proteins and CXCR4 which is important to identify pathways by which HIV-1 may become resistant to this class of antiviral agents. To date none of CXCR4 blockers has successfully proceeded into clinical practice due to their severe side effects. Generally, CXCR4-based blocking agents are less attractive due to the crucial role of CXCR4 in many biological processes. However, agents that aim at down-modulating CXCR4 expression may provide some benefits to HIV-positive patients. Antagonism of CXCR4 has been shown to significantly improve survival from lethal infection through enhanced intraparenchymal migration of West Nile Virus-specific CD8+ T cells within the brain, leading to reduced viral loads and decreased immunopathology at affected sites.

38. Small-molecule CCR5 antagonists

The CCR5 antagonists act on a wide spectrum of viruses with affinity or tropism for this receptor. They are absorbed orally and have powerful antiviral activity through interaction with amino acids from the pocket formed by the transmembrane (TM) domains of CCR5. Mechanism of action is through allosteric effects, altering extracellular CCR5 conformation after binding to a hydrophobic pocket of CCR5, formed by transmembrane helices. Mutations within transmembrane domains are associated with impaired activity. Small molecule CCR5 antagonists such as maraviroc, vicriviroc, aplaviroc, TAK-779, and TAK-220) have been found to fit in the same binding pocket. Other small-molecule CCR5 antagonists include:

Tak-652, spirodiketopiperazine derivatives such as E913 and SCH-C/SCH-351125. Spirodiketopiperazine derivatives have been associated with severe hepatotoxicity, leading to the cancellation of their development. SCH351125 or SCH-C was the first CCR5 antagonist to enter clinical efficacy studies but has been dropped out due to variable antiviral effect and provocation of prolonged QTc interval. To counter these setbacks Vicriviroc was developed which was much more potent than SCH-C, safer and better oral bioavailability.

Two agents, maraviroc and vicriviroc, are the agents within this family that have passed the final stages of clinical development. These agents have their scientific names ending in "–viroc", to denote their action of "viral receptor occupancy". Since these drugs show activity against R5 viruses only, viral tropism testing should be made before their prescription and eventually during treatment in order to exclude the presence of X4 viruses. They are less expensive to produce and have good oral bioavailability. Their half maximal inhibitory concentrations (IC50) are in the nanomolar ranges.

39. Maraviroc

A success story has been the introduction CCR5 antagonist, Maraviroc, trade name Selzentry or Celsentri into clinical practice. Maraviroc is a non-competitive CCR5 antagonist that selectively binds to the human CCR5, present on the cell membrane, preventing the interaction with HIV-1 env gp 120. CCR5 is necessary for CCR5-tropic HIV-1 to enter cells. It is metabolized in the liver. Drug plasma concentrations are likely to be increased in patients with hepatic impairment. Route of metabolism is through Cytochrome P450 3A4 (CYP3A). The drug has shown potent activity against multidrug-resistance CCR5-tropic HIV-1 strains. It has antiviral activity *in vitro* against CCR5 tropic HIV-1 isolates from various subtypes. However, Maraviroc has no activity against CXCR4-tropic and dual tropic HIV-1. It has been found to be effective, efficient and safe to use in combination with other antiretroviral agents such as with lopinavir/ritonavir plus efavirenz or saquinavir/ritonavir plus efavirenz in adult patients with exclusive CCR5 tropic HIV-1 isolates. Maraviroc was developed by Pfizer Inc. (Kent, UK).

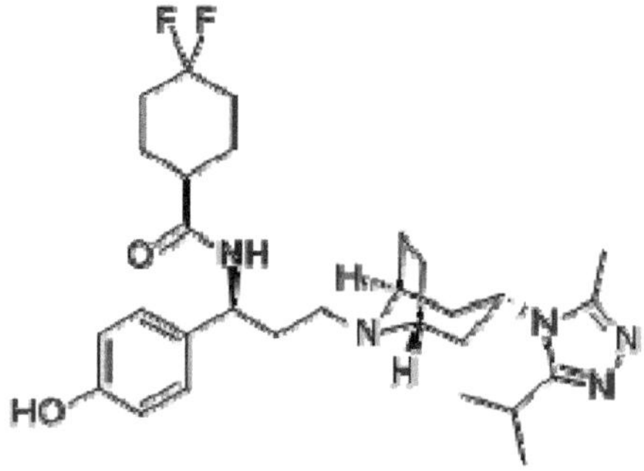

Figure 5. Structure of Maraviroc adopted from chemicalbook.com

Maraviroc inhibit CCR5 binding and signaling at nanomolar (nM) concentrations (IC_{90} of 2 nM). It is well tolerated with most common mild to moderate side-effects including headache, asthenia, dizziness, gingivitis and nausea. It is known that before starting on a coreceptor antagonist, patients need to determine their viral tropism. The introduction of the CCR5 antagonist, maraviroc for HIV-1 therapy has increased the research interest in the epidemiology of tropism and its relationship with HIV-1 subtype. A greater understanding of the tropism of non-B subtypes is key for the optimal use of CCR5 antagonists in the treatment of these infections in the developing world and HIV-1 prevention strategies. There is no food effect as it can be taken with or without food and can be stored at room temperature. Hence it is very suitable for resource poor settings which also bear the brunt of the HIV scourge with predominant R5 variants.

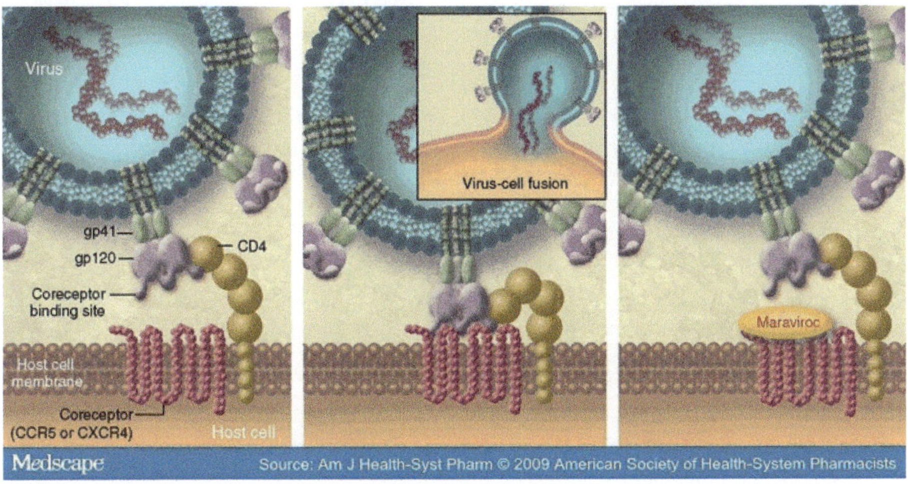

Figure 6. Mode of action of maraviroc, adopted from Qian K, 2008.

40. Challenges of CCR5 antagonists

The CCR5-to-CXCR4 switch represents a concern because while CCR5 inhibitors suppress R5 viruses they may allow the emergence of CXCR4-tropic viruses. Efforts to develop HIV entry inhibitors are hampered by problems associated with rapid evolution of the virus, leading to drug resistance. Blocking only one of the pathways for HIV entry into cells has resulted in the opening of the other pathways potentially accelerating disease progression by promoting the evolution of more virulent CXCR4-dependent variants. In this view, AnorMED Company has announced the discovery and development of a joint CXCR4/CCR5 antagonist although little is known about the binding mechanism at this time.

41. Future of coreceptor antagonists

There have been speculations that new, safe and effective chemokine receptor inhibitors should facilitate CCR5 and CXCR4 internalization independent of the cellular signaling. The most anticipated eventual combination of CXCR4 and CCR5 inhibitors would be beneficial, since selective pressure could direct the virus to use less productive coreceptors, avoiding the progression of the disease. In addition leveraging new technologies capable of detecting low-level minority species may provide the most significant advances in ensuring that individuals with low levels of dual/mixed tropic virus are not inadvertently prescribed CCR5 antagonists.

Author details

Kerina Duri
University of Zimbabwe, College of Health Sciences, Department of Immunology, Harare, Zimbabwe

42. References

[1] Asjo B, Morfeldt-Manson L, Albert J, Biberfeld G, Karlsson A, Lidman K, et al. Replicative capacity of human immunodeficiency virus from patients with varying severity of HIV infection Lancet 1986 Sep 20;2(8508):660-2.

[2] Hoffman TL and Doms RW (1999). HIV-1 envelope determinants for cell tropism and chemokine receptor use. Mol Membr Biol 16: 57-65.

[3] Sundaravaradan V, Das SR, Ramakrishnan R, Sehgal S, Gopalan S, Ahmad N and Jameel S (2007). The role of HIV-1 subtype C V3 to C5 region in viral entry, coreceptor utilization and replication efficiency in primary T- lymphocytes and monocyte derived macrophages. Virology Journal, 4:126

[4] Johnston ER, Zijenah LS, Mutetwa S, Kantor R, Kittinunvorakoon C and Katzenstein DA (2003). High frequency of syncytium–inducing and CXCR4–Tropic viruses among human Immunodeficiency virus type 1 subtype C infected patients receiving antiretroviral treatment. J. Virol 77(13): 7682-7688.

[5] Moyle GJ, Wildfire A Mandalia S. (2005) Epidemiology and predictive factors for chemokine receptor use in HIV-1 infection. J. Infect Dis 191: 866-872.

[6] Casper CHE, Clevestig P, Carlenor E, Leitner T, Anzen B, Lidman K, Belfrage E, Albert J, Bohlin AB, Naver L, Lindgren S, Fenyo EM and Ehrnst AC (2002). Link between the X4 phenotype in Human Immunodeficiency Virus Type 1 infected mothers and their children, despite the early presence of R5 in the child. JID 186: 914-921

[7] Regoes RR and Bonhoeffer S (2005) The HIV coreceptor switch: a population dynamics perspective. Trends Microbiol.13: 269-277.

[8] Huang W, Toma J, Stawiski E, Frasen S, Wrin T, Parkin N, Whitcomb JM, Coakley E, Hecht FM, Deeks SG, Gandhi RT, Eshleman SH and Petropoulos CJ (2009). Characterisation of Human Immunodeficiency virus type 1 population containing CXCR4- using variants from recently infected individuals. AIDS Research and Human Retroviruses 25(8): 795-802.

[9] Huang W, Eshleman SH, Toma J, Stawiski E, Whitcomb JM (2007). Coreceptor tropism in human immunodeficiency virus type 1 subtype D: high prevalence of CXCR4 tropism and heterogeneous composition of viral population. J. Virol 81: 7885-7893).

[10] Sayana and Homayoon Khanlou, (2008). Maraviroc: a new CCR5 antagonistic. Expert Rev. Anti Infect Ther 7(1): 9-19.

[11] Hunt JS and Romanelli F (2009). Maraviroc, a CCR5 coreceptor antagonist that blocks entry of Human Immunodeficiency Virus type 1. Pharmacotherapy 29(3):295-304

[12] Delobel P, Nugeyre MT, Cazabat M, Pasquier C, Marchou B, Massip P (2007). Population based sequencing of the V3 region of *env* for predicting the coreceptor usage of human immunodeficiency virus type I quasispecies. J Clin Microbiol: 45: 1572-1580.

[13] Raymond S, Delobel P, Mavigner M, Cazabat M, Souyris C, Sandres-Saune K, Cuzin L, Marchou B, Massip P and Izopet J (2008). Correlation between genotype predictions based V3 sequences and phenotypic determination of HIV-1 tropism. AIDS 22: F11-F16.

[14] Jensen MA, Coetzer M, van't Wout AB, Morris L. and Mullins JI (2006). A reliable phenotype predictor for Human Immunodeficiency virus type 1 subtype C based on envelope v3 sequences. J of Virol: 80: 4698-4704.

[15] Moore JP, Kitchen SG, Pugach P, Zack JA. The CCR5 and CXCR4 coreceptors: central to understanding the transmission and pathogenesis of human Immunodeficiency virus type 1 infection. AIDS Res Hum Retroviruses 2004: 20: 111-126.

[16] Clerici M, Butto S. and Lukwiya M (2000). Immune activation in Africa is environmentally –driven and is associated with up-regulation of CCR5. Italian-Ugandan AIDS Project. AIDS 14: 2083-2092.

[17] Poveda E, Briz V, de Mendoza C, Benito JM, Corral A, Zahonero N, Lozano S Gonzalez-Lahoz and Soriano V (2007). Prevalence of X4 tropic HIV-1 variants in patients with differences in disease stage and exposure to antiretroviral therapy. J Med virology 79: 1040-1049.

[18] Huang W, Eshleman SH, Toma J, Stawiski E, Whitcomb JM, Jackson JB, Guay L, Musoke P, Parkin N and Petropoulos CJ (2009). Vertical transmission of X4 tropic and dual tropic HIV-1 in five Ugandan mother-infant pairs. AIDS: 23 (14): 1903-1908.

[19] Fitzgibbon JE, Gaur S, Gavai M, Gregory P, Frenkel LD, John JF Jr. (1998) Effect of the HIV-1 syncytium- inducing phenotype on disease stage in vertically–infected children. J. Med Virol 55: 56-63.

[20] Coetzer M, Cilliers T, Ping L, Swanstrom R and Morris L (2006) Genetic characteristics of the V3 region associated with CXCR4 usage in HIV-1 subtype C isolates. Virology 356: 95-105.

[21] Nabatov AA, Pollakis G, Linnemann T, Kliphius A, Chalaby MI, Paxton WA (2004). Intra-patient alteration in the human immunodeficiency virus type 1 gp120 V1V2 and V3 regions differentially modulate coreceptor usage, virus inhibition by CC7CXC chemokines, soluble CD4 and b12 and 2G12 monoclonal antibodies. J Virol 78(1): 524-530.

[22] Mild M, Kvist A, Esbjornsson J, Karlsson I Fenyo EM and Medstrand P (2009). Differences in molecular evolution between switch (R5 to R5X4/X4-tropic) and non switch (R5 tropic only) HIV-1 populations during infection. Infection, Genetic & evolution MEEGID- 584: 1-9

[23] Imai T, Hieshima K, Haskell C, Baba M, Nagira M, Nishimura M, Kakizaki M, Takagi S, Nomiyama H, Schall TJ, Yoshie O (November 1997). "Identification and molecular

characterization of fractalkine receptor CX3CR1, which mediates both leukocyte migration and adhesion". *Cell* 91 (4): 521–30

[24] Imai T, Hieshima K, Haskell C, Baba M, Nagira M, Nishimura M, Kakizaki M, Takagi S, Nomiyama H, Schall TJ, Yoshie O (November 1997). "Identification and molecular characterization of fractalkine receptor CX3CR1, which mediates both leukocyte migration and adhesion". *Cell* 91 (4): 521–30

[25] Duri K, Soko W, Gumbo F, Kristiansen K, Mapingure M, Stray-Pedersen B, Muller, F and the BHAMC Group. ARHR 2010; 27(4):411-419.Genotypic analysis of Human Immunodeficiency Virus type 1 (HIV-1) env V3 loop sequences: Bioinformatics prediction of coreceptor usage among 28 infected mother-infant pairs in a drug-naive population.

[26] Duri K, Gumbo FZ, Kristiansen KI, Mapingure MP, Munjoma M, Rusakaniko S, Chirenje MZ, Stray-Pedersen B and Muller F. ARHR 2011 Dec [Epub ahead of print].Phylogenetic Analysis of Human Immunodeficiency Virus type 1 (HIV-1) Subtype C Env gp 120 sequences among four drug naïve families following subsequent heterosexual and vertical transmissions.

[27] Pillai SK, Good B, Pond SK, Wong JK, Strain MC, Richman DD, et al. Semen-specific genetic characteristics of human immunodeficiency virus type 1 env. J Virol 2005 Feb;79(3):1734-42.

[28] Typical chemokine receptor structure showing seven transmembrane domains and a characteristic "DRY" motif in the second intracellular domain. In *Wikipedia, the free encyclopedia*, vol. 29 KB; 2006.

[29] Mild M, Esbjornsson J, Fenyo EM, Medstrand P: Frequent intra-patient recombination between human immunodeficiency virus type 1 R5 and X4 envelopes: implications for coreceptor switch. *J Virol* 2007, 81: 3369-3376.

[30] Qian K, Morris-Natschke SL, Lee KH: HIV entry inhibitors and their potential in HIV therapy. *Med Res Rev*2008.

[31] Salazar-Gonzalez JF, Salazar MG, Learn GH, Fouda GG, Kang HH, Mahlokozera T, et al. Origin and evolution of HIV-1 in breast milk determined by single-genome amplification and sequencing. J Virol 2011 Mar;85(6):2751-63.

Chapter 11

HIV-Infected Patients and Potential Impact on Thrombotic Events

Hortensia Álvarez Díaz, Ana Mariño Callejo and
José Francisco García Rodríguez

Additional information is available at the end of the chapter

1. Introduction

There is increasing evidence that infection with HIV may be associated with a hypercoagulate state.

The incidence of thrombotic events in Human Immunodeficiency Virus (HIV)-infected patients is rising as suggested in recent retrospective cohort studies (1%- 2%, which is 10 times that expected among people without HIV) [**1**], but the underlying etiology remains uncertain.

2. Procoagulant mechanisms underlying HIV infection

Several mechanisms associated with HIV infection that may lead to predispose to a hypercoagulate state, in the absence of classic thrombophilic risk factors [**2**], are emerging.

More than one "hit" seems to be involved [**3**]:

2.1. Host risk factors

2.1.1. Age

HIV-infected patients are older than their chronological age, experiencing the so-called "*premature aging* ", with persistent immunological defects and inflammation, even after years of treatment mediated viral suppression (similar to those seen in normal ageing, but they occur at an earlier age than normal): low CD4: CD8 ratio, low *naïve*: memory cell ratio and reduced responsiveness to vaccines. In addition, longevity and life expectancy is increasing due to effective antiretroviral therapy (ART), making HIV infection a chronic disorder.

In a Nederland cohort [4] of 109 patients with HIV, the annual incidences of venous and arterial thrombosis were 5- to 16-fold higher and 2- to 8-fold higher, respectively, than in the healthy population. The median age at the onset of venous thrombosis was 45 years, 17 years earlier than the median age of onset for venous thrombosis in non-HIV- infected patients; and the median age for arterial thrombosis onset was 53 years, a decade earlier than that documented in the Framingham study.

2.1.2. Hypercoagulate state - Primary prothrombotic abnormalities boosted by direct effect of HIV

- Protein S (PS) deficiency (27-76%): decreased synthesis by the endothelial cells, hepatocytes and megakariocytes injured in HIV infection; antibodies to PS and low levels of circulating free antigen; tumor necrosis-factor alpha (TNF α) can lower the levels of active protein S, down-regulating the protein S synthesis in the endothelial cells; and loss of protein S in urine in HIV-related nephropathy [5].
- Protein C (PC) deficiency (0-14%): altered synthesis and metabolism of PC, as well as low-grade disseminated intravascular coagulation (DIC) with consumptive coagulopathy, in the setting of HIV infection with severe immunosuppression [5].
- Presence of Factor V Leiden (activated protein C resistance) [6].
- Antithrombin deficiency: decreased protein synthesis (liver diseases and malnutrition), protein-losing nephropathies or enteropathies, consumptive states (malignancy, surgery, DIC).
- Antiphospholipid antibodies: Anticardiolipin antibodies (aCL) and lupus anticoagulant (LA) have been reported in HIV-infected patients with a prevalence ranging from 7 to 94% and 0 to 72%, respectively. They have been implicated with antiphospholipid syndrome features (mainly avascular bone and cutaneous necrosis) or playing a limited role beside the multifactorial origin of HIV-related thrombosis [7]. HIV infection induces destruction of CD4 lymphocytes, which leads to polyclonal stimulation of B cells and hypergammaglobulinemia, resulting in antibodies against damaged endothelial cells (phospholipids exposed) and inhibition of protein S synthesis [5]. It is thought that LA activity in these patients might be an epiphenomenon secondary to chronic immune stimulation in HIV infection and no pathogenic correlation has been found with thromboses.
- Tissue Factor (TF): TF expression on circulating monocytes has been postulated in the setting of driving immune activation by translocation of microbial products through the damaged gut. In addition, HIV- associated gp120 causes release of TF via activation of arterial smooth muscle cells [2].
- Microparticles (MP): The MP are generated from endothelial cells, platelets and apoptotic CD4 lymphocytes.
- HIV-associated autoimmune haemolytic anemia has been related with an increased risk of thromboembolism during the acute phase of hemolysis [5].
- Homocysteine: Mild to moderate hyperhomocysteinemia (11-29%), related to a homozygous C677T mutation of the methylenetetrahydrofolate reductase gene [8],

especially in the setting of ART. It is not sufficient alone to cause thrombosis, but it may add an additional risk among patients with other risk factors for venous clots.

- Endothelial dysfunction: A dysfunctional venous endothelium, induced by HIV, may express heparin cofactor II deficiency and increased amounts of P-selectin, von Willebrand factor, TF, plasminogen activator inhibitor-1 and factor V, all of which may promote blood clotting. Biomarkers of endothelial dysfunction [**9**] (P-selectin, D-dimer and hyaluronic acid), coagulation, and tissue fibrosis may help identify HIV-infected patients at elevated risk of venous thromboembolism (VTE). Other endothelial dysfunction biomarker is asymmetric dimethylarginine (ADMA), a competitive inhibitor for endothelial nitric oxide synthase (eNOS) which seems to be related to an increased immune activation pathways in HIV-1 infection [**10**].

  In addition, intravenous drug use (IDU) can induce endothelial injury [**11**]. From a Danish HIV cohort [**12**], the 5-year risk of VTE was 8.0% [95% confidence interval (CI) 5.78-10.74%] in IDU HIV-infected patients, 1.5% (95% CI 1.14-1.95%) in non-IDU HIV-infected patients and 0.3% (95% CI 0.29-0.41%) in the population comparison cohort. In non-IDU HIV-infected patients, adjusted incidence rate ratios (IRRs) for unprovoked and provoked VTE were 3.42 (95% CI 2.58-4.54) and 5.51 (95% CI 3.29-9.23), respectively, compared with the population comparison cohort. In IDU HIV-infected patients, the adjusted IRRs were 12.66 (95% CI 6.03-26.59) for unprovoked VTE and 9.38 (95% CI 1.61-54.50) for provoked VTE. Low CD4 cell count had a minor impact on these risk estimates, while ART increased the overall risk (IRR 1.93; 95% CI 1.00-3.72).

- High density lipoprotein (HDL). A prospective study from South Africa [**13**] compared thrombotic profiles of 30 HIV-positive and 30 HIV-negative patients with acute coronary syndrome (ACS). Patients with HIV were younger; and besides smoking (73% vs 33%) and low HDL (0.8 ± 0.3 vs 1.1 ± 0.4), they had fewer traditional risk factors. Thrombophilia was more common in HIV-positive patients with lower protein C (PC; 82 ± 22 vs 108 ± 20) and higher factor VIII levels (201 ± 87 vs 136 ± 45). Patients with HIV had higher frequencies of aCL 47% vs 10%) and antiprothrombin antibodies (87% vs 21%).

  In addition to promoting cholesterol efflux from lipid-filled macrophages (foam cells) and reverse cholesterol transport, HDL protects low density lipoprotein (LDL) from oxidation and decreases expression of adhesion molecules on endothelial cells (including E-selectin and sICAM-1). HDL also improves endothelial function via stimulation of nitric oxide synthase activity, increases prostacyclin production by endothelial cells and inhibits endothelial TF expression, all of which enhance endothelium-dependent vasodilation and down-regulate thrombotic pathways. In this way, HDL possesses anti-inflammatory and antithrombotic properties. A cross-sectional study [**14**] was designed to assess large and small high density lipoprotein particle (HDLp) concentrations in persons with untreated HIV infection. Lower small HDLp (primarily responsible for HDL's anti-inflammatory properties and inhibition of endothelial activation) concentrations and higher IL-6, sICAM-1 and D-dimer levels were found. The relationship of these markers to HIV-mediated atherosclerotic risk requires further study. The Strategies for Management of AntiRetroviral Therapy (SMART) trial demonstrated a 60% increased relative risk for cardiovascular disease (CVD) with a strategy of CD4+ cell count–guided interruption of ART, and adverse changes in HDL after stopping ART may explain some of the excess CVD risk. IL-6 and D-dimer levels increased after discontinuation of ART, and this was associated with increases in HIV RNA levels. In addition, baseline HDLp, but not low density lipoprotein particle (LDLp), predicted CVD risk in SMART.

2.2. HIV disease state

2.2.1. CD4 cell count

CD4 cell count at the time of the thrombotic event, is the strongest predictor in some multivariate models. Protein C and protein S deficiencies [**5**] and increased von Willebrand factor and fibrinogen concentrations [**4**], have been correlated with immunossuppresion, evidenced by reduced CD4 cell counts. Although the frequency of thrombosis is higher in the presence of lower CD4, there are reports of thrombosis occurring with higher CD4 [**15**].

2.2.2. Viral load

High HIV RNA level is predictive of progression of HIV infection and higher risk of thrombosis.

The frequencies of thrombophilic abnormalities (described above), increases with the progression to AIDS [**2**].

2.3. Comorbidities - Secondary prothrombotic abnormalities

2.3.1. Infections

A link between infection and thrombosis via endothelial activation [**2**] has been suggested, through up-regulation of some cytokines (the same ones that activate the coagulation system and appear during HIV infection), such as TNFα, IL-1, IL-6, factor VIII and fibrinogen, as well as down-regulation of fibrinolytic proteins, protein C (consumption as an antiinflammatory mediator) and free protein S concentrations. Deficiency of free protein S appears during an acute inflammatory process, such as opportunistic infections: C4b binding protein is increased up to 400% of its typical concentration [**4**] and binds free protein S, which is the active component as anticoagulant [**5**].

HIV-associated infections, including syphilis, *Pneumocystis jiroveci, Mycobacterium tuberculosis and avium intracellulare* [**3**] and hepatitis C [**5**], have been related to the induction of antiphospholipid antibodies (molecular mimicry between infectious agent and beta2-glycoprotein I). Furthermore, cytomegalovirus induces thrombotic events via endo- thelial damage [5]. In a cross-sectional study [16] of 104 consecutive HIV- infected patients, active cytomegalovirus infection (defined as patients who had anti - cytomegalovirus antibody levels above the 75th percentile, > 209IU/ml), was associated with hypercoagulability independently of stage of HIV disease. It was observed higher levels of anticoagulant factors (antithrombin and total protein S levels) and higher procoagulant factors (factor VIII and fibrinogen levels), with a balance shifted to a procoagu- lant state. The majority of thrombosis have been associated with gastroin-testinal-related disease [3].

2.3.2. *HIV-associated malignancy*

Kaposi´s sarcoma and non-Hodgkin lymphoma (B cell), via abnormalities of lymphatic flow and stasis; and anal and cervical carcinoma, via production of procoagulants, invasion of vascular space or secretion of vascular permeability factors from tumor cells [5].

2.4. Hospitalization

Hospitalization in the past 3 months, was the risk factor more strongly associated with thrombosis in patients with HIV/AIDS, in a case-control study by Ahonkhai et al. [1].

2.5. Therapy

- Protease Inhibitors (PI), in highly active ART (HAART), above all indinavir and saquinavir, are thought to interfere with hepatic metabolism, specifically cytochrome P450, and regulation of thrombotic proteins: increasing of the expression of CD36, receptor for oxidized LDL, inducing, in addition, increased absorption of cholesterol [2].
- HIV-positive individuals with lipodistrophy and fat redistribution induced by ART, may be at increased risk for developing an abnormal coagulation profile, such as increased fibrinogen, D-dimer, plasminogen activator inhibitor-1 or protein S deficiency.
- Some authors recommend that clinicians must remain aware about the possibility of the occurrence of a thromboembolic event, especially during [17] the first few months after introduction of the ART.
- However, other authors [18] have observed that ART or PI therapy does not appear to play a significant role in the occurrence of thrombotic events; advanced HIV disease is the most relevant risk factor for development of thromboses, possibly due to an increased inflammatory state or the presence of concurrent comorbidities such as infections.

  The Nederland cohort of 109 patients with HIV, previously referred above [4], showed that ART may improve thrombophilic abnormalities and lead to a decreased risk of venous and arterial thrombosis.

In other study [19], the incidence of VTE in patients with HIV in the post - protease inhibitor era (after 1996) was higher than in HIV patients before 1996. However, the higher incidence since 1996 is small, probably not clinically significant, and not necessarily because of protease inhibitors.

Moreover, another study [20] analyzed levels of von Willebrand factor, D-dimer and factor VIII, in 160 HIV-infected and homosexual patients with a median age of 46 years, of whom 92% were male, 70% using ART, 74% Caucasian, 11% African American, 9% Hispanic, and 6% Asian. Significant lower levels of these parameters were observed in HIV-infected patients on ART compared to patients not on ART. Significant lower levels of protein C and free protein S, and increased activated protein C sensitivity ratio (APCsr) were found in the HIV-infected patients not on ART. However, *although the prevalence of coagulation abnormalities was lower in HIV- infected patients using ART, a considerable proportion of HIV - infected patients on ART showed endothelial cell activation and increased APCsr, suggestive of a persistent procoagulant state.*

Immune depletion contributes to HIV – related inflammation, and ADMA concentrations decrease in patients with HIV infection under ART, slowing down endothelial activation. However, ADMA levels (or changes) did not consistently correlate with HIV RNA levels (or changes) [21].

Otherwise, some drugs from ART show more favourable profile related to decrease immune activation. Switching from ritonavir - boosted protease inhibitors to raltegravir (integrase inhibitor), appeared to de- crease biomarkers of inflammation (high sensitivity C reactive protein, osteoprotegerin, IL-6, TNFα, insulin and D-dimer) [22].

- Megestrol acetate (progestational agent), used widely to stimulate appetite and weight gain in patients with AIDS-related anorexia and/or cachexia, could increase risk of VTE [3].

The data referred above, support the hypothesis that HIV-infected individuals are more likely to have clinically detected thromboembolic disease as opposed to non-HIV-infected individuals. One study performed by Malek et al. [23] revealed up to a 43% increase in developing a pulmonary embolism (PE), 10% increase in developing a deep venous thrombosis (DVT), and 40% increase in developing PE or DVT, in an HIV-infected individual over the 9-year study period. This increase differed by age group, with age group 21 to 50 years having the highest odds for PE among HIV+ individuals (OR, 1.58; 95% CI, 1.54-1.63).

Also, other study by Kiser et al. [24], showed patients with HIV had higher rate of VTE, being younger than 50 years (3.31% vs 0.53% in age-matched healthy controls, $p < 0.0001$), had a CD4(+) cell count less than 200 cells/mm^3, or a diagnosis of acquired immunodeficiency syndrome.

Anyway, many authors propose the need to perform long-term, prospective studies assessing the factors associated with thrombotic events in patients with HIV.

3. Case reports

[25] In a previous published letter, we described 9 patients with HIV infection and thrombotic event, defined as thrombosis involving an artery or a deep or splanchnic vein. Here, we included 2 patients more as follows.

All of them were heterosexual patients, and one of them was an intravenous drug user. Median age was 38 years (range, 35-58 years). Seven of them were male. Only one patient had a family history of thrombosis (stroke). Four patients were coinfected with hepatitis C virus. The most frequent Centers for Disease Control and Prevention (CDC) HIV stage was 3 [**26**]. There were neither AIDS-related malignancies or autoimmune disorders nor concurrent opportunistic infections at the time of the thrombotic event. Six patients were on ART, and only two patients were undergoing protease inhibitor therapy. Basic coagulation assays were unremarkable and only one patient was evaluated for hypercoagulate state and was found to have low protein C and S values.

- Misdiagnosis of thromboembolism as a *Pneumocystis jiroveci* pneumonia (diagnosed by computed tomographic pulmonary angiogram) delayed anticoagulant treatment in a patient. Several months after this event, the same patient developed yugular vein thrombosis associated with a catheter placement.
- Four patients had a diagnosis of lower extremity DVT, as confirmed by venous duplex ultrasonography. One of them had recurrent DVT, in the setting of progressive multifocal leukoencephalopathy. Another one, a young woman, developed a DVT in the setting of malabsorption syndrome by *Giardia lamblia;* she had been diagnosed with non-B HIV infection a few months before, and she showed high CD4 cell counts, high viral load, as well as increasing aCL antibodies and probably decreasing C protein and antithrombin-III (enteral loss); she was not receiving ART.
- One male patient felt pain in the lower back since several weeks before admission, and his condition was diagnosed by abdominal computed tomography (CT), as inferior vena cava thrombosis (the patient had a congenital double inferior vena cava system). He was receiving interferon and ribavirin for the treatment of chronic hepatitis C.
- A man was admitted to the hospital complaining of pain in the epigastric area. His condition was diagnosed by CT as alcoholic chronic pancreatitis and mesenteric vein thrombosis.
- A woman was attended in the emergency unit because of massive hematemesis, and a portal vein thrombosis was documented by splanchnic angiography. A portocaval shunt was performed and the patient survived and went well.
- Two patients died, and a suspicious diagnosis of pulmonary embolism was made on the basis of a clinical approach (pleuritic chest pain, cough and shortness of breath) in the setting of septic shock (an autopsy was not available) in one case, and by high-probability ventilation/perfusion lung scanning, in another one.
- A young man developed severe pulmonary hypertension secondary to recurrent pulmonary embolism, in the presence of aCL antibodies and high CD4 cells count, but high viral load, without ART.

4. Specific settings for thrombotic events

4.1. Autoimmune background

Autoimmune disturbances have emerged in the setting of immunological reconstitution and constant antigenic viral stimulation in HIV-infected patients. Different types of autoantibodies have been observed, including aCL, anti-Beta2-glycoprotein I and antiprothrombin antibodies [**27**]. Clinical challenges can arise when the two conditions coexist.

Lupus anticoagulants were first described in AIDS and asymptomatic HIV-infected individuals (in whom they could be transient), by Bloom et al. in 1986. The association between aCL and HIV infection in men who have sex with men was reported in 1991. Falco et al., in 1993, found that, on the contrary to systemic lupus erythematosus (SLE), in the HIV-positive serum samples, reduced aCL binding capacity was evident if the cofactor (beta2-glycoprotein I) was added. Canoso et al. reported in 1997, aCL positivity in association with human T cell lymphotropic virus type 3 infection.

The presence of SLE and HIV infection in the same individual is being increasingly reported, particularly in Africa and Asia. This coexistence has been associated with remissions or amelioration of SLE symptoms, with advancing HIV infection during pre-Highly Active ART (HAART) era (before 1996 and introduction of protease inhibitors); or with flares in immune reconstitution, during effective HAART, through a cross-reactive mechanism between inflammatory factors and common nuclear antibodies.

Overlapping features between SLE and HIV infection can include: arthralgias and arthritis, polyclonal B cell activation, antibodies against double-stranded DNA, anti-Smith antibodies, antiphospholipid antibodies and autoimmune haemolytic anemia with positive Coombs test; however, low complement has not been detected in HIV infection. In addition, patients with SLE without previous exposure to retroviral infection may express antibodies against retroviral proteins, including gag, env, nef and p24 of HIV-1, with false-positive results of ELISA and Western blot for detection of HIV. Some authors have suggested that these antibodies directed against HIV proteins may protect SLE subjects from exogenous infection.

4.2. Immune reconstitution inflammatory syndrome (IRIS)

When ART is started, a striking immune restoration inflammatory response can appear. In this setting, there could be a predisposition to thrombotic events, as in the case reported as follows [**28**]. A 26-year-old HIV-infected man who had started HAART a few months earlier, developed multiple linear nodules following the superficial veins in both legs. Histopathologic examination demonstrated a mostly septal panniculitis with features of superficial thrombophlebitis. Authors propose that superficial thrombophlebitis should be added to the list of clinical manifestations of this newly observed immune reconstitution disease.

4.3. Acute coronary artery disease and non-bacterial thrombotic endocarditis

In addition to the issues referred above, protease inhibitors [**29**] have also been implicated in direct endothelial damage, which may be mediated by reduced nitric oxide production or release. The development of CVD risk factors such as insulin resistance, hyperlipidemia and fat redistribution syndrome, may exacerbate already existing underlying atherosclerotic risk in patients using these medications. However, necropsy studies de- monstrated *premature CVD in HIV-infected patients even before the advent of protease inhibitors*, indicating that other mechanisms might be involved independent of these drugs.

Other authors could not demonstrate relation between a patient's human immunodeficiency virus status and valve thrombosis [**30**] or non-bacterial thrombotic endocarditis [**31**].

4.4. Non cirrhotic portal hypertension

A multifactorial mechanism has been proposed to explain the pathogenesis of non-cirrhotic portal hypertension (NCPH) in HIV-infected patients, and we have reviewed it and described two cases, in a previous published paper [**32**]: prothrombotic state, by HIV as a direct cause or through anti-protein S antibodies, leading to protein S deficiency; as well as didanosine, an ARTdrug, adenosine analogue, which has been postulated as an independent predictor of developing NCPH through cumulative dosing or idiosyncratic mechanisms. It results in an obliteration of the small portal venules and liver regenerative hyperplasia. Considering the data regarding prothrombotic abnormalities in HIV-infected patients, we wondered if patients with HIV and NCPH should be evaluated for hypercoagulate state.

4.5. Pregnancy-puerperium

Annual incidence of VTE within 3 months postpartum in a cohort of 41 consecutive HIV-infected pregnant women [33], was 313 per 1000 person-years (95% CI, 65- 915). This risk is 120-fold higher than in HIV-positive controls, whereas the risk is 157-fold higher compared to HIV-negative pregnant women.

4.6. Other settings

Thrombophilia might have a limited role in the development of osteonecrosis in HIV-positive, according a case - control study [34], being only significantly associated with osteonecrosis: nadir of CD4(+) < 60 cells/microL and steroid use.

5. Management

Notably, the 2008 American College of Chest Physicians (ACCP) guidelines on antithrombotic and thrombolytic therapy, are silent regarding HIV-infected patients [**35**]. Anyway, the management of proven VTE should be the same as for the non HIV-patients [**3**].

Some special issues must be considered:

5.1. Antiretroviral therapy and warfarin drug interaction

Interactions between warfarin and ART (non-nucleoside reverse transcriptase inhibitors-NNRTIs and protease inhibitors-PIs), are through influence of ART on CYP2C9, the enzyme responsible for the metabolism of the more active S-enantiomer of warfarin [3]. Among the NNRTIs, induction of warfarin metabolism is likely with nevirapine. Inhibition of warfarin metabolism may occur with efavirenz o etravirine. Interactions involving ritonavir-boosted PIs are most frequent when warfarin is initiated in patients receiving concurrent efavirenz therapy [**36**]. International Normalized Ratio (INR) response should be used to guide warfarin dosage requirements; otherwise, low-molecular-weight heparin (LMWH) could be considered as a safer choice, although always keeping in mind that HIV infection may be an independent risk factor for the development of heparin-induced thrombocytopenia (HIT).

5.2. Warfarin-induced skin necrosis (WISN)

The presentation of WISN, a condition due to decrease protein C levels by warfarin, in HIV-1 infected patients, is a novel clinical entity, reported recently [**37**]. Six cases of WISN occurred in 973 patients receiving warfarin therapy for venous thrombosis (0.62%, 95% CI 0.25 - 1.37%) at a referral hospital in Cape Town, South Africa. All 6 cases occurred in HIV-1-infected women (median age 30 years, range 27 - 42) with microbiologically confirmed tuberculosis (TB) and venous thrombosis. All were profoundly immunosuppressed (median CD4+ count at TB diagnosis 49 cells/microl, interquartile range 23 - 170). Of the 3 patients receiving combination ART, 2 had TB-IRIS. The occurrence of 6 WISN cases in a 40-month period may be attributed to: hypercoagulability secondary to HIV-1(above all if associated to decreased protein C levels) and TB, short concurrent heparin and warfarin therapy and high loading doses of warfarin. Active prevention and appropriate management of WISN are likely to improve the morbidity and mortality of this unusual condition.

6. Questions and remarks arised from clinical practice [3, 25]

- Should young patients (especially men) who develop thromboembolic events, in the absence of classic thrombophilic risk factors, be evaluated for HIV infection?
- Given the overlapping features between SLE and HIV-infection, should be mandatory to rule out HIV infection in black South African patients with SLE (above all if they are not females of childbearing age), who present an unsatisfactory course?.
- Should patients with HIV with severe immunosuppression be screened for prothrombotic abnormalities?
- Venous thromboembolism can mimic opportunistic lung infection in patients with HIV; so, the former should be considered in differential diagnosis of lung diseases in this setting, above all when patients have unexplained dyspnea or hypoxemia.

- Should patients with HIV with low CD4 cell count receive prophylactic anticoagulation?
- Appropriate prophylactic measures should be instituted, including low-molecular weight heparin on hospitalization and for high-risk HIV-infected outpatients.
- HIV infection may be an independent risk factor for the development of heparin-induced thrombocytopenia (HIT). Should be considered any special caution regarding it?
- Finally, considering the absence of specific recommendations or guidelines on antithrombotic and thrombolytic therapy directed to VIH-infected patients, are traditional screening methods and management strategies applicable in HIV?

Author details

Hortensia Álvarez Díaz, Ana Mariño Callejo and José Francisco García Rodríguez
Infectious Diseases Unit, Department of Internal Medicine, Hospital Arquitecto Marcide-Profesor Novoa Santos, Sanitary Area of Ferrol, A Coruña, Spain

7. References

[1] Ahonkhai AA, Gebo KA, Streiff MB et al. Venous thromboembolism in patients with HIV/AIDS: a case-control study. J. Acquir Immune Defic Syndr 2008; 48 (3): 310-4.
[2] Jacobson MC, Dezube BJ, Aboulafia DM et al. Thrombotic complications in patients infected with HIV in the era of Highly Active Antiretroviral Therapy: a case series. CID 2004; 39: 1214-1222.
[3] Bibas M., Biava G. and Antinori A. HIV-associated venous thromboembolism. Mediterr J Hematol Infect Dis 2011; 3; Open Journal System.
[4] Lijfering WM, Sprenger HG, Georg RR et al. Relationship between progression to AIDS and thrombophilic abnormalities in HIV infection. Clin Chem 2008; 54 (7): 1226-33.
[5] Saif M and Greenberg B. HIV and thrombosis: a review. Aids Patient Care STDS 2001; 15 (1): 15-24.
[6] Santos JL, Cruz I, Martín F et al. Trombosis coronaria recurrente, síndrome antifosfolípido primario, factor V Leiden y virus de la inmunodeficiencia humana. Rev Esp Cardiol 2004; 57 (10): 997-9.
[7] Ramos-Casals M, Cervera R, Lagrutta M et al. Clinical features related to antiphospholipid syndrome in patients with chronic viral infections (hepatitis C virus/HIV infection): description of 82 cases. CID 2004; 38: 1009-1016.
[8] Bernasconi E, Uhr M, Magenta L et al. Homocysteinaemia in HIV-infected patients treated with highly active antiretroviral therapy. AIDS 2001;15 (8): 1081-1082.

[9] Musselwhite LW, Sheikh V, Norton TD et al. Markers of endothelial dysfunction, coagulation and tissue fibrosis independently predict venous thromboembolism in HIV. AIDS. 2011 Mar 27; 25 (6): 787-95.

[10] Kurz K, Teerlink T, Sarcletti M et al. Plasma concentrations of the cardiovascular risk factor asymmetric dimethylarginine (ADMA) are increased in patients with HIV-1 infection and correlate with immune activation markers. Pharmacol Res 2009 Dec; 60 (6): 508-14.

[11] Saif M, Bona R, Greenberg B et al. AIDS and thrombosis: retrospective study of 131 HIV-infected patients. Aids Patient Care STDS 2001; 15 (6): 311-320.

[12] Rasmussen LD, Dybdal M, Gerstoft J et al. HIV and risk of venous thromboembolism: a Danish nationwide population-based cohort study.HIV Med. 2011 Apr; 12(4):202-10. doi: 10.1111/j.1468-1293.2010.00869.x. Epub 2010 Aug 18.

[13] Becker AC, Jacobson B, Singh S et al. The thrombotic profile of treatment-naive HIV-positive Black South Africans with acute coronary syndromes. Clin Appl Thromb Hemost. 2011 Jun; 17 (3):264-72. Epub 2010 May 11.

[14] Baker J, Ayenew W, Quick H et al. High-density lipoprotein particles and markers of inflammation and thrombotic activity in patients with untreated HIV infection. JID 2010; 201: 285-292.

[15] Basavanagowdappa H, Babu MS, Karuturi S. HIV infection and thromboembolism.J Assoc Physicians India. 2011 Jun; 59:380-2.

[16] Mulder R, Tichelaar YI, Sprenger HG et al. Relationship between cytomegalovirus infection and procoagulant changes in human immunodeficiency virus-infected patients. Clin Microbiol Infect. 2011 May; 17(5):747-9.

[17] Lyonne L, Magimel C, Cormerais L et al.Thromboembolic events at the time of highly active antiretroviral therapies against human immunodeficiency virus.Rev Med Interne. 2008 Feb;29(2):100-4. Epub 2007 Nov 26.

[18] Crum-Cianflone NF., Weekes J. and Bavaro M. Thromboses among HIV-infected patients during the highly active antiretroviral therapy era. AIDS Patient Care STDS. 2008 Oct; 22 (10): 771-8.

[19] Mata F., Yaekoub AY and Stein PD. Human immunodeficiency virus infection and risk of venous thromboembolism. Am J Med Sci. 2008 Nov; 336 (5): 402-6.

[20] Jong E, Louw S, Meijers JC et al. The hemostatic balance in HIV-infected patients with and without antiretroviral therapy: partial restoration with antiretroviral therapy. AIDS Patient Care STDS. 2009 Dec;23(12):1001-7.

[21] 19th Conference on Retroviruses and Opportunistic Infections, March 5-8, 2012, Seatle. Zangerle R., Parikh R. Posters 831, 832, 833.

[22] 19th Conference on Retroviruses and Opportunistic Infections, March 5-8, 2012, Seatle. Martínez E. Poster 834 (SPIRAL study)

[23] Malek J, Rogers R, Kufera J, Hirshon JM. Venous thromboembolic disease in the HIV-infected patient. Am J Emerg Med. 2011 Mar; 29 (3): 278-82. Epub 2010 Mar 26.

[24] Kiser KL, Badowski ME. Risk factors for venous thromboembolism in patients with human immunodeficiency virus infection. Pharmacotherapy. 2010 Dec; 30 (12): 1292-302.

[25] Álvarez Díaz H, Mariño Callejo A and García Rodríguez JF. Non-cirrhotic portal hypertension in Human Immunodeficiency Virus-Infected patients: a new challenge in antiretroviral therapy era. The Open AIDS Journal 2011, 5: 59-61.

[26] Schneider E., Whitmore S, Glynn KM et al.; Centers for Disease Control and Prevention (CDC). Revised surveillance case definitions for HIV infection among adults, adolescents, and children aged < 18 months and for HIV infection and AIDS among children aged 18 months to < 13 years-United States, 2008.MMWR Recomm Rep. 2008 Dec 5; 57 (RR-10): 1-12.

[27] Asherson R.A., Gómez-Puerta J.A. and Marinopoulos G. Recurrent pulmonary thromboembolism in a patient with systemic lupus erythematosus and HIV-1 infection associated with the presence of antibodies to prothrombin: a case report. CID 2005; 41: 89-92.

[28] Alcaraz I, Revelles JM, Camacho D et al. Superficial thrombophlebitis: A new clinical manifestation of the immune reconstitution inflammatory syndrome in a patient with HIV infection. Am J Dermatopathol. 2010 Dec;32(8):846-9.

[29] Cilingiroglu M, Lather N, Youseff A et al. ST-elevation myocardial infarction due to a spontaneous thrombus in the left anterior descending artery in a young HIV-infected patient. Arch Turk Soc Cardiol 2011; 39 (4): 308-311.

[30] Achouh P, Jemel A, Chaudeurge A et al. Aortic biological valve thrombosis in an HIV positive patient. Ann Thorac Surg. 2011 Jun; 91(6): e90-1.

[31] Jedlinski I, Baralkiewicz G and Poprawski K. Acute coronary syndrome in a patient with acquired immunodeficiencysyndrome and non-bacterial thrombotic endocarditis. Eur Heart J (2010) 31 (8): 935.

[32] Álvarez Díaz H, Mariño Callejo A and García Rodríguez JF. Non-cirrhotic portal hypertension in Human Immunodeficiency Virus-Infected patients: a new challenge in antiretroviral therapy era. The Open AIDS Journal 2011, 5: 59-61.

[33] Jansen JM, Lijfering WM, Sprenger HG et al. Venous thromboembolism in HIV-positive women during puerperium: a case series. Blood Coagul Fibrinolysis. 2008 Jan; 19(1): 95-7.

[34] De Larrañaga G, Bottaro E, Martinuzzo M et al. Thrombophilia in human immunodeficiency virus-infected patients with osteonecrosis: Is there a real connection? The first case-control study. Clin Appl Thromb Hemost. 2009 May-Jun; 15(3): 340-7. Epub 2007 Dec 26.

[35] Hirsh J., Guyatt G, Albers GW. et al. Antithrombotic and thrombolytic therapy: American College of Chest Physicians Evidence-Based Clinical Practice Guidelines (8th Edition). Chest 2008 Jun; 133: 71S-105S.

[36] Welzen ME, van den Berk GE, Hamers RL et al. Interaction between antiretroviral drugs and acenocoumarol. Antivir Ther. 2011; 16 (2): 249-52.

[37] Bhaijee F, Wainwright H, Meintjes G et al. Warfarin-induced skin necrosis in HIV-1-infected patients with tuberculosis and venous thrombosis. S Afr Med J. 2010 Jun 1; 100(6): 372-7.

Chapter 12

The Role of Liver Transplantation in HIV Positive Patients

Deepak Joshi and Kosh Agarwal

Additional information is available at the end of the chapter

1. Introduction

1.1. Burden of liver disease

In developed countries, the management and treatment of HIV-1 infection was revolutionised after the introduction of combined anti-viral therapy (cART) in 1996. The major outcome was the reduction of AIDS and AIDS-related deaths (1). Such was the success of cART, that now more than 50% of deaths in HIV positive patients on cART are not directly related to HIV infection or AIDS (1-3). The D:A:D (data collection on adverse events of anti-HIV drugs) study demonstrated that liver disease had become the commonest cause of a non-AIDS related death overtaking cardiovascular disease (2). Given the similar transmission routes, unsurprisingly nearly two-thirds of deaths were secondary to chronic hepatitis C virus (HCV) infection, 17% secondary to chronic hepatitis B virus (HBV) infection and 3% due drug-induced liver injury related to cART (2). Other liver-related aetiologies amongst HIV positive individuals include alcohol, non-alcohol related liver disease (NAFLD), hepatocellular carcinoma (HCC) (Table 1). HIV positive patients present with the same clinical sequelae of chronic liver disease as their HIV negative counterparts but tend to present at a younger age but with a markedly reduced survival rate after the first episode of decompensation (4). In HIV-positive patients with compensated cirrhosis an increased mortality rate is associated with age > 50 years, MELD score > 11 and poor control of HIV disease (5).

1.2. Viral aetiologies

One third of patients with HIV infection are co-infected with chronic HCV, and the majority of deaths in HIV-positive patients with ESLD can be attributable to HCV infection(6). HCV is transmitted via contaminated blood or blood products. At-risk groups include intravenous drug users, patients with haemophilia who were exposed to contaminated infusions of plasma derived factor VIII or X concentrate, men who have sex with men (MSM) and individuals who have sex with IVDUs (7). Vertical transmission is also possible and is more likely if the mother is HIV-positive. A more recent trend is the increase in the number of new cases of acute HCV in MSM who are HIV-positive acquired via sexual transmission (8, 9).

HIV infection clearly affects HCV-related liver disease. The combination of HIV/HCV co-infection is associated with a reduced rate of spontaneous HCV RNA clearance and therefore an increased likelihood of developing chronic HCV infection (10). Once HCV infection is established then a more rapid fibrosis progression rate is evident (11). The development of cirrhosis tends to occur on average 15 years earlier than in HCV mono-infected individuals (12). Predictors of fibrosis progression include detectable HIV viraemia, low CD4+ counts, baseline necro-inflammatory activity on liver biopsy and increased alcohol consumption (>50g per day) (13, 14). HIV/HCV co-infected patients have a poorer survival following the first episode of decompensation; median estimated survival of only 13 months (4). Mechanisms for this accelerated fibrosis rate appear to be multi-factorial and include a weaker adaptive immune response of CD8+ cells, the increased number of the pro-fibrogenic CD8+ cells and relative reduction in CD4+ cells, the presence of insulin resistance and reduction of interleukin – 10 expression(15-19, 19, 20). The HIV virus cannot enter hepatocytes directly but it can upregulate pro-fibrotic pathways e.g. transforming growth factor B-1 which further activates hepatic stellate cells (10).

Treatment of HCV in patients with HIV is more difficult compared to HCV-monoinfected patients and is associated with an increased side-effect profile. At present pegylated interferon and ribavirin are the only licensed medications for the treatment of HCV in HIV/HCV co-infected patients. Compared to HCV mono-infected patients, end-of-treatment (29-62%) and sustained virological response rates (SVR) are inferior (17-35%) (21-26). The use of the newer protease inhibitors in the treatment of HCV in HIV-positive patients has only been limited to the trial arena. Preliminary data from the 110 Phase 2 study demonstrate similar outcomes to monoinfection with 74% SVR 12 in telaprevir triple therapy group (n=38) vs 45% standard of care (n=22); with no breakthrough in HIV RNA and similar side effect profile to monoinfection treated with telaprevir.

HIV-positive patients commonly exhibit evidence of previous HBV infection, whereas 10% of the HIV-positive population have evidence of chronic HBV infection (27). Vertical transmission of HBV remains the most common route of infection worlwide, whilst sexual transmission and percutaneous transmission is more likely in Europe and North America (28, 29). HIV-positive patients that contract HBV infection are less likely to clear the virus, a quarter of patients will develop chronic HBV infection, especially those with low CD4+ cell counts (30). HIV/HBV co-infected patients also have increased HBV DNA viral loads compared to HBV mono-infected patients, which also translates into an increased risk of developing HCC (31).

HIV/HBV co-infection related – morbidity is considerably less when compared to HIV/HCV co-infected patients. This is due to the use of nucleoside and nucleotide reverse-transcriptase inhibitors (lamivudine, emtricitabine and tenofovir) that are used in cART regimens and have both anti-HIV and anti-HBV activity.

Given that co-infection with HBV and HCV are the leading causes of liver disease amongst HIV-positive patients, the incidence of hepatocellular carcinoma (HCC) is expected to rise and the MORTAVIC and French Mortalite studies have both demonstrated an increasing number of deaths attributable to HCC (6, 32). HIV-positive patients presenting with HCC are younger at presentation (52 versus 64 years, $p<0.0001$), are more likely to be symptomatic at presentation, have multiple tumours at presentation, and have advanced disease compared to HIV-negative patients (31, 33).

1.3. Non-viral aetiologies

Awareness of drug-induced liver injury or cART-induced hepatotoxicity is increasing. Deciding on the culprit drug is often difficult because of the use of combination therapies. Recognised patterns of liver injury include hypersensitivity, idiosyncratic hepatotoxicity, mitochondrial toxicity, an immune reconstitution syndrome and hepato-steatosis (34-38). Acute liver failure resulting from cART is uncommon. The development of non-cirrhotic portal hypertension (NCPH) secondary to cART in particular to didanosine is an emerging disease entity (39). The pathogenesis of NCPH appears to be linked to a pro-thrombotic state, an acquired protein S deficiency. The spectrum of histological findings include nodular regenerative hyperplasia, hepatoportal sclerosis, peri-portal fibrosis and sclerosing portal venopathy (40-42).

The D:A:D study also highlighted that the prevalence of the metabolic syndrome has increased over the last decade from 19% in 2000-2001 to 42% in2006-2007 (43). This is likely to result in an increase in the prevalence of NAFLD, given that NAFLD is the hepatic manifestation of the metabolic syndrome. There is limited data available on the risk factors for NAFLD in HIV-positive patients but attention has focused on the role of cART because of its negative effects of insulin resistance, glucose metabolism and lipid metabolism. Central adiposity, male sex, low serum high-density lipoprotein levels, raised triglycerides levels and an increased ratio of alanine aminotransferase to aspartate aminotransferase have been suggested as risk factors for the development of NAFLD (44).

1.4. Selection criteria for liver transplantation

Irrespective of liver aetiology, HIV-positive patients with liver disease need to be managed in a multi-disciplinary environment by an experienced HIV physician and Hepatologist. Given their rapid disease kinetic, HIV-positive patients with end stage liver disease (ESLD) need to be identified early. Specific guidelines for LT in HIV-positive patients evolved as our understanding of the specific issues faced by this cohort improves. Current US National

Institutes of Health multi-center trial guidelines for LT in HIV positive patients with chronic liver disease are listed in Table 2. UK guidelines have similar requirements.

The Model for End-Stage Liver Disease (MELD) score has been adopted by transplant centers across Europe and North America to ensure the appropriate allocation of organs to those at the highest risk of death (45). Although MELD has been well validated in the HIV-negative patients, there have been mixed reports on its sensitivity in HIV-positive patients with ESLD (46). One prospective study reported similar MELD scores at the initial LT assessment for HIV-positive and HIV negative patients despite those with HIV having a significantly shorter cumulative survival time (880 versus 1427 days, $p=0.04$) (47). Another observation made by the same study was that the MELD score did not differentiate between survivors and non-survivors (13 versus 15, $p = 0.6$). Two more recent studies, both prospective, however have suggested that the MELD score may actually be a sensitive predictor of patient outcome (47, 48). Multivariate analysis of predictive factors of mortality demonstrated that the MELD score was independently associated with death (HR per 5-U increase 1.53, $p<0.001$). The MELD score also remained predictive of death on subgroup analysis of HIV/HCV patients (without HCC) and on comparison with HIV negative historical controls, the mortality rates were significantly higher for HIV-positive patients in each MELD category (48). In the second study, which matched 167 HIV-positive patients with 792 HIV-negative patients the baseline MELD score was the only significant predictor of pre-LT mortality in HIV-positive patients after controlling for $CD4^+$ counts and HIV RNA levels (47).

Optimal control of HIV disease is an important prerequisite for HIV-positive patients undergoing consideration for LT. In patients with portal hypertension, splenic sequestration of T lymphocytes can lead to a fall in the CD4+ T cell count. In such cases a CD4+ cell count > 100 cells/uL is acceptable. A fall in the $CD4^+$ cell count can also be precipitated by the use of pegylated interferon. In our opinion, CD4+ T cell percentages may represent a more sensitive indicator of immune reconstitution in HIV-positive patients with portal hypertension. HIV-positive patients undergoing evaluation for LT also require an undetectable HIV viral load (< 50 copies/mL) except for those that presently acutely. The inability to achieve an undetectable HIV RNA viral load before LT has been associated with an increased mortality rate (HR 3.5, p<0001)(48). In addition to good therapeutic options available in the pre-transplant period, HIV-positive patients require future cART options based upon their previous regimens and HIV phenol- genotype resistance testing. It is not inconceivable that certain HIV-positive patients may not be able to tolerate cART medications pre-LT due to brittle liver synthetic function. This group should not be automatically excluded from LT as long as HIV control is deemed possible post LT by the multidisciplinary team. cART intolerance post-LT, however has been identified as an important predictor of survival (49).

A thorough knowledge of past opportunistic infections is required. A distant history of an opportunistic infection in a patient that was not taking cART is not a contraindication to LT unless there is no effective treatment available for possible recurrence post-LT. Absolute contra-indications include multidrug resistant HIV, resistant fungal infections, chronic intestinal cryptosporidiosis, progressive multi-focal leukoencephalopathy and central nervous system lymphoma.

2. Post liver transplantation

Standard surgical techniques with conventional arterial, venous and biliary anastomosis are recommended. One concern highlighted is the possible risk of transmission of HIV to the surgical team. The risk of HIV however is low and is substantially lower than the risk of transmission of HBV and HCV (50). In the event of HIV exposure, current regimens provide effective prophylaxis (51). As HIV infection is associated with a pro-thrombotic state, concerns have been raised regarding an increased risk of vascular complications post transplantation (52). Recent data from our Institution demonstrated an increased an increased incidence of hepatic artery thrombosis compared to HIV negative patients (12% vs. 3.2%, p=0.016) (53). Given the increased pro-thrombotic risk, the introduction of prophylactic subcutaneous heparin (5000 units every 8 hours) is recommended once the international normalised ration (INR) is below 1.5 and the platelet count is greater than 50 x 10^9 cells/L.

Immunosuppression should be tailored to the individual taking into account aetiology of liver disease, renal function, risk factors for the metabolic syndrome and specifically to HIV patients the possible interactions with combined anti-viral therapy (cART) medications. Dual immunosuppression with calcineurin inhibitors (CNIs) and cortico-steroids is recommended post-LT. Target trough levels in the first 3 months should be the same as HIV negative patients (cyclosporin, 100-250 ng/ml; tacrolimus, 8-10ng/ml). Utilising data from HCV mono-infected patients post-LT, rapid withdrawal of cortico-steroids should be avoided due to the association of a more severe recurrence of HCV (54). We therefore recommend that prednisolone, which is usually commenced at 20mg daily, be withdrawn by a slow taper at 3 months. Anti-fungal prophylaxis (fluconazole 50mg daily) should be given for a minimum of 3 months post-LT. Episodes of acute cellular rejection (ACR) should also be managed as one would in HIV negative patients namely moderate-severe episodes be treated with a 3-day course of intravenous methylprednisolone (1g daily). Consideration of the introduction of mycophenalate mofetil (MMF) after the 2nd episode of ACR is recommended.

Both tacrolimus and cyclosporin are metabolised via the P450 cytochrome. In addition, non-nucleoside reverse-transcriptase inhibitors (NNRTIs) and protease inhibitors (PIs), which are commonly part of cART regimens, are also metabolised by the same pathway, therefore increasing the risk of drug – drug interactions. NNRTIs (e.g. efavirenz) decrease serum CNI concentrations by induction of the P450 cytochrome whilst PIs (e.g. ritonavir and lopinavir) are inducers resulting in increased CNI concentrations (55). We have used tacrolimus doses as low as 1mg per week in certain individuals. Raltegravir, a novel HIV-1 integrase inhibitor, is not metabolised via the P450 cytochrome and has been used successfully post transplantation in combination with nucleoside reverse-transcriptase inhibitors and standard CNI doses (56). Meticulous monitoring and surveillance is required to reduce the possibility drug-drug interactions and toxicity.

2.1. Outcomes post liver transplantation

Initial case series of HIV positive patients undergoing liver transplantation were associated with poor outcomes (57, 58). It is important to note that this was before the introduction of cART regimens. Retrospective data since has however demonstrated an increasing understanding of the complexities faced by this unique patient cohort. To date, the largest study analysed data provided by the US United Network for Organ Sharing LT database (1997-2006) and identified 138 HIV-positive patients (59). Overall survival rates were inferior in the HIV positive cohort compared to a comparative HIV negative cohort ($n = 30.520$) at 2- and 3-years post transplant (70% and 60% vs 81% and 77%, $p < 0.047$). Considerable data however was missing from the HIV cohort raising the possibility that HIV infection may not have been optimally treated prior to LT.

2.2. Hepatitis C co-infection

The present literature clearly demonstrates that outcomes in HIV/HCV co-infected patients is suboptimal when compared to other aetiologies. Studies to date have only described small numbers from single centres. Survival rates have ranged between 64-88% at 1 year and 33-51% at 5 years (49, 60-62). The only prospective cohort study of 89 HIV/HCV co-infected patients and 235 HCV mono-infected controls performed at 17 US centers which was recently published, warrants further analysis (63). The authors evaluated the 2 cohorts for a median 2.7 years and 2.4 years respectively (ref). Compared to HCV controls, HIV/HCV co-infected patients were younger (49 vs. 54 years, $p<0.0001$), had lower BMI at listing (25 vs. 28 kg/m^2, $p<0.0001$), more HBV co-infection (6% vs. 1%, $p=0.02$), were more likely to receive a non-heart beating graft (17% vs. 4%, $p = 0.0002$), longer median warm ischaemia time (41 vs. 21 minutes, $p =0.001$) and less use of tacrolimus-based (versus cyclosporine) initial immunosuppression (58% vs. 80%, $p<0.0001$). 1- and 3-year patient survival rates were 76% and 60% in HIV/HCV cohort compared to 92% and 79% in the HCV cohort ($p<0.001$). Graft loss was also significantly higher in the HIV/HCV cohort ($p<0.001$). Multivariate analysis identified HIV infection as the only baseline factor associated with increased risk of death (HR 2.3, $p = 0.002$) and graft loss (HR 1.9, $p = 0.01$). Analysis of the HIV/HCV co-infected cohort only identified that receipt of a combined kidney-liver transplant (HR 3.8, $p=0.003$), BMI<21 kg/m^2 at enrolment (HR = 3.2, $p=0.01$), receipt of an anti-HCV positive donor (HR 2.5, $p=0.03$), and older donor age (HR 1.3 per decade, $p=0.04$) were significant predictors of reduced graft survival. A previous study identified a MELD score > 20, intolerance of cART post transplantation and high post-transplant HCV viral loads as predictors of mortality post-LT (49). The cumulative incidence of acute cellular rejection (ACR) requiring treatment was significantly higher in HIV/HCV patients compared to HCV-mono-infected patients (39% vs. 24% at year 3, HR 2.1, $p=0.01$)(63). 50% of the cases of ACR occurred within the first 21 days following LT.

Recurrence of HCV post-LT is universal but an accelerated disease course is well recognised in HIV/HCV co-infected patients (62, 64). HCV recurrence, especially the aggressive severe fibrosing cholestatic variant of recurrent hepatitis C (FCH) and sepsis are the leading causes of death post-LT amongst HIV/HCV co-infected patients (61, 62, 65-68). Although no reliable markers are available to identify patients who will develop FCH, higher HCV viral loads immediately after LT at week 1 and week 2 may be an indicator for those at risk (69). A French study highlighted the rapid fibrosis progression rates in HIV/HCV co-infected patients (2.4 versus 1.4 score, $p=0.01$) at 24 months post-LT (62). The likelihood of progression to a fibrosis score ≥ 2 was also significantly higher in HIV/HCV co-infected patients ($p<0.0001$).

Re-treatment of HCV recurrence post-LT is associated with an increased side-effect profile and poorer treatment outcomes compared to HCV patient's pre-LT. Pegylated interferon and ribavirin remain the 'standard of care' for a minimum of 48 weeks irrespective of viral genotype. Treatment for recurrent HCV post-LT in our institution is instigated when histological disease is demonstrable ($F\geq 2$) although some groups have commenced treatment within 90 days of LT (70, 71). The concurrent use of didanosine and ribavirin is not recommended due to increased risk of mitochondrial toxicity (72). cART regimens that contain abacavir should also be avoided due to the impairment of ribavirin phosphorylation (73).

2.3. Hepatitis B co-infection and non-viral aetiologies

Patients co-infected with HBV and non-viral aetiologies including those that present with acute liver failure, have excellent short and long-term outcomes post LT. Reported median survival at 1 year ranges between 75-100% and 100% at 5 years (74)(75). The largest prospective study to date in HIV/HBV co-infected patients was conducted in 21 patients for a median of 42 months with no patient suffering graft loss (76).

The key difference between HIV/HBV and HIV/HCV co-infected patients is the presence of highly potent anti-viral agents against HBV in the therapeutic armamentarium. Patients co-infected with HBV and receiving cART will undoubtedly be receiving an oral nucleoside/nucleotide analogue that will have anti-viral actions against both HIV and HBV. Tenofovir in conjunction with emtricitabine (Truvada) is recommended (76, 77). The use of these highly efficacious, potent oral agents results in the majority of patients undergoing LT with an undetectable HBV viral load. Immuno-prophylaxis with Hepatitis B Immunoglobulin (HBIg) is also recommended in the post LT period indefinitely. Reported data on the use of HBIg and oral anti-viral agents has demonstrated that this combination is highly effective at preventing HBV recurrence even in those who have a detectable HBV viral load at the time of LT (78). Data on patients with HIV and non-viral liver disease undergoing LT is limited. Our experience suggests that these patients have similar survival rates as HIV negative patients (74).

2.4. Hepatocellular carcinoma

Studies specifically evaluating outcomes of LT in HIV positive patients with HCC have been limited. One such study compared 21 HIV positive patients with 65 HIV negative patients (79). The authors demonstrated a trend towards a higher drop-out rate on the waiting-list amongst HIV positive patients (23% vs 10%, $p = 0.08$) with 16 HIV positive and 58 HIV negative patients eventually undergoing LT. HIV positive patients were younger at the time of LT (50 versus 58 years, $p<0.002$) and following LT, observed survival was comparable at 1 and 3 years (81% and 74% versus 93% and 85%, $p=0.07$). HCC recurred in 5 HIV positive patients (31%) and in 9 HIV negative patients (15%) at a median time of 11 and 18 months respectively. Predictive factors for HCC recurrence before LT included Child Pugh C ($p=0.003$), being outside the Milan criteria radiologically ($p=0.0008$) and AFP progression > 15 ug/L per month on the waiting list ($p=0.005$). Factors predictive of HCC recurrence post LT which took into account pathological factors included those outside the Milan criteria ($p=0.01$), those outside the UCSF criteria ($p=0.03$) and those with evidence of satellite nodules ($p=0.03$) and microscopic ($p=0.005$) or macroscopic vascular invasion ($p=0.001$). Further studies are required to evaluate the influence of HIV infection on the impact of HCC post-LT but this indication in the HIV population will become more relevant.

2.5. HIV disease post transplant

At present no standardised cART regimen is utilised, but instead is tailored to the individual patient reflecting known resistance and mutations. The re-introduction of cART post-LT also varies between individual centers, with some continuing cART throughout the transplant period whilst others re-introduce the medication between 4-14 days. We recommend that cART medication should be re-introduced once liver graft function has normalised thereby avoiding the possibility of confusion with the other causes of graft dysfunction immediately post-LT.

In a recent study of HIV/HCV patients bacterial infections were identified as the principal aetiological agents of post-LT infections and viral infections were secondary to uncomplicated herpes simplex virus (HSV) infections (80). Risk factors associated with severe infections included a pre-LT MELD score of > 15 (HR 3.5, 95% CI 1.7-7.1, $p = 0.001$), history of category C AIDS-defining events (HR4.0, 1.9-8.6, $p<0.001$) and non-tacrolimus based immunosuppression (HR 2.5, 1.3-4.8, $p=0.006$). The same study also suggested that opportunistic infections namely CMV disease, disseminated HSV, invasive fungal infections and tuberculosis were increased in HIV positive patients, affecting 11% of their cohort. It is important to note these 'opportunistic' infections however can occur in HIV negative patients post LT. This study also did not have a HIV negative comparative group therefore not allowing the authors to be able to demonstrate that these deemed opportunistic infections were due to HIV infection only. Reassuringly reported data from other studies fails to demonstrate a higher incidence of opportunistic infections in comparison to HIV negative patients (81).

• **Viral:** **Hepatitis A, Hepatitis B, Hepatitis C, Hepatitis D, Hepatitis E** **CMV** **HSV**
• **Non-viral:** **Alcohol** **cART induced liver injury (e.g. NNRTI, NRTI, PI)** **Immune reconstitution** **Non-alcohol related fatty liver disease** **Non-cirrhotic portal hypertension** **Opportunistic infections**

cART, combined anti-retroviral therapy; CMV, cytomegalovirus; HSV, herpes simplex virus; NNRTI, non-nucleoside reverse transcriptase inhibitor; NRTI, nucleoside reverse transcriptase inhibitor; PI, protease inhibitor

Table 1. Causes of liver disease in HIV-positive individuals

• **The criteria for liver transplantation are met**
• **$CD4^+$ cell count > 100 cells/uL (> 200 cells/uL with a previous history of opportunistic complications).**
• **HIV viral load < 50 copies/mL (using ultrasensitive Amplicor Monitor PCR assay)**
• **Absence of AIDS-defining illness**
• **Absence progressive multi-focal leukoencephalopathy, chronic intestinal cryptosporidiosis (> 1 month) or primary CNS lymphoma**

Table 2. Criteria for Liver Transplantation in HIV-positive individuals

3. Conclusion

HIV-positive patients established on cART are expected to have good long-term outcomes. Given the success of cART, more patients are likely to present with the long-term sequelae of ESLD. In an era of organ/donor shortage, more of these patients are likely to present as potential candidates for liver transplantation. Our understanding of the issues faced by this patient cohort both pre- and post-liver transplantation continues to improve but challenges remain in the management of HIV-HCV coinfection. The data discussed in this article certainly represents a learning curve of the experience of this patient cohort. Liver transplantation in HIV-positive patients is a viable option and should be considered for carefully selected patients in transplant units with multi-disciplinary expertise.

Abbreviations

AIDS – Acquired immunodeficiency syndrome
cART – Combined anti-retroviral therapy
DILI – Drug induced liver injury
HBV – Hepatitis B virus
HCV – Hepatitis C virus
HCC – Hepatocellular carcinoma
HIV – Human immunodeficiency virus
LT – Liver transplantation
NAFLD – Non-alcohol related fatty liver disease

Author details

Deepak Joshi* and Kosh Agarwal
Institute of Liver Studies, King's College Hospital, Denmark Hill, London, UK

4. References

[1] Mocroft A, Brettle R, Kirk O, Blaxhult A, Parkin JM, Antunes F, et al. Changes in the cause of death among HIV positive subjects across Europe: results from the EuroSIDA study. AIDS 2002 Aug 16;16(12):1663-1671.
[2] Weber R, Sabin CA, Friis-Moller N, Reiss P, El-Sadr WM, Kirk O, et al. Liver-related deaths in persons infected with the human immunodeficiency virus: the D:A:D study. Arch Intern Med 2006 Aug 14;166(15):1632-1641.
[3] Salmon-Ceron D, Lewden C, Morlat P, Bevilacqua S, Jougla E, Bonnet F, et al. Liver disease as a major cause of death among HIV infected patients: role of hepatitis C and B viruses and alcohol. J Hepatol 2005 Jun;42(6):799-805.
[4] Pineda JA, Romero-Gomez M, Diaz-Garcia F, Giron-Gonzalez JA, Montero JL, Torre-Cisneros J, et al. HIV coinfection shortens the survival of patients with hepatitis C virus-related decompensated cirrhosis. Hepatology 2005 Apr;41(4):779-789.
[5] Tuma P, Jarrin I, Del AJ, Vispo E, Medrano J, Martin-Carbonero L, et al. Survival of HIV-infected patients with compensated liver cirrhosis. AIDS 2010 Mar 13;24(5):745-753.
[6] Rosenthal E, Pialoux G, Bernard N, Pradier C, Rey D, Bentata M, et al. Liver-related mortality in human-immunodeficiency-virus-infected patients between 1995 and 2003 in the French GERMIVIC Joint Study Group Network (MORTAVIC 2003 Study). J Viral Hepat 2007 Mar;14(3):183-188.
[7] Bollepalli S, Mathieson K, Bay C, Hillier A, Post J, Van Thiel DH, et al. Prevalence of risk factors for hepatitis C virus in HIV-infected and HIV/hepatitis C virus-coinfected patients. Sex Transm Dis 2007 Jun;34(6):367-370.

* Corresponding Author

[8] Fox J, Nastouli E, Thomson E, Muir D, McClure M, Weber J, et al. Increasing incidence of acute hepatitis C in individuals diagnosed with primary HIV in the United Kingdom. AIDS 2008 Mar 12;22(5):666-668.
[9] Wang CC, Krantz E, Klarquist J, Krows M, McBride L, Scott EP, et al. Acute hepatitis C in a contemporary US cohort: modes of acquisition and factors influencing viral clearance. J Infect Dis 2007 Nov 15;196(10):1474-1482.
[10] Graham CS, Baden LR, Yu E, Mrus JM, Carnie J, Heeren T, et al. Influence of human immunodeficiency virus infection on the course of hepatitis C virus infection: a meta-analysis. Clin Infect Dis 2001 Aug 15;33(4):562-569.
[11] Bonnard P, Lescure FX, Amiel C, Guiard-Schmid JB, Callard P, Gharakhanian S, et al. Documented rapid course of hepatic fibrosis between two biopsies in patients coinfected by HIV and HCV despite high CD4 cell count. J Viral Hepat 2007 Nov;14(11):806-811.
[12] Soto B, Sanchez-Quijano A, Rodrigo L, del Olmo JA, Garcia-Bengoechea M, Hernandez-Quero J, et al. Human immunodeficiency virus infection modifies the natural history of chronic parenterally-acquired hepatitis C with an unusually rapid progression to cirrhosis. J Hepatol 1997 Jan;26(1):1-5.
[13] Benhamou Y, Bochet M, Di M, V, Charlotte F, Azria F, Coutellier A, et al. Liver fibrosis progression in human immunodeficiency virus and hepatitis C virus coinfected patients. The Multivirc Group. Hepatology 1999 Oct;30(4):1054-1058.
[14] Haydon GH, Flegg PJ, Blair CS, Brettle RP, Burns SM, Hayes PC. The impact of chronic hepatitis C virus infection on HIV disease and progression in intravenous drug users. Eur J Gastroenterol Hepatol 1998 Jun;10(6):485-489.
[15] Woitas RP, Rockstroh JK, Beier I, Jung G, Kochan B, Matz B, et al. Antigen-specific cytokine response to hepatitis C virus core epitopes in HIV/hepatitis C virus-coinfected patients. AIDS 1999 Jul 30;13(11):1313-1322.
[16] Garba ML, Pilcher CD, Bingham AL, Eron J, Frelinger JA. HIV antigens can induce TGF-beta(1)-producing immunoregulatory CD8+ T cells. J Immunol 2002 Mar 1;168(5):2247-2254.
[17] Safadi R, Ohta M, Alvarez CE, Fiel MI, Bansal M, Mehal WZ, et al. Immune stimulation of hepatic fibrogenesis by CD8 cells and attenuation by transgenic interleukin-10 from hepatocytes. Gastroenterology 2004 Sep;127(3):870-882.
[18] Graham CS, Curry M, He Q, Afdhal N, Nunes D, Fleming C, et al. Comparison of HCV-specific intrahepatic CD4+ T cells in HIV/HCV versus HCV. Hepatology 2004 Jul;40(1):125-132.
[19] Blackard JT, Komurian-Pradel F, Perret M, Sodoyer M, Smeaton L, St Clair JB, et al. Intrahepatic cytokine expression is downregulated during HCV/HIV co-infection. J Med Virol 2006 Feb;78(2):202-207.
[20] Shintani Y, Fujie H, Miyoshi H, Tsutsumi T, Tsukamoto K, Kimura S, et al. Hepatitis C virus infection and diabetes: direct involvement of the virus in the development of insulin resistance. Gastroenterology 2004 Mar;126(3):840-848.
[21] Cargnel A, Angeli E, Mainini A, Gubertini G, Giorgi R, Schiavini M, et al. Open, randomized, multicentre italian trial on PEG-IFN plus ribavirin versus PEG-IFN

monotherapy for chronic hepatitis C in HIV-coinfected patients on HAART. Antivir Ther 2005;10(2):309-317.

[22] Torriani FJ, Rodriguez-Torres M, Rockstroh JK, Lissen E, Gonzalez-Garcia J, Lazzarin A, et al. Peginterferon Alfa-2a plus ribavirin for chronic hepatitis C virus infection in HIV-infected patients. N Engl J Med 2004 Jul 29;351(5):438-450.

[23] Laguno M, Cifuentes C, Murillas J, Veloso S, Larrousse M, Payeras A, et al. Randomized trial comparing pegylated interferon alpha-2b versus pegylated interferon alpha-2a, both plus ribavirin, to treat chronic hepatitis C in human immunodeficiency virus patients. Hepatology 2009 Jan;49(1):22-31.

[24] Chung RT, Andersen J, Volberding P, Robbins GK, Liu T, Sherman KE, et al. Peginterferon Alfa-2a plus ribavirin versus interferon alfa-2a plus ribavirin for chronic hepatitis C in HIV-coinfected persons. N Engl J Med 2004 Jul 29;351(5):451-459.

[25] Carrat F, Bani-Sadr F, Pol S, Rosenthal E, Lunel-Fabiani F, Benzekri A, et al. Pegylated interferon alfa-2b vs standard interferon alfa-2b, plus ribavirin, for chronic hepatitis C in HIV-infected patients: a randomized controlled trial. JAMA 2004 Dec 15;292(23):2839-2848.

[26] Moreno A, Barcena R, Garcia-Garzon S, Moreno L, Quereda C, Muriel A, et al. Viral kinetics and early prediction of nonresponse to peg-IFN-alpha-2b plus ribavirin in HCV genotypes 1/4 according to HIV serostatus. J Viral Hepat 2006 Jul;13(7):466-473.

[27] Kellerman SE, Hanson DL, McNaghten AD, Fleming PL. Prevalence of chronic hepatitis B and incidence of acute hepatitis B infection in human immunodeficiency virus-infected subjects. J Infect Dis 2003 Aug 15;188(4):571-577.

[28] Chapman LE, Sullivent EE, Grohskopf LA, Beltrami EM, Perz JF, Kretsinger K, et al. Recommendations for postexposure interventions to prevent infection with hepatitis B virus, hepatitis C virus, or human immunodeficiency virus, and tetanus in persons wounded during bombings and other mass-casualty events--United States, 2008: recommendations of the Centers for Disease Control and Prevention (CDC). MMWR Recomm Rep 2008 Aug 1;57(RR-6):1-21.

[29] Gilson RJ, Hawkins AE, Beecham MR, Ross E, Waite J, Briggs M, et al. Interactions between HIV and hepatitis B virus in homosexual men: effects on the natural history of infection. AIDS 1997 Apr;11(5):597-606.

[30] Colin JF, Cazals-Hatem D, Loriot MA, Martinot-Peignoux M, Pham BN, Auperin A, et al. Influence of human immunodeficiency virus infection on chronic hepatitis B in homosexual men. Hepatology 1999 Apr;29(4):1306-1310.

[31] Brau N, Fox RK, Xiao P, Marks K, Naqvi Z, Taylor LE, et al. Presentation and outcome of hepatocellular carcinoma in HIV-infected patients: a U.S.-Canadian multicenter study. J Hepatol 2007 Oct;47(4):527-537.

[32] Salmon-Ceron D, Rosenthal E, Lewden C, Bouteloup V, May T, Burty C, et al. Emerging role of hepatocellular carcinoma among liver-related causes of deaths in HIV-infected patients: The French national Mortalite 2005 study. J Hepatol 2009 Apr;50(4):736-745.

[33] Puoti M, Bruno R, Soriano V, Donato F, Gaeta GB, Quinzan GP, et al. Hepatocellular carcinoma in HIV-infected patients: epidemiological features, clinical presentation and outcome. AIDS 2004 Nov 19;18(17):2285-2293.

[34] Bourezane Y, Salard D, Hoen B, Vandel S, Drobacheff C, Laurent R. DRESS (drug rash with eosinophilia and systemic symptoms) syndrome associated with nevirapine therapy. Clin Infect Dis 1998 Nov;27(5):1321-1322.

[35] de Maat MM, ter HR, van Gorp EC, Mulder JW, Mairuhu AT, Beijnen JH. Case series of acute hepatitis in a non-selected group of HIV-infected patients on nevirapine-containing antiretroviral treatment. AIDS 2003 Oct 17;17(15):2209-2214.

[36] Bossi P, Colin D, Bricaire F, Caumes E. Hypersensitivity syndrome associated with efavirenz therapy. Clin Infect Dis 2000 Jan;30(1):227-228.

[37] Laguno M, Milinkovic A, de LE, Murillas J, Martinez E, Blanco JL, et al. Incidence and risk factors for mitochondrial toxicity in treated HIV/HCV-coinfected patients. Antivir Ther 2005;10(3):423-429.

[38] Vrouenraets SM, Treskes M, Regez RM, Troost N, Smulders YM, Weigel HM, et al. Hyperlactataemia in HIV-infected patients: the role of NRTI-treatment. Antivir Ther 2002 Dec;7(4):239-244.

[39] Maida I, Nunez M, Rios MJ, Martin-Carbonero L, Sotgiu G, Toro C, et al. Severe liver disease associated with prolonged exposure to antiretroviral drugs. J Acquir Immune Defic Syndr 2006 Jun;42(2):177-182.

[40] Sandrine PF, Sylvie A, Andre E, Abdoulaye D, Bernard L, Andre C. Nodular regenerative hyperplasia: a new serious antiretroviral drugs side effect? AIDS 2007 Jul 11;21(11):1498-1499.

[41] Schiano TD, Kotler DP, Ferran E, Fiel MI. Hepatoportal sclerosis as a cause of noncirrhotic portal hypertension in patients with HIV. Am J Gastroenterol 2007 Nov;102(11):2536-2540.

[42] Mallet V, Blanchard P, Verkarre V, Vallet-Pichard A, Fontaine H, Lascoux-Combe C, et al. Nodular regenerative hyperplasia is a new cause of chronic liver disease in HIV-infected patients. AIDS 2007 Jan 11;21(2):187-192.

[43] Worm SW, Friis-Moller N, Bruyand M, D'Arminio MA, Rickenbach M, Reiss P, et al. High prevalence of the metabolic syndrome in HIV-infected patients: impact of different definitions of the metabolic syndrome. AIDS 2010 Jan 28;24(3):427-435.

[44] Guaraldi G, Squillace N, Stentarelli C, Orlando G, D'Amico R, Ligabue G, et al. Nonalcoholic fatty liver disease in HIV-infected patients referred to a metabolic clinic: prevalence, characteristics, and predictors. Clin Infect Dis 2008 Jul 15;47(2):250-257.

[45] Kamath PS, Wiesner RH, Malinchoc M, Kremers W, Therneau TM, Kosberg CL, et al. A model to predict survival in patients with end-stage liver disease. Hepatology 2001 Feb;33(2):464-470.

[46] Ragni MV, Eghtesad B, Schlesinger KW, Dvorchik I, Fung JJ. Pretransplant survival is shorter in HIV-positive than HIV-negative subjects with end-stage liver disease. Liver Transpl 2005 Nov;11(11):1425-1430.

[47] Subramanian A, Sulkowski M, Barin B, Stablein D, Curry M, Nissen N, et al. MELD score is an important predictor of pretransplantation mortality in HIV-infected liver transplant candidates. Gastroenterology 2010 Jan;138(1):159-164.

[48] Murillas J, Rimola A, Laguno M, de LE, Rascon J, Aguero F, et al. The model for end-stage liver disease score is the best prognostic factor in human immunodeficiency virus

1-infected patients with end-stage liver disease: a prospective cohort study. Liver Transpl 2009 Sep;15(9):1133-1141.

[49] de Vera ME, Dvorchik I, Tom K, Eghtesad B, Thai N, Shakil O, et al. Survival of liver transplant patients coinfected with HIV and HCV is adversely impacted by recurrent hepatitis C. Am J Transplant 2006 Dec;6(12):2983-2993.

[50] Goldberg D, Johnston J, Cameron S, Fletcher C, Stewart M, McMenamin J, et al. Risk of HIV transmission from patients to surgeons in the era of post-exposure prophylaxis. J Hosp Infect 2000 Feb;44(2):99-105.

[51] Henderson DK. Postexposure chemoprophylaxis for occupational exposures to the human immunodeficiency virus. JAMA 1999 Mar 10;281(10):931-936.

[52] Ahonkhai AA, Gebo KA, Streiff MB, Moore RD, Segal JB. Venous thromboembolism in patients with HIV/AIDS: a case-control study. J Acquir Immune Defic Syndr 2008 Jul 1;48(3):310-314.

[53] Cherian PT, Alrabih W, Douiri A, Quaglia A, Heneghan MA, O'Grady J, et al. Liver transplantation in human immunodeficiency virus-infected patients: procoagulant, but is antithrombotic prophylaxis required? Liver Transpl 2012 Jan;18(1):82-88.

[54] Berenguer M, Royuela A, Zamora J. Immunosuppression with calcineurin inhibitors with respect to the outcome of HCV recurrence after liver transplantation: results of a meta-analysis. Liver Transpl 2007 Jan;13(1):21-29.

[55] Frassetto LA, Browne M, Cheng A, Wolfe AR, Roland ME, Stock PG, et al. Immunosuppressant pharmacokinetics and dosing modifications in HIV-1 infected liver and kidney transplant recipients. Am J Transplant 2007 Dec;7(12):2816-2820.

[56] Tricot L, Teicher E, Peytavin G, Zucman D, Conti F, Calmus Y, et al. Safety and efficacy of raltegravir in HIV-infected transplant patients cotreated with immunosuppressive drugs. Am J Transplant 2009 Aug;9(8):1946-1952.

[57] Tzakis AG, Cooper MH, Dummer JS, Ragni M, Ward JW, Starzl TE. Transplantation in HIV+ patients. Transplantation 1990 Feb;49(2):354-358.

[58] Dummer JS, Erb S, Breinig MK, Ho M, Rinaldo CR, Jr., Gupta P, et al. Infection with human immunodeficiency virus in the Pittsburgh transplant population. A study of 583 donors and 1043 recipients, 1981-1986. Transplantation 1989 Jan;47(1):134-140.

[59] Mindikoglu AL, Regev A, Magder LS. Impact of human immunodeficiency virus on survival after liver transplantation: analysis of United Network for Organ Sharing database. Transplantation 2008 Feb 15;85(3):359-368.

[60] Ragni MV, Belle SH, Im K, Neff G, Roland M, Stock P, et al. Survival of human immunodeficiency virus-infected liver transplant recipients. J Infect Dis 2003 Nov 15;188(10):1412-1420.

[61] Schreibman I, Gaynor JJ, Jayaweera D, Pyrsopoulos N, Weppler D, Tzakis A, et al. Outcomes after orthotopic liver transplantation in 15 HIV-infected patients. Transplantation 2007 Sep 27;84(6):697-705.

[62] Duclos-Vallee JC, Feray C, Sebagh M, Teicher E, Roque-Afonso AM, Roche B, et al. Survival and recurrence of hepatitis C after liver transplantation in patients coinfected with human immunodeficiency virus and hepatitis C virus. Hepatology 2008 Feb;47(2):407-417.

[63] Terrault NA, Roland ME, Schiano T, Dove L, Wong MT, Poordad F, et al. Outcomes of liver transplantation in HCV-HIV coinfected recipients. Liver Transpl 2012 Feb 12.

[64] Gane EJ, Portmann BC, Naoumov NV, Smith HM, Underhill JA, Donaldson PT, et al. Long-term outcome of hepatitis C infection after liver transplantation. N Engl J Med 1996 Mar 28;334(13):815-820.

[65] Vennarecci G, Ettorre GM, Antonini M, Santoro R, Perracchio L, Visco G, et al. Liver transplantation in HIV-positive patients. Transplant Proc 2007 Jul;39(6):1936-1938.

[66] Castells L, Escartin A, Bilbao I, Len O, Allende H, Vargas V, et al. Liver transplantation in HIV-HCV coinfected patients: a case-control study. Transplantation 2007 Feb 15;83(3):354-358.

[67] Roland ME, Barin B, Carlson L, Frassetto LA, Terrault NA, Hirose R, et al. HIV-infected liver and kidney transplant recipients: 1- and 3-year outcomes. Am J Transplant 2008 Feb;8(2):355-365.

[68] Di BF, Di SS, De RN, Berretta M, Montalti R, Guerrini GP, et al. Human immunodeficiency virus and liver transplantation: our point of view. Transplant Proc 2008 Jul;40(6):1965-1971.

[69] Antonini TM, Sebagh M, Roque-Afonso AM, Teicher E, Roche B, Sobesky R, et al. Fibrosing cholestatic hepatitis in HIV/HCV co-infected transplant patients-usefulness of early markers after liver transplantation. Am J Transplant 2011 Aug;11(8):1686-1695.

[70] Castells L, Esteban JI, Bilbao I, Vargas V, Allende H, Ribera E, et al. Early antiviral treatment of hepatitis C virus recurrence after liver transplantation in HIV-infected patients. Antivir Ther 2006;11(8):1061-1070.

[71] Wojcik K, Vogel M, Voigt E, Speidel N, Kalff JC, Goldmann G, et al. Antiviral therapy for hepatitis C virus recurrence after liver transplantation in HIV-infected patients: outcome in the Bonn cohort. AIDS 2007 Jun 19;21(10):1363-1365.

[72] Lafeuillade A, Hittinger G, Chadapaud S. Increased mitochondrial toxicity with ribavirin in HIV/HCV coinfection. Lancet 2001 Jan 27;357(9252):280-281.

[73] Mira JA, Lopez-Cortes LF, Barreiro P, Tural C, Torres-Tortosa M, de Los SG, I, et al. Efficacy of pegylated interferon plus ribavirin treatment in HIV/hepatitis C virus co-infected patients receiving abacavir plus lamivudine or tenofovir plus either lamivudine or emtricitabine as nucleoside analogue backbone. J Antimicrob Chemother 2008 Dec;62(6):1365-1373.

[74] Joshi D AVBAea. Liver transplantation for HIV: analysis of outcomes suggest HIV/HCV co-infected patients have prohibitively poor survival at 5 years. 59th Annual Meeting of the American Association for the Study of Liver Diseases; San Francisco, CA, USA; Oct 31-Nov 4, 2008. Abstract 6. 2012.

[75] Tateo M, Roque-Afonso AM, Antonini TM, Medja F, Lombes A, Jardel C, et al. Long-term follow-up of liver transplanted HIV/hepatitis B virus coinfected patients: perfect control of hepatitis B virus replication and absence of mitochondrial toxicity. AIDS 2009 Jun 1;23(9):1069-1076.

[76] Terrault NA, Carter JT, Carlson L, Roland ME, Stock PG. Outcome of patients with hepatitis B virus and human immunodeficiency virus infections referred for liver transplantation. Liver Transpl 2006 May;12(5):801-807.

[77] Gazzard BG, Anderson J, Babiker A, Boffito M, Brook G, Brough G, et al. British HIV Association Guidelines for the treatment of HIV-1-infected adults with antiretroviral therapy 2008. HIV Med 2008 Oct;9(8):563-608.
[78] Coffin CS, Stock PG, Dove LM, Berg CL, Nissen NN, Curry MP, et al. Virologic and clinical outcomes of hepatitis B virus infection in HIV-HBV coinfected transplant recipients. Am J Transplant 2010 May;10(5):1268-1275.
[79] Vibert E, Duclos-Vallee JC, Ghigna MR, Hoti E, Salloum C, Guettier C, et al. Liver transplantation for hepatocellular carcinoma: the impact of human immunodeficiency virus infection. Hepatology 2011 Feb;53(2):475-482.
[80] Moreno A, Cervera C, Fortun J, Blanes M, Montejo E, Abradelo M, et al. Epidemiology and outcome of infections in human immunodeficiency virus/hepatitis C virus-coinfected liver transplant recipients: a FIPSE/GESIDA prospective cohort study. Liver Transpl 2012 Jan;18(1):70-81.
[81] Neff GW, Bonham A, Tzakis AG, Ragni M, Jayaweera D, Schiff ER, et al. Orthotopic liver transplantation in patients with human immunodeficiency virus and end-stage liver disease. Liver Transpl 2003 Mar;9(3):239-247.

Chapter 13

Hodgkin's Lymphoma and Human Immunodeficiency Virus Infection

Moosa Patel

Additional information is available at the end of the chapter

1. Introduction

Hodgkin's lymphoma is a lymphoid neoplasm first described by Thomas Hodgkin in 1832 and subsequently by Samuel Wilks in 1865 (1,2). Greenfield (1878), Sternberg (1879) and Reed (1902) are credited with the earliest descriptions of the pathological characteristics of the disease (3,4,5). In has now become clear that the Reed-Sternberg cell is derived from clonal B-cells, more specifically post-germinal center B-cells, giving credence to the malignant nature of the disease, and hence the preferred term of Hodgkin's lymphoma –HL, instead of Hodgkin's disease (6).

Major and striking advances have been made in the biology and management of HL. More than 70% of patients with HL are curable (especially those presenting with early stage disease). Better insight has been gained with regard to the acute and long term toxicities of chemotherapy and radiotherapy. Furthermore, the advent of new imaging techniques such as PET (positron emission tomography)-scans are allowing therapy to be individualized and tailored in a risk adapted and response adapted fashion (7).

The incidence of HL varies widely throughout the world (approximately 1-3.5/100 000), based on geographical and ethnic factors. The highest rates of HL are seen in the United States, Canada and Europe, with much lower rates occurring in Japan, Korea and China. HL is more common in males compared to females, with a male to female ratio of 1.5:1. HL occurs most often in young adults, with a peak frequency in the third decade of life. A bimodal age distribution may be seen, with a second age peak noted in the 6th to 8th decades (8,9,10,11).

The exact aetiology of HL is unknown. An increased risk of HL is seen with Epstein-Barr Virus (EBV) infection, congenital and acquired immunodeficiency states (such as Human Immunodeficiency Virus – HIV infection/AIDS- Acquired Immunodeficiency Syndrome, post solid organ and haematopoietic stem cell transplantation) and autoimmune disease (12-18). There is also an increased risk of familial aggregation of HL (19).

HIV infection is known to be associated with an increased risk of HL, based on linkage and cohort studies. The relative risk is now 10-15 fold higher compared with the general population (13-15,17,18,20-22). This review will focus on HL in southern Africa, and describe the differences compared to HL in developed countries, highlighting the emerging increase in HL in the HIV seropositive population/people living with HIV/AIDS (PWHA).

2. General aspects of HIV lymphoma

Lymphomas are known to occur with an increased frequency in PWHA (20,21,23). NHL (Non-Hodgkin's Lymphoma) is the commonest malignancy in the post cART (combination antiretroviral therapy) era in PWHA. The incidence of NHL in resource-rich settings has decreased in the post cART era compared to the pre cART era (23-24). However, the contrary is true in resource-poor settings, with a noticeable increase in NHL incidence (24-26). This is particularly true of sub-Saharan Africa - the epicenter of the HIV pandemic. The increase in NHL incidence is due mainly to the high prevalence and heavy burden of HIV in sub-Saharan Africa, a region in which two thirds of PWHA reside, and additionally, in many countries in sub-Saharan Africa, there has been a lack of availability of, or delay in initiation of cART. In South Africa, which is home to over 5 million PWHA, the rollout of cART occurred in 2004, 8 years later than in the Western world (introduced in developing countries during the end of 1996 and the beginning of 1997) and until recently, cART was generally only available to individuals with CD4 counts of <200/ul. Although this practice has changed in the last two years, with access/availability of cART to individuals with a higher CD4 count of <350/ul, the burden of diseases related to the immunodeficiency state (with notable exceptions such as Kaposi's sarcoma) appear to be on the increase (17,25,26,27).

In Africa, the HIV/AIDS epidemic was first reported in 1984 (28). The major risk of HIV in Africa occurs in/with heterosexual relationships, and accounts for an approximately equal male to female ratio, as compared to the Western world in which the major risk groups involve intravenous drug use and homosexual relationships, thus predominantly affecting males. Furthermore, early in the HIV epidemic, there was no marked increase in the incidence of NHL compared to the USA. This was attributed to PWHA dying earlier in the course of their disease possibly from infectious complications such as pneumonia and tuberculosis. The decreased longevity prevented the subsequent or later development of NHL. In addition, there may be underreporting of lymphoma or the missed diagnosis of lymphoma, with a diagnosis of an infective cause of lymphadenopathy (such as tuberculosis) being favoured over lymphoma, in the absence of performing a fine needle aspirate or lymph node biopsy (28-30).

At Chris Hani Baragwanath Academic Hospital (CHBAH) – a tertiary, public sector, University of the Witwatersrand linked hospital located in Soweto, Johannesburg, studies in the 1990's with respect to HIV-NHL showed only a modest increase of NHL in seropositive individuals, with an odds ratio of 4.8, 5 and 5.9 respectively (31-33). The first patient at this hospital with HIV-NHL was seen in 1993. Since then, there has been a steady increase in HIV-NHL up to 2000. However, since 2001, the percentage seropositivity of NHL has exceeded 50% (approximately between 60 – 80%), and since 2002, there has additionally been a significant increase in the total number of patients diagnosed with NHL at CHBAH (from 20-30 new patients per year to 70-80 patients per year) (see Table 1 and Figure 1) (25). Indeed, NHL is now the commonest haematological malignancy in South Africa, in the current HIV/AIDS era and the number of seropositive patients continues to increase.

With respect to Hodgkin's lymphoma (HL), the data is less dramatic, but is becoming more significant. In a study by Stein et al, 2008 (33), the percentage seropositivity of HL in a South African cohort (which included patients from CHBAH) was 19.5% (OR=1.6, 95% CI=1.0-2.7), during the period 1995-2004. The first patient with HIV-HL was seen in 1994 at CHBAH. Since then, there has been a modest increase in HIV-HL up to 2006. However, in the last 5 years (2007 - 2011) at our single institution, the percentage seropositivity is greater than 50% (see Figure 2) and the number of patients over the years are gradually increasing (doubled compared to an earlier series in the late 1980's and early 1990's – (17,34)(see Figure 3). Thus, the focus of this review relates to the emerging problem of Hodgkin's lymphoma in the setting of HIV in southern Africa.

Year	Total Number of Patients	Number of Seronegative Patients	Number of Seropositive Patients	% Seropositive
1993	20	19	1	5%
1994	20	18	2	10%
1995	18	15	3	16.7%
1996	28	25	3	10.7%
1997	18	14	4	22.2%
1998	34	18	16	47.1%
1999	22	14	8	36.4%
2000	30	16	14	46.7%
2001	24	4	20	83.3%
2002	40	15	25	62.5%
2003	44	17	27	61.4%
2004	58	23	35	60.3%
2005	54	15	39	72.2%
2006	72	17	55	76.4%
2007	72	19	53	73.6%
2008	76	10	66	86.8%

Table 1. Patients with non-Hodgkin's Lymphoma seen at Chris Hani Baragwanath Academic Hospital from 1993 to 2008

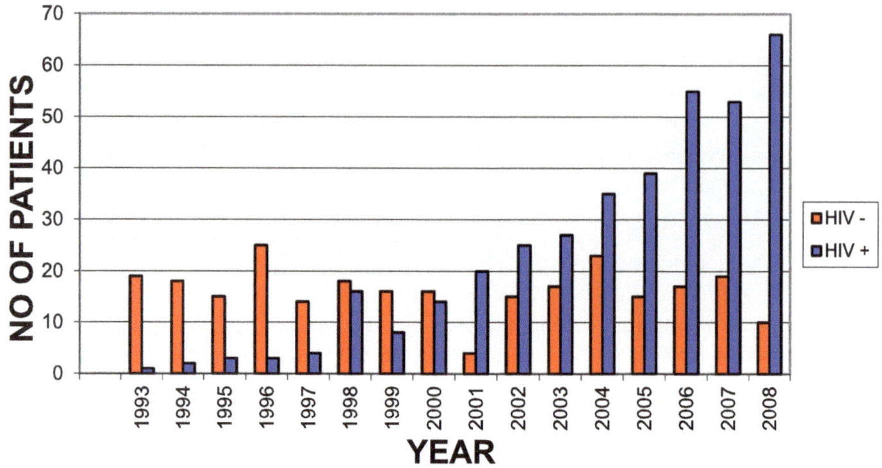

Figure 1. HIV seropositive and HIV seronegative patients with non-Hodgkin's Lymphoma from 1993 to 2008 seen at Chris Hani Baragwanath Academic Hospital

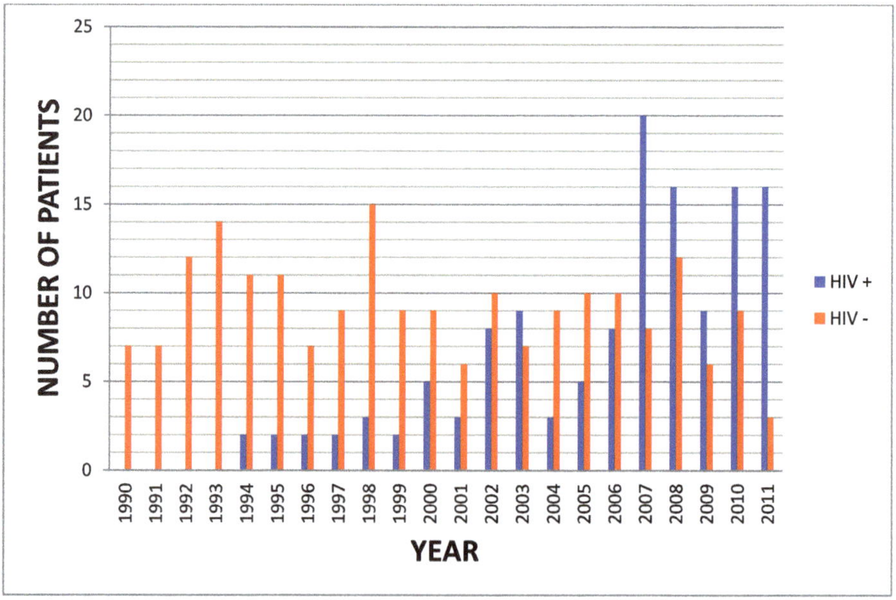

Figure 2. HIV seropositive and HIV seronegative patients with Hodgkin's Lymphoma from 1990 to 2011 seen at Chris Hani Baragwanath Academic Hospital

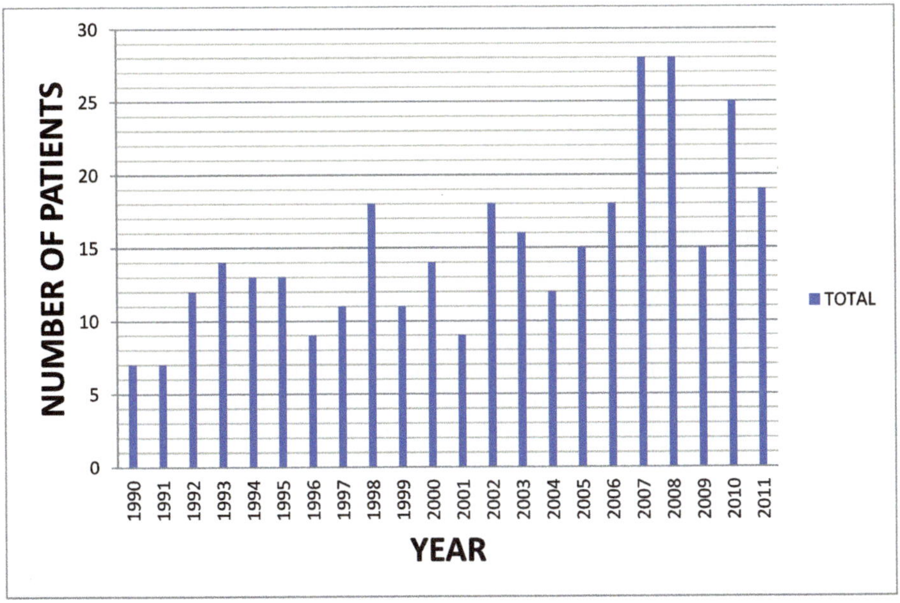

Figure 3. Total number of patients with Hodgkin's Lymphoma seen at Chris Hani Baragwanath Academic Hospital from 1990 - 2011

3. Hodgkin's lymphoma and HIV

3.1. Introduction and epidemiology

HL occurring in the setting of immunodeficiency (with particular reference to HIV/AIDS) is generally aggressive, presents with advanced stage disease, frequent constitutional ('B') symptoms, less favourable histology, more frequent bone marrow involvement and a poorer prognosis compared to immunocompetent individuals (17,18).

With the advent of HAART (highly active antiretroviral therapy), now referred to as cART (combination antiretroviral therapy), the AIDS related morbidity, particularly with respect to opportunistic infections has decreased and the survival of HIV/AIDS patients has increased (35,36). In the post cART era, ADCs (AIDS-defining cancers) continue to fall, but the rates of NADCs (non-AIDS defining cancers) such as HL, anal carcinoma, lung carcinoma and skin cancers are on the increase (37). With HL, there is a noticeably increasing relative risk of approximately 10 - 15 fold, compared with the general population (13-15,17,18,20-22).

Several epidemiological studies conducted in the last two decades, and summarised in the article by Carbone et al, 2009 (22) strongly support the evidence that HIV positive individuals have a higher risk of developing HL compared to their HIV negative counterparts. This is in contrast to HIV-NHL or HIV-Kaposi's sarcoma (where the incidence of the disease has decreased significantly after the introduction of cART). cART has allowed the use of standard therapeutic options to be delivered to seropositive patients in a more optimal manner, bringing about renewed optimism in the management of such patients. cART use is associated with higher CD4 T cell counts and enhanced immunity. Thus, despite the benefit of cART, which improves immunity and decreases the risk of opportunistic infections, there is a paradoxical increased risk of HL (22). The authors conclude that the improved CD4 T cell count that occurs post cART use, provides anti-apoptotic pathways and mechanisms for immune escape by tumour cells, thus resulting in an increased risk of HL (22).

However, in contrast to this, a 20-year cohort study has shown that with the advent of antiretroviral therapy, ADCs (AIDS-defining cancers) continue to fall, but the rates of NADCs (non-AIDS defining cancers) are on the increase. The authors suggest that this increase appears to be more related to the aging of the HIV population (i.e. increased longevity allowing a greater risk of developing lymphoma) rather than the antiretroviral therapy and its effect on the CD4 T cell count (37).

3.2. Pathogenesis

Histologically, HL is characterized by a population of neoplastic Reed-Sternberg (RS) cells, which constitute <1-2% of the cellular component, admixed with a reactive, mixed inflammatory infiltrate of lymphocytes, plasma cells, eosinophils and histiocytes. Cytokines and chemokines are produced by either the RS cells or the reactive cells in the background micro-environment of the tissue. The cytokine production may explain the presence and maintenance of an impaired immune response, while the chemokines (cytokines with chemoattractant properties) play a role in leucocyte trafficking, attract chemokine receptor CCR4-expressing Th-2 cells and T regulatory cells, and allow a favourable environment for survival of RS cells (38-40). Cross talk between the RS cells and reactive cells mediated by cytokines such as IL-13, IL-17, IL-10, transforming growth factor-beta and chemokines - principally CCL17 (thymus and activation-regulated chemokine, TARC) and CCL22 (macrophage-derived chemokine, MDC), lead to an environment where RS cells are able to proliferate, escape from apoptosis and survive host anti-tumour defense (38-40). The CD4+ T cells surrounding the neoplastic cells in HL are CD45RO+/CD45RA-/CD45RB^{dim}, suggesting a memory Th2 phenotype (41).

HIV-associated immunosuppression is a state that permits the unchecked and uncontrolled proliferation of Epstein-Barr virus (EBV) infection. EBV has been implicated in the etiopathogenesis of classic HL, with a high frequency of EBV association (80-100%) noted in tissues of patients with HIV-HL (42,43). EBV transforming proteins, such as latent membrane protein-1 (LMP-1), is expressed in virtually all HIV-HL patients (43-45). The expression of EBV-LMP-1 is important in the pathogenesis of HIV-HL. LMP-1 expression by EBV-infected RS cells represents the principal mechanism for constitutive NF (nuclear factor) -κB activity, which confers an apoptosis resistant phenotype to the RS cells (43,45). EBV-immortalized B cells also produce CCL17 and CCL22 through LMP-1 mediated activation of NFκB (46).

RS cells of classical HL represent transformed B cells (post germinal center B cells) that originate from preapoptotic germinal center B cells. They express CD15 and CD30 as well as LMP-1 and display a BCL6-/CD138+/MUM1/IRF4+ (Interferon Regulatory Factor-4) phenotype (43,47,48). In addition, LMP2A and EBNA-1 may also contribute to the development of the RS cells and are expressed in the RS cells of this tumour (44,45). LMP2A may promote the survival of the 'crippled' germinal center B cells, thereby aiding in their development (49).

3.3. Clinical presentation and management

In general, HIV-seropositive patients with HL tend to have a more aggressive clinical course than their seronegative counterparts. The behaviour of the disease is different, and based on a number of studies (22,50-57), the following characteristics were noted: more frequent constitutional 'B' symptoms – 70-96%, more advanced stage disease (III and IV) – 74-92%, , more frequent involvement of extranodal sites – 17-62%, with bone marrow involvement being the most common extranodal site – 40-59%, followed by involvement of the liver – 17-40% and spleen – 20-30%. The vast majority (>80%) of the patients were males. The median age at presentation was approximately 34 years. The median CD4 count was mostly in the intermediate range of 240-306/µl (22,50-57). Compared to HIV negative HL, where nodular sclerosis is the dominant histological subtype, mixed cellularity is most commonly encountered in HIV-HL – 33-53% (17,22,34,56-57). Nodular sclerosis is the second most common histological subtype in HIV-HL – 24-31%. However, with more severe immunosuppression, nodular sclerosis becomes infrequent (38). There is also an increasing number of patients with lymphocyte depleted histology - 14-20% in HIV-HL (17,22,56-57).

Based on the Italian Cooperative Group on AIDS and Tumors (GICAT) study, in comparison with patients who were cART naive, patients receiving cART before the onset of HL are older, have less B symptoms, have higher leukocyte and neutrophil counts and have a higher haemoglobin level (56).

In a recent review of 43 patients with HIV associated HL seen at CHBAH over a 2 year period (July 2008 – June 2010) a number of striking similarities and differences were noted when comparing this cohort with other published studies outside of Africa (17). The median age at presentation of 38 years was similar to other series. There was no striking male predominance. Conversely, the male to female ratio is almost equal at 1.1:1. All the patients had heterosexual acquisition of HIV. None of the patients acquired their HIV through intravenous drug use or homosexual contacts. This is different to other series where homosexuality and intravenous drug use are significant, documented risk groups (15,20,22,50,56,57). The presentation with advanced stage disease (82%), more frequent 'B' symptoms (93%), more frequent involvement of extranodal sites (bone marrow-38%; liver-45%; spleen-28%) and 'true' extranodal sites (17%) and the histological pattern of disease (mixed cellularity being the most common) is similar to that reported in the literature. The median CD4 count of 176/µl is generally lower, although there are series reported of HIV-HL with median CD4 counts of <200/µl (51). In this series 12/29 (41%) of the patients had newly diagnosed HIV at the time of the diagnosis of HL. In 62% of the patients, the duration of the diagnosis of HIV (including new patients was < 1 year). Only 45% of the patients were on antiretroviral therapy at diagnosis of HL, compared to 71-80% in other series (22,56,57). A further striking difference is the high proportion of patients with Tuberculosis in this series – 59% (38% with active disease and 21% with past, documented disease). The high prevalence of tuberculosis may be a reflection of the more severe immunosuppression in the patients, the delay in diagnosis of HIV and hence the absence of antiretroviral therapy use at diagnosis and the very common occurrence of tuberculosis in the general population. The presence of tuberculosis, often in a disseminated fashion, has an adverse impact on the clinical outcome of the patients. In general, the outcome of the HIV-HL patients was less favourable than the HIV seronegative patients (17).

In another local study from CHBAH, covering a fifteen period from 1990 to 2004, the clinical characteristics of 163 patients with Hodgkin's lymphoma are reviewed (58). Table 2 depicts the differences between the HIV seropositive and HIV seronegative patients in this study.

HIV Status	Seropositive	Seronegative
Total Number of Patients = 163	47 (29%)	116 (71%)
Median Age (Range) in Years	30 (13-59)	29 (13-87)
M:F Ratio	1.8:1	1.2:1
CD4 Count at Presentation (/ul)	186 (32-769)	N/A
'B' Symptoms	77%	78%
Advanced Stage (III & IV) Disease	78%	67%
'True' Extranodal Disease	13%	12%
Histological Subtype:		
Mixed Cellularity	61%	42%
Nodular Sclerosis	17%	41%
Other	22%	13%
Tuberculosis		
Prevalence	27%	23%
Active Disease	19%	17%
Treatment Response		
Complete Response	38%	57%
Partial Response	8%	21%

Table 2. Clinical characteristics of HIV seropositive and HIV seronegative patients seen over a fifteen year period (1990 - 2004) at Chris Hani Baragwanath Academic Hospital (adapted from Fazel, 2012)

Based on the findings of this study, HIV seronegative patients compared to HIV seropositive patients have more advanced stage disease, a higher frequency of mixed cellularity subtype, a slightly higher risk of tuberculosis and 'true' extranodal disease and a poorer response to treatment (58).

The management of HIV-HL is challenging because of the frequency of infections, likelihood of organ dysfunction due to HIV, more frequent involvement of the bone marrow, increased myelosuppression, potential drug-drug interactions of the antiretrovirals and anti-infectives with chemotherapy, the advanced and widespread nature of the disease at presentation and the preponderance of less favourable histological subtypes. Treatment approaches include vigorous supportive care (HAART, antivirals, antifungals, neutrophil-stimulating growth factors), together with standard multiagent chemotherapy.

Chemotherapy regimens for HIV-HL such as EBV, EBVP, ABVD and MOPP/ABV hybrid are feasible and can be delivered with concomitant cART. The AIDS Clinical Trials Group (ACTG) treated 21 patients with ABVD for 4-6 cycles with G-CSF support. Antiretroviral therapy was not used. The complete remission rate (CR) was 43% with a median overall survival of 18 months (59). In a more recent Spanish study (GESIDA – Groupo de Estudia de SIDA), 62 patients with HIV-HL received the standard, full-dose ABVD and cART with 87% of the patients achieving a CR. The 5-year overall survival (OS) and event-free survival (EFS) probabilities were 76 and 71% respectively. The immunological response to HAART had a positive impact on OS (p=0.002) and EFS (p=0.001) (60). Use of cART substantially improves the overall survival in HIV associated HL. This is due to a decrease in the incidence of opportunistic infections, the ability to deliver more appropriate and aggressive chemotherapy on schedule and to the less aggressive presentation of lymphoma in patients on cART, in comparison with those lymphomas that arise in patients who never received cART (50-53). In the study of Hentrich et al, 2006, 34/59 patients receiving cART (n=34) had a significantly better 2-year overall survival than those not receiving cART (74% versus 30%, p<0.001) (61). The advent of cART also allows for more aggressive treatment options such as VEBEP (62), BEACOPP (63), Stanford V (64) and the use of high-dose chemotherapy and autologous stem cell transplantation (ASCT) in selected patients (65,66). However, in general, response rates and cure rates are lower than in HIV seronegative patients, despite the substantial progress made in the last decade. The challenge at present is to optimise the use of standard approaches as used in HIV negative HL. Once this is established, evaluation of experimental and newer therapies should follow.

4. Conclusion

HIV is associated with an increased risk of developing HL, a risk that has not lessened despite the introduction and benefit of cART. HL is now being regarded among the most common NADCs, which have clearly increased in the post cART era. The association from being largely coincidental (overlapping and similar age group for both HL and HIV) may now be increasingly causal, with the most plausible explanation being attributed to the pathogenetic role of Epstein Barr virus infection.

The recognition of an increasing trend of HIV-HL in resource-poor settings needs to be further highlighted, so that early diagnosis, early recourse to cART and appropriate supportive therapy and specific therapy such as chemotherapy can be administered to improve survival.

Therapy of HIV associated HL entails using the same therapeutic approaches as in seronegative HL, including standard chemotherapy regimens such as ABVD, and in the salvage setting, autologous stem cell transplantation in selected patients. In general, the prognosis and overall survival still remains poorer in HIV-HL compared to HIV negative HL. Importantly, the concomitant use of anti-retroviral agents has allowed for the delivery of full-dose and dose-intensive chemotherapy given on schedule, as well as prophylaxis against certain opportunistic infections such as Pneumocystis jirovecii pneumonia, and the liberal use of growth factors (granulocyte colony stimulating factor) and other supportive measures, constitutes an important aspect of supportive therapy and has contributed to an improvement in prognosis. The early recognition and treatment of tuberculosis cannot be overemphasized in settings where tuberculosis is endemic. Newer specific treatment approaches for HL may become necessary in the future to improve survival. However, for the present, HIV-associated HL appears to be on the increase and remains an emerging and ongoing challenge.

Author details

Moosa Patel
Clinical Haematology Unit, Department of Medicine, Chris Hani Baragwanath Academic Hospital and Faculty of Health Sciences, University of the Witwatersrand, Johannesburg, South Africa

Acknowledgement

I thank all the medical, nursing and allied healthcare professionals who were involved in the diagnosis, management and follow up of the patients with Hodgkin's lymphoma. In particular, I extend my sincere gratitude to the staff of the Clinical Haematology Unit, Department of Medicine, CHBAH, and all the patients whose data has been used in this study.

5. References

[1] Hodgkin T. On some morbid appearances of the absorbent glands and spleen. *Medico-Chirug Trans* 17:68, 1832.
[2] Wilks S. Cases of the enlargement of the liver and spleen (or Hodgkin's disease) with remarks. *Guys Hosp Rep* 11:56, 1865.
[3] Greenfield WS. Specimens illustrative of the pathology of lymphadenoma and leucocythemia. *Trans Pathol Soc Lond* 29:272, 1878.
[4] Sternberg C. Uber eine eigenartige unter dem Bilde der Pseudoleukamie verlaufende Tuberculose des lymphatischen Apparates. *Ztschr Heilk* 19:21, 1879.
[5] Reed D. On pathological changes in Hodgkin's disease, with special reference to its relation to tuberculosis. *Johns Hopkins Hosp Rep* 10:133, 1902.
[6] Marafioti T, Hummel M, Foss H-D, et al. Hodgkin and Reed-Sternberg cells represent an expansion of a single clone originating from a germinal center B-cell with functional immunoglobulin gene rearrangement but defective immunoglobulin transcription. *Blood* 95:1443-50, 2000.

[7] Evens AM and Horning SJ. Hodgkin lymphoma: epidemiology, diagnosis, and treatment. In Management of Hematologic Malignancies. Ed. S O'Brien, JM Vose and HM Kantarjian. Cambridge University Press pp 367-403, 2011.
[8] Katanoda K and Yako-Suketomo H. Comparison of time trends in Hodgkin and Non-Hodgkin lymphoma incidence (1973-97) in East Asia, Europe and USA, from cancer incidence in five continents, Vol. IV-VIII. *Jpn J Clin Oncol* 38:391-3, 2008.
[9] http://www.seer.cancer.gov/csr/1975_2005/results_single/sect_01_table.01.pdf.
[10] Correa P and O'Connor GT. Epidemiologic patterns of Hodgkin's disease. *Int J Cancer* 8:192-201, 1971.
[11] Macfarlane GJ, Evstifeeva T, Boyle P, et al. International patterns in the occurrence of Hodgkin's disease in children and young adult males. *Int J Cancer* 61:165-9, 1995.
[12] Brousset P, Knecht H, Rubin B, et al. Demonstration of Epstein-Barr virus replication in Reed-Sternberg cells of Hodgkin's disease. *Blood* 82:872-6, 1993.
[13] Herida M, Mary-Krause M, Kaphan R, et al. Incidence of non-AIDS-defining cancers before and during the highly active antiretroviral therapy era in a cohort of human immunodeficiency virus-infected patients. *J Clin Oncol* 21:3447-53, 2003.
[14] Biggar RJ, Jaffe ES, Goedert JJ, et al. Hodgkin lymphoma and immunodeficiency in persons with HIV/AIDS. *Blood* 108:3786-91, 2006.
[15] Hessol NA, Katz MH, Liu JY, et al. Increased incidence of Hodgkin disease in homosexual men with HIV infection. *Annals of Internal Medicine* 117(4):309-11, 1992.
[16] Landgren O, Engels EA, Pfeiffer RM, et al. Autoimmunity and susceptibility to Hodgkin lymphoma: a population-based case-control study in Scandinavia. *J Natl Cancer Inst* 98;1321-30, 2006.
[17] Patel M, Philip V and Fazel F. Human immunodeficiciency virus infection and Hodgkin's Lymphoma in South Africa – An emerging problem. Advances in Hematology Volume 2011 (2011), doi:10.1155/2011/578163, 2011.
[18] Spina M, Carbone A, Gloghini A, et al. Hodgkin's Disease in Patients with HIV infection. *Advances in Hematology* Volume 2011 (2011), doi:10.1155/2011/402682, 2011.
[19] Hjalgrim H, Rasmussen S, Rostgaard K, et al. Familial clustering of Hodgkin lymphoma and multiple sclerosis. *J Natl Cancer Inst* 96:780-4, 2004.
[20] Lyter D, Bryant J, Thackeray R, et al. Incidence of human immunodeficiency virus related and non related malignancies in a large cohort of homosexual men. *J Clin Oncol* 13:2540-6, 1995.
[21] Goedert J, Cote T, Virgo P, et al. Spectrum of AIDS-associated malignant disorders. *Lancet* 351:1833-9, 1998.
[22] Carbone A, Gloghini A, Serraino D, et al. HIV-associated Hodgkin lymphoma. *Current Opinion in HIV and AIDS* 4:3-10, 2009.
[23] Ziegler JL, Drew WL and Miner RC. Outbreak of Burkitt's-like lymphoma in homosexual men. *The Lancet* 2(8299):631-33, 1982.
[24] Ulrickson M, Press OW and Casper C. Epidemiology, Diagnosis, and Treatment of HIV-Associated Non-Hodgkin's Lymphoma in Resource Limited Settings. *Advances in Hematology* Volume 2012(2012), doi:10.1155/2012/932658, 2012.

[25] Patel M, Philip V, Turton D, et al. The impact of HIV on Non-Hodgkin's Lymphoma at Chris Hani Baragwanath Hospital. *Haematologica* 92(s1):273, 2007.
[26] UNAIDS. Report on the global AIDS epidemic. Geneva: UNAIDS, 2008.
[27] Casper C. The increasing burden of HIV-associated malignancies in resource-limited regions. *Annual Review of Medicine* 62:157-170, 2011.
[28] Clumeck N, Sonnet J and Taelman H. Acquired immunodeficiency syndrome in African patients. *NEJM* 310(8):492-97, 1984.
[29] Parkin DM, Wabinga S, Nambooze S, et al. AIDS-related cancers in Africa: maturation of the epidemic in Uganda. *AIDS* 13(18):2563-70, 1999.
[30] Adeniji KA and Anjorin AS. Peripheral lymphadenopathy in Nigeria. *African Journal of Medicine and Medical Sciences* 29(3-4):233-37, 2000.
[31] Sitas F, Bezwoda WR, Levin V, et al. Association between human immunodeficiency type 1 infection and cancer in the black population of Johannesburg and Soweto, South Africa. *Br J Cancer* 75:1704-07, 1997.
[32] Sitas F, Pacella-Norman R, Carrara H, et al. The spectrum of HIV-1 related cancers in South Africa. *Int J Cancer* 88,489-92, 2000.
[33] Stein L, Urban MI, O'Connell D, et al. The spectrum of human immunodeficiency virus associated cancers in a South African black population: Results from a case-control study, 1995-2004. *Int J Cancer* 122:2260-2265, 2008.
[34] Patel M. Haematology. In: Baragwanath Hospital 50 years – A Medical Miscellany. Eds. K Huddle and A Dubb. Ultra Litho. 173-190, 1994.
[35] Ribera JM, Navarro JT, Oriol A, et al. Prognostic impact of highly active antiretroviral therapy in HIV-related Hodgkin's disease. *AIDS* 16(14):1973-6, 2002.
[36] Gerard L, Galicier L, Boulanger E, et al. Improved survival in HIV-related Hodgkin's lymphoma since the introduction of highly active antiretroviral therapy. *AIDS* 17(1):81-87, 2003.
[37] Crum-Cianflone N, Hullsiek KH, Marconi V et al. Trends in the incidence of cancers among HIV-infected persons and the impact of antiretroviral therapy: a 20-year cohort study. *AIDS* 23:41-50, 2009.
[38] Takegawa S, Jin S, Nakayama T et al. Expression of CCL17 and CCL22 by latent membrane protein 1-positive tumor cells age-related Epstein-Barr virus-associated B lymphoproliferative disorder. *Cancer Sci* 99:296-302, 2008.
[39] Niens M, Visser L, Nolte IM et al. Serum chemokine levels in Hodgkin lymphoma patients: highly increased levels of CCL17 and CCL22. *British Journal of Haematology* 140:527-536, 2008.
[40] Maggio E, van den Berg A, Diepstra A et al. Chemokines, cytokines and their receptors in Hodgkin's lymphoma cell lines and tissues. *Annals of Oncology* 13(Suppl. 1):52-56, 2002.
[41] Poppema S, Lai R, Visser L et al. CD45 (leucocyte common antigen) expression in T and B lymphocyte subsets. *Leuk Lymphoma* 20:217-222, 1996.
[42] Rezk SA and Weiss LM. Epstein-Barr virus-associated lymphoproliferative disorders. *Human Pathology* 38(9):1293-1304, 2007.

[43] Carbone A, Gloghini A, Larocca LM, et al. Human immunodeficiency virus-associated Hodgkin's disease derives from postgerminal center B cells. *Blood* 93:2319-2326, 1999.

[44] Young LS and Rickinson AB. Epstein-Barr virus: 40 years on. *Nat Rev Cancer* 4:757-768, 2004.

[45] Carbone A, Gloghini A, Dotti G. EBV-associated lymphoproliferative disorders: classification and treatment. *Oncologist* 13:577-585, 2008.

[46] Nakayama T, Hieshima K, Nagakubo D et al. Selective induction of Th2-attracting chemokines CCL17 and CCL22 in human B cells by latent membrane protein1 of Epstein-Barr Virus. *J Virol* 78:1665-74, 2004.

[47] Klein U and Dalla-Favera R. Germinal centres: role in B-cell physiology and malignancy. *Nat Rev Immunol* 8:22-33, 2008.

[48] Carbone A, Gloghini A, Larocca LM, et al. Expression profile of MUM1/IRF4, BCL-6, and CD138/syndecan-1 defines novel histogenic subsets of human immunodeficiency virus-related lymphomas. *Blood* 97:744-751, 2001.

[49] Mancao C and Hammerschmidt W. Epstein-Barr virus latent membrane protein 2A is a B-cell receptor mimic and essential for B-cell survival. *Blood* 109:2597-2603, 2007.

[50] Tirelli U, Errante D, Dolcetti R, et al. Hodgkin's disease and human immunodeficiency virus infection: clinicopathologic and virologic features of 114 patients from the Italian Co-operative group on AIDS and Tumors. *J Clin Oncol* 13:1758-1767, 1995.

[51] Tirelli U, Vaccher E, Serraino D, et al. Comparison of presenting clinical and laboratory findings of patients with persistent generalized lymphadenopathy (PGL) syndrome and malignant lymphoma (ML). *Haematologica* 72:563-565, 1987.

[52] Andrieu JM, Roithmann S, Tourani JM, et al. Hodgkin's disease during HIV-1 infection: the French registry experience. *Ann Oncol* 4:635-641, 1993.

[53] Rubio R. Hodgkin's disease associated with human immunodeficiency virus infection. A clinical study of 46 cases. *Cancer* 73:2400-2407, 1994.

[54] Garcia-Noblejas A, Nieto S, Liberal R, et al. Intracerebral Hodgkin's lymphoma in a patient with human immunodeficiency virus. *Haematologica* 92:e72-e73, 2007.

[55] Vaccher E, Spina M, Talamini R, et al. Improvement of systemic human immunodeficiency virus-related NHL in the era of HAART. *Clin Infect Dis* 37:1556-1564, 2003.

[56] Chimienti E, Spina M, Gastaldi R, et al. Clinical characteristics and outcome of 290 patients (pts) with Hodgkin's disease and HIV infection (HD-HIV) in pre and HAART (highly active antiretroviral therapy) era (abstract 168). *Ann Oncol* 19:iv136, 2008.

[57] Berenguer J, Miralles P, Ribera JM, et al. Characteristics and outcome of AIDS-related Hodgkin's lymphoma before and after the introduction of highly active antiretroviral therapy. *J Acquir Immune Defic Syndrome* 47:422-428, 2008.

[58] Fazel FB. Hodgkin's Lymphoma at Chris Hani Baragwanath Hospital. A fifteen year review. MMed dissertation. University of the Witwatersrand 2012.

[59] Levine AM, Li P, Cheung T, et al. Chemotherapy consisting of doxorubicin, bleomycin, vinblastine and dacarbazine with granulocyte-colony-stimulating-factor GCSF in HIV infected patients with newly diagnosed Hodgkin's disease: a prospective, multi-

institutional AIDS Clinical Trials Group Study (ACTG 149). *J Acquir Immune Defic Syndr* 24:444-450, 2000.

[60] Xicoy B, Ribera JM, Miralles P, et al. Results of treatment with doxorubicin, bleomycin, vinblastine and dacarbazine and highly active antiretroviral therapy in advanced stage human immunodeficiency virus-related Hodgkin's lymphoma. *Haematologica* 92:191-198, 2007.

[61] Hentrich M, Maretta L, Chow JR, et al. Highly active antiretroviral therapy (HAART) improves survival in HIV-associated Hodgkin's disease: results of a multicentre study. *Annals of Oncology* 17:914-919, 2006.

[62] Spina M, Rossi G, Antinori A, et al. VEBEP regimen and highly active antiretroviral therapy (HAART) in patients (pts) with HD and HIV infection (HD-HIV) (abstract 227). *Ann Oncol* 19:iv152, 2008.

[63] Hartmann P, Rehwald U, Salzberger B, et al. BEACOPP therapeutic regimen for patients with Hodgkin's disease and HIV infection. *Ann Oncol* 14:1562-1569, 2003.

[64] Spina M, Gabarre J, Rossi G, et al. Stanford V regimen and concomitant HAART in 59 patients with Hodgkin disease and HIV infection. *Blood* 100:1984-1988, 2002.

[65] Krishnan A, Molina A, Zaia J, et al. Durable remission with autologous stem cell transplantation for high-risk HIV-associated lymphomas. *Blood* 105:874-878, 2005.

[66] Spitzer TR, Ambinder RF, Lee JY, et al. Dose-reduced busulfan, cyclophosphamide, and autologous stem cell transplantation for human immunodeficiency virus-associated lymphoma: AIDS Malignancy Consortium Study 020. *Biol Blood Marrow Transplant* 14:59-66, 2008.

Chapter 14

What I Knew was What I Learnt on the Street! Irish Drug Using Sex Workers Accounts of How They Contracted HIV and Hepatitis C

Teresa Whitaker, Paul Ryan and Gemma Cox

Additional information is available at the end of the chapter

1. Introduction

This paper draws from a larger piece of research conducted by the authors [1] for the National Advisory Committee on Drugs (NACD) whose remit is to provide advice to the Irish government on problematic drug use in Irish society. Under Action 98 of the Irish National Drug Strategy [2] the NACD was required to carry out research on drug misuse amongst groups who were considered 'at risk'. Prostitutes were identified as one such group. Because of the negative connotations and stigma associated with the word 'prostitute' the research team used the term 'sex-worker', the term favored by the World Health Organisation [3-6] and the United Nations [6].

The objectives of this paper are:

- To briefly review research on the links between HIV and sex work, internationally
- To describe the prevalence of HIV among sex workers in Ireland
- To explore the Irish policy response to HIV prevention in relation to this population
- To explore the risk environment of drug using sex workers in Dublin

The aim of this paper is to understand the myriad ways in which HIV was contracted and managed by drug-using sex workers.

2. Literature review

The relationship between HIV and sex work is well documented. In 2009 the UNAIDS Advisory Group[7] was established to provide guidance and advice on issues to do with HIV and sex work, while at the same time emphasizing the human rights of female, male, and transgender sex workers and the importance of universal access to HIV prevention, treatment, care and support.

The overall growth of the HIV global AIDS epidemic seems to have stabilized. There has been a steady decline in the number of new HIV infections since the late 1990s; and due to antiretroviral therapy fewer AIDS-related deaths have occurred. The UNAIDS vision is zero new HIV infections, zero discrimination and zero AIDS-related deaths. That said, new HIV infections are still high and worldwide there has been an increase in the number of people living with HIV. The population under discussion in this paper remain at particularly high risk [7].

The UNAIDS report (2010) states that there are three high risk behaviours associated with the spread of HIV are injecting drug use, practising unprotected paid sex, and men having sex with men [7]. There are also risks in discordant heterosexual relationships where one partner is HIV positive and risks transmitting the virus to the other partner in a long term relationship. It emphasizes the importance of couples testing for HIV. Becoming sexually active at a young age is also a risk factor; the report states that young people still lack the information and the necessary tools to practice HIV risk-reduction strategies. There is a lack of provision of harm reduction materials such as condoms and lubrication, and sterile needles. It argues that in order to protect women and girls from HIV they need to be protected against gender-based violence.

The UNAIDS Advisory Group Report [7] noted that sex workers often face widespread and interconnected human rights violations which impede both their effective participation in HIV responses and their right to access HIV and other health and social services. It stated that societal stigma and discrimination against sex workers results in repressive laws, policies and practices, and the economic disempowerment of sex workers. The Report warns countries against the persecution of sex workers and the conflation of trafficking with sex work.

3. Irish government policy response to HIV

In Ireland, in response to the HIV epidemic in the 1980s the then Eastern Health Board [1] (now the Eastern Region Health Service Executive) established two specialised drugs intervention clinics (one for female sex workers and one for gay men and male sex workers) in the capital city, Dublin. These clinics provide free HIV screening and other harm reduction services such as needle exchanges and methadone maintenance for intra-venous drug users. In 1987 the Dublin Aids Alliance (DAA), a voluntary non-governmental organisation with charitable status, was set up to improve conditions for people living with or affected by HIV and AIDS. DAA is; provides front line services, such as counselling, outreach and condom distribution. It is the representative for the eastern region of Ireland on the Department of Health and Children's National AIDS Strategy Committee (NASC) and its Education and Prevention Subcommittee. NASC was established in 1991 and published its first Strategic Report in 1992. It took a multi-disciplinary approach involving statutory and non-statutory sectors and people living with HIV and AIDs. In 2000 it published an AIDS Strategy 2000 [8] which promoted prevention, treatment and care. In 2008 NASC [9] published a 4-year plan for HIV and AIDS Education and Prevention in Ireland with the aim of reducing infection through education, awareness raising and prevention measures. The action suggests that best practice measures targeting sex workers and those buying sex should be integrated into sexual health campaigns. It recommends that there should be appropriate and innovative approaches to HIV screening and treatment including mobile services and new technology. In 2010 a mobile health clinic entitled Safetynet Network for Homeless Health Services was established in Dublin targeting homeless people and sex workers [10]. It provides primary health care and harm reduction services.

4. Prevalence of HIV in Ireland

Figures published by the Health Protection Surveillance Centre [11] on newly diagnosed HIV infections in Ireland in 2011 showed that there were 152 new HIV diagnoses in the first six months of 2011 (less than the 166 cases reported in Q1&2 2010 and the 164 in Q3&4 2010). This brought the cumulative total number of HIV infections reported in Ireland to more than 6,120. The HPSC notes that, as regards new cases:

- The highest proportion (39.5%) was among men who have sex with men.
- Heterosexual contact accounted for 27.6%.
- Females accounted for 25.0%.
- People in the 15-24 year old age band comprised 9.2%.
- Intravenous drug users accounted for 7.9%.
- Of these newly identified cases, 9.2% were diagnosed with an AIDS defining illness at the time of their HIV diagnosis, and 41.4% were asymptomatic.
- Of the heterosexual cases, 35.7% were individuals originating from countries with generalised epidemics, and a further 19% were individuals with a partner originating from a country with a generalised epidemic, or with a partner known to be HIV positive or a partner who is an injecting drug user.

5. Risk environment

The 'risk environment' is a simple model or explanatory framework developed by Tim Rhodes [12] to examine the multiple environmental factors that produce health and other types of risk. There are four types of environmental influences: physical, social, economic and policy in the context of three levels of environmental influence – micro, meso and macro. The risk environment is made up of the risk factors that are external to the individual; these risks can mediate the individual's capacity to reduce the risk of harm. For example, if a country provides free needle exchange programs or opiate substitution programs they help the individual user to reduce the harms associated with intravenous opiate use.

Although harm reduction is most commonly applied to reducing harms related to drug use (especially intravenous drug use), harm reduction principles are increasingly being applied to sex work. The harms associated with sex work include the vulnerabilities that may lead to sex work, the harms that are introduced by engaging in sex work such as stigma [13], criminalisation, and the mutually reinforcing harms such as problem drug use and in particular injecting drug use [14]. The nature and extent of harms associated with sex work varies with the type of sex market they work in e.g. brothels, massage parlours, escorts, street work, however, the harms are greatest in street-based sex markets [15] and where sex workers' pre-existing vulnerabilities can be exploited [16].

There are a number of layers in the risk environment in Ireland. In terms of sex work, there is the legal environment which criminalizes sex workers if they work in brothels or if they solicit sex on the streets[17]. Due to policing, risks are increased because sex workers cannot take time to negotiate with clients and assess the safety aspect of the transaction. To decrease their visibility on the street, there is the added risk of sex workers working in badly lit and remote areas where they are more likely to be victims of violent clients. Due to the societal disapproval of sex work, there is the risk of stigma[13] or public disclosure. The use of crack cocaine has been shown to be associated with street sex working in Dublin [18].

In response to the heroin epidemic in the 1980s in Dublin drug treatment clinics and harm reduction services (methadone maintenance, needle exchange programs etc.) were established [19] within a risk environment where illicit drug use is criminalized[17]. Despite the criminality associated with drug use, reported levels of cocaine use in Ireland are above the European average [20] and Ireland also reports the highest estimate of opioid use in the European Union [20]. The Irish Health Service Executive [21] reports that there are 9,264 people in methadone maintenance treatment, whilst it is estimated that there are another 10,000 heroin users who are not in treatment [22]. In the past heroin use was concentrated in Dublin however now it is spreading all over Ireland. Disadvantaged communities are hardest hit.

A tragic consequence of illicit drug use is early death. In Ireland in 2009 (the latest figures available) there were 357 deaths due to illicit drug use. Cocaine was implicated in 52 of these, heroin was implicated in 108 and methadone in 66 [23]. Poly substance (heroin and methadone) use was implicated in 117 deaths. The majority of those who died were aged between 25 and 44 years; the median age was 38 years. Delays in service provision are clearly a factor: drug users seeking treatment have to wait an average of three to 18 months for opioid substitute treatment depending on the area of Ireland they live in [20].

Although there are adequate health services available for sex workers in Dublin, sex workers are stigmatized [13] on many levels (due to injecting drug use, HIV or HCV infections, and sex working) and may hide their work from health personnel. There is also a high incidence of HCV (70%) among injecting drug users in Ireland [13]. Whilst it is not possible to ascertain the prevalence of HIV among drug using sex workers in Ireland and it is certainly unjust to consider them as vectors of disease, one fifth of the sex workers in our study [13] self-reported as being HIV positive.

6. Methods

The focus of this research was to gain an understanding of drug-using sex workers' lived experience of risk, in order to understand how the local risk environment (i.e. the physical, social, economic and policy environment) produces risks in their daily life and work contexts, and how drug-using sex workers implement strategies to manage and reduce the risk of harm. A qualitative methodology was chosen as being the most appropriate to answer the research question. Ethical permission for the study was sought and granted from the Drug Treatment Centre Board in Dublin and also from the Prison services.

7. Sample

A purposive sample (4 men and 31 women: n=35) of drug-using sex workers was selected. They were located for the research by key service providers and by an agency which offers specialist support to drug using sex workers. In order for sex workers to be eligible for inclusion in the study they had to self identify as a problematic drug user as defined by the Irish National Drug Strategy – i.e. their drug use caused them social, psychological, physical or legal difficulties, and they were involved in sex work or had recently given up sex work after a prolonged period of sex working.

8. Research instruments

Two research instruments were utilised to register these sex workers' accounts. A topic guide was designed for use in in-depth face-to-face interviews, and a short survey was used to gather biographic and demographic information and to record current drug use frequency and any associated criminal activity over the previous 90 days. The interviews were conducted in a number of different venues: some in rooms provided by an agency, some in cars, some in prison and some in cafés. In keeping with NACD policy all participants were recompensed for their time with a voucher for a local chain store.

In order to comply with ethical guidelines, prior to conducting the interview, the research was explained to the participant, who signed a consent form and was assured that they could withdraw from the study at any time and that all information was confidential and anonymous. Their permission to audio record the interview was also sought; all agreed to be recorded.

The interviews lasted 45 minutes to an hour and the data quality was good. Generally speaking, the sex workers were very open and viewed the interview as a way of helping out, or doing the researcher a favor. Ethical guidelines were complied with in relation to storage of the data on a password protected computer; all personal identifiers were removed from the data. The data were anonymized, each sex worker was given a pseudo-name (in alphabetical order). Hard copies of the data were stored in a locked filing cabinet. Data was only used for the purpose of the research.

9. Data analysis

The researchers fully immersed themselves in the data by listening repeatedly to the recordings. All interviews were fully transcribed. Emerging themes and trends were identified in the data as were comparative data. Inductive analysis of the qualitative data was facilitated by the use of QSR NVivo software, and quantitative data were analysed using the statistical package for the social sciences (SPSS). In the following accounts, I denotes 'Interviewer' and R denotes 'Respondent'.

10. Findings

The women and men interviewed were white indigenous Irish people; the vast majority were from Dublin, and all, but one, were living in Dublin at the time of interview. In addition many respondents reported other vulnerabilities such as being homeless, two had spent many years in residential care systems, four were in prison at the time of the interview either serving a sentence or on remand; four women had recently been released from prison and were living in transitional accommodation (specifically for women released from prison). Nine were living in emergency accommodation, most in city centre hostels and nine were living in the private rented sector. Four were living in the parental home or were staying with friends. In many cases, their marginality was compounded by the loss of their children, many were parents (24 women and one man) but the majority had put their children into care which substantially added to their distress and to their drug use. A brief outline of participants' reported drug use sets the context for reading their accounts of managing risk in their daily lives and work.

11. Illicit drug use and treatment experience

Research participants [were asked about their use of a range of substances in the 90 days prior to interview. Although 88 per cent of participants were on prescribed methadone, 65 per cent also reported recent heroin use, 29 per cent reported cocaine use, and 15 per cent reported crack cocaine use. Participants who were actively involved in sex work at the time of interview were more likely to report the use of all substances [1].

All 35 participants had a history of injecting drug use: 53 per cent reported injecting in the 90 days preceding interview, and seven were high frequency injectors (they reported daily injecting in the preceding 90 days, with five of them injecting more than four times per day in that period). Four of these high frequency injectors were injecting cocaine daily [1].

Participants reported a high level of contact with healthcare services: 64.7 per cent reported having had a health check in the 90 days prior to interview. Almost all also reported having been tested for HIV (figures for reported infection have been given above). Over three-quarters of the study participants (78.1 per cent) had had a positive HCV diagnosis; 26.7 per cent said that they had received information about the virus, 36.7 per cent reported having received an onward referral; however, only 13.3 per cent (n=4) reported having ever received treatment for HCV. Less than half the sample (43.8 per cent) reported having received the hepatitis B vaccine, and 17.2 per cent had received it in the last three months; 19.4 per cent had received confirmation that the vaccine had worked. Only one of the study participants reported receiving the combination interferon and ribavirin HCV treatment and three of the women were receiving HIV triple therapy treatment; all three commenced treatment while in prison [1].

12. Risk and risk management in participants' accounts

While all participants reported using needle exchanges to access sterile injecting equipment, most admitted to engaging in unsafe injecting practices in the past. Because they had commenced illicit drug use at a young age, many were unaware of the attendant risks of contracting HIV/HCV at the time and in any case were unable to access sterile injecting equipment, because there were limited harm reduction interventions in Dublin at the time.

Some spoke about recent occasions where they put themselves at risk by sharing injecting equipment or accidentally using another's equipment, for example, Eileen explained:

> *R: I have shared works and that's how I got the hepatitis. And then one day last year I was with a girl and she has the HIV. We were actually out one night and we got cocaine off somebody. And I actually brought her home back to the hostel. And we went to IV cocaine, and she was after putting her needle, her works into me and she only realised, or so she said, she only realised that she put the wrong needle in, that it was hers. And it was after being used already because she had HIV. So my head was wrecked, for the whole three months I had to wait for the antibodies and all to come back.*

Despite having access to sterile needles, Úna explained how she unwittingly used a friend's equipment because she was in the throes of withdrawal. This account highlights the struggle to maintain safe practices in a very risky, unsafe environment with an irresponsible drug using friend who was HIV positive. This detailed narrative has been tabulated to facilitate reading. Úna's account is presented in the left hand column where it is broken into numbered blocks to highlight the main topic focus in each. In the right hand column the author's accompanying analysis and interpretation is presented.

In the above account Úna describes how she always accessed sterile needles (1), and would always put an identifier on them (6), dispose of them carefully (14) and would not inject in a public space (15). She expresses her horror (9) and disappointment at discovering that she had used another's works and had thus contracted HIV (13). This narrative also emphasizes other risks such as homelessness (4), sex working (3) to fund a cocaine habit (13) and the dangers of social drug (3) use with a treacherous drug buddy who did not alert her to his HIV positive status. She received her HIV diagnosis in prison (12), given her marginalized position she may never had had a blood test for in a treatment service.

Úna's account		Analysis
1.	I used to go up to [Drugs Treatment Service] and get them [sterile needles]. I always did yea, but then	Commitment to safe drug use
2.	I ended up meeting a fella [boy]. He was only a friend ... like, he wasn't a boyfriend or that. He was more like a drug buddy. We used to just go off and get drugs together and	Drug buddy enabling and sharing in use
a.	he'd give me a lift up to [...] Street every night and he would wait in the car for me and I'd go off, do whatever and come back and he would give me a lift back up to get the drugs. But I was buying drugs for the two of us. He would go up to the park and have a turn-on and then we'd go back out and make more money and that's the way it was going then, every day. And	Enabled to do sex work to fund shared drug use
3.	I was living on the streets, and we were sleeping in the car, like he was letting me sleep in the car. It was a robbed car but he was sleeping in it as well.	Buddy enabling shared marginalisation, sleeping in a stolen car
4.	So I didn't know that he had HIV. He had it for 14 years, but he never told me and	Risky relationship
5.	we ended up going up to the Park one night to have a turn-on [inject drugs] and I used to burn the end of me works so I'd know that was MY works.	Concern for safe injecting by putting identifier on own syringe
6.	And I was dying sick that day and we were just basically rushing to get the drugs into us like, 'cause I was dying sick.	Hunger and hurry and impaired judgement due to being in the throes of withdrawal
7.	And he ended up anyway taking my works and giving me his works. And I didn't know. I didn't cop it until I had my turn-on and then until he was having his turn-on and I copped that the works that he had was my works and I looked and I had his works and	Using the other's contaminated syringe
8.	I nearly died. I went mad over it like and a few days later his ex-girlfriend called me, and she was saying to me "I hope you're not using after him, 'cause did he not tell you that he has HIV?". And I said, "No". She said "He has it for the last 14 years". She said, "Don't use after him".	Awful horror at discovering that her drug buddy was HIV positive
9.	I was getting real agitated because I knew that I was after using his works. I didn't use his works knowing that it was his works. I didn't know that it was his works. Like, he gave me I thought it was my works,	Reemphasizes that she would not knowingly use another's works
10.	and he thought – well, I don't know if he knew that he was using my works and I think he did know that I was using his works but he didn't open his fuckin' mouth	Treacherous, reckless buddy
11.	I came in here [prison] then and I found out then a few weeks later that I was HIV positive.	HIV diagnosis done in prison

Úna's account	Analysis
12. I knew that I was after catching it from him. I was after being stopped [cocaine] for a while and I was after getting back on the coke then and he was the only one then I was hanging around with and that I was going and getting drugs with. He was the only one that I knew I was after using after because	Links between cocaine use and sex working
13. I was always careful about my needles and all. And I'd always clean up after myself and I'd wrap them up well and I'd throw them out, you know like. I'd never leave them around or	Pride in strict hygiene practices
14. I'd never, like, up in X Apartment Block they'd all sit round the stairs and you'd come up, they'd have their trousers down banging [injecting] their groins and all.	Rejects reckless practices of those who inject in public spaces such as the stairs in apartment blocks
15. I'd never do anything like that.	Asserts own carefulness

Table 1.

Yolanda has also contracted HIV and Hep C from sharing needles.

R: I don't know, I just think I shared with other people.

I: Do you think that you might have accidentally used other peoples?

R: I don't know. I knew some of the times.

Carol talked about her lack of knowledge and ignorance of how blood borne viral infections were transmitted

I: But at that time, because you were very young did you know anything about needles?

R: I knew nothing about nothing. What I knew was what I learnt on the street. That's where I learned how to inject from someone else showing me. I knew nothing at the time. I didn't know anything really about hepatitis till I went in for clinics to get off methadone, to get clean completely and that was seven years ago. Other than that I knew nothing about nothing. I knew nothing. Nobody tells you anything. You have Hep C and that's the end of it. There's no one telling you what hepatitis is, or anything like and to get to the doctor, now you ring the doctor and you have to wait three months to see the doctor. When you go into the doctor you're only in there and you could have a list of questions and they only want you in and out real quick because of the way it runs; so many behind you. It's ridiculous.

I: So thinking back to that period, would you have shared needles?

R: Yes. But I was very fussy, a fussy junkie, people say, but I was. I'd only share with X [my sister] and Y [my child's father] father at the time. Anybody else, no I wouldn't. I was fussy. Even with the prostitution when I had had enough. The last time I had a right cry was when I came home and I was on my knees crying. I never had to score drugs for a few days. I was actually asked to work three or four days non-stop at that time. I was more crying, you know that kind of way. I said I'll never do this again. I'd rather go sick. I'd never try prostitution again.

Having a baby was a turning point in Yseult's life in that she decided to discontinue the use of illicit substances and stopped engaging in sex work.

> I: *And what about blood test for HIV or Hepatitis C?*
>
> R: *Yes I have Hepatitis C. And the last blood test I had was after I had him. But I haven't turned on [injected] or used or anything like that since then, so I don't think I have HIV and I didn't go for any other blood tests. But when he was born I was HIV negative and Hep C positive.*
>
> I: *When was that last test?*
>
> R: *Well he is two now, so it was about two years ago. I don't go into all the risks that I would have taken when I was using.*

Florence felt that using cocaine was the factor which precipitated her throwing caution to the wind and asked her friend to inject her with equipment that turned out to be contaminated.

> R: *… the time I got the hepatitis C, 'cause when I was on the coke, I, it's like, with gear you have a conscience, but with coke you don't and this young fella, now, I wasn't going out with him, we were just friends, but I couldn't get meself, so I needed him to get me, and that's how, I got hepatitis from him. I knew he had hepatitis and I still used, we just threw the works on the table and whichever …*

Mary was unsure as to whether or not she was HIV positive, one doctor had said she was and another had said she wasn't.

> R: *... when he told me, I nearly collapsed, because at the time I wasn't sleeping around. When I was working I wore condoms. I never shared a needle in my life. I was always scrupulous clean, spotless like. If I had a turn on, I'd have everything ready down to tissue, water, and you know the way if you're injecting with a few friends, and they say do you want me to clean that out, I say oh Jesus, no. I don't know whether I'm sick or not. What do you mean, sick or not? I say I don't know if I have the virus or not I'd say. I'd have a tissue, I'd have a bag. I'd have a tissue in the bag for squirting the watery blood into. I don't know if I have or not. I'm not in denial.... they just told me that they were sorry, because I was after giving 3 signatures for Hepatitis A, B and C. And then it came back with like a print, except it was writ in pen, but photocopied and HIV. But I didn't sign for any HIVs to be done. They told me, "Sorry you haven't any hepatitis (s) but it's very unusual for you to be HIV" because when I went to the hospital they told me they couldn't detect any virus in my body. So that's why I was to get it re-checked because I am still convinced that I haven't got it. And that's why I don't like answering questions about because I'm not sure if I have it or not. One place told me I had it and the other place told me I hadn't. And that's why I went up to James's Hospital*

Angels contracted HIV as a result of being raped.

R: I still got HIV from the time I was raped down there. You know like. Every time like I came in here and they asked me: 'Did I have hepatitis C test? And they asked me, "Did I want a HIV test? I don't need a HIV test! The only person I used after was me partner". Other than that I never had unsafe sex apart from three times, I was raped. And it comes back and they told me that I had HIV, I couldn't believe it. I asked for another test just to make sure. And then I accused my partner, they wanted to know what I had done. But I asked him for his results, his results came back negative. So the only other person I could lead it to was that ... creep...

Twelve of the research participants lived in city centre hostels, refuges or emergency accommodation and had experienced homelessness in the past. Due to the lack of a private space, they used semi-public or public environments to administer their injections which increased their risks of unhygienic injecting practices. For example:

R: … sometimes I have to take them [drugs] in the toilets of – [drug service]. You're not meant to, you're not allowed to, but people do it, you know what I mean, but I'd use, most of the time I'd use in public toilets. I'd do it on my own … most of the people that I know are on the streets and you're not going to be going with a group of people somewhere to have a turn on. So you go into the discretion of a toilet where no one sees what you are doing. (Laura)

… With me like, I'd have to go to a restaurant toilet or sometimes and do it [inject], or like if I was in a car and drive somewhere to the Park or somewhere and do it, but I wouldn't dare do it on a stairs or just anywhere. (Úna)

13. Condom use

All the men and women interviewed were aware of the risk of contracting and transmitting a range of sexually transmitted infections, including HIV and HCV infection if they did not use condoms. The vast majority reported always using condoms while working. However, most said that although they did not have sex with a customer without a condom, they were aware that other sex workers did. For example, Iseult said:

R: … like you'd get a fella that would come up to you: 'Will you have sex without a condom?' and I'd say, 'No way!' and next of all, say a girl that was standing down there, a couple of yards away, she would jump into the car, but I know what he is after asking, and I do be thinking: 'Jesus Christ, she is going to bring that home' and he is bringing that [HIV] home, and then he is going to come back out here next week. And the next stupid girl that gets in the car with him is going to.

Among the few who reported having unprotected sex with a paying customer, the enticement was always the prospect of getting more money.

R: But I never ended up catching anything else 'cause I used to say, if they wanted to do it without a johnnie [condom], I used to put up the price. But they'd have to be sorta clean, or if there was someone who sorta that has a bird [girl friend] or something. … I even let some young fellas use without a condom, but I used to put the price up, sure, they used to think it was worth it … (Carmel)

Zoë said she had sex once without a condom with a customer (for €200), but bitterly regretted it afterwards: 'It was the worst thing I ever done because I had to get tests after that.'

Although sex workers may use condoms with their customers, there is also the danger that they will not use condoms in intimate relations with their partners. Pauline reported that her partner would not use condoms thus increasing the risk of transmission of HIV.

> R: *My partner hasn't got HIV, only Hepatitis.*
>
> I: *And so do you use condoms when you are having sex with him?*
>
> R: *No to be honest and he said, 'No, he won't!'*

Some participants reported being overpowered by a customer and being raped, and said that this was the only time they had sex without a condom. Angela said, 'I never had unsafe sex apart from three times when I was raped.' Similarly, Molly said, 'I always used my condoms, except for the times that I was either beaten up or whatever.'

14. Men who have paid sex with men

Four men -- Alan, Barry, Colm and Darragh (three were gay and one was heterosexual) -- were interviewed in this study. All were illicit drug users and were either having paid sex with other men, or had discontinued to do so. Men who have sex with men are at risk of contracting HIV (as are those who start having sexual relations in their adolescent (15 years) [24].

Despite embodying all these risk factors, Alan had not contracted any blood borne viral infections. He was working as an escort, and had been homeless since the age of 15. He started smoking cannabis at the age of 12, progressed to ecstasy and then used heroin as a 'come down'. At the time of the interview he was injecting heroin. His choice of drugs was: 'If money was no object, heroin and LSD or cocaine mixed in with heroin and LSD. That would be definitely the choice of drugs'. He was fully cognisant of the dangers of injecting drug use: 'I'd be very, very worried about contracting certain diseases such as hepatitis virus and HIV virus'. Consequently he always uses the needle exchange for sterile needles and ensured to dispose of his needles in a responsible way:

> R: *Yes, definitely go to [X needle exchange] and get clean needles. We have "puncture bins". We call them "sin bins". I always carry one of them around with me to make sure that, you know I'd hate the idea of any syringe being left around or the thought of a child pricking themselves on a syringe, you know that kind way. I'd always have a sin bin with me as I call them.*

He describes how he started injecting drugs and sex working.

> I: *In terms of the start of that – when do you appear to have started?*

R: I'd say about 15, 16. I couldn't get any money off the Government whatsoever. ... I was homeless. I couldn't get any cash. No cash whatsoever. I was unprepared to go out to one of those fucking boys' homes and be locked up; you know that kind of way. It wasn't an option for me at the time. And plus I was dealing with my sexual orientation as well on top of it which is not an easy task. And to deal with your sexual orientation and actually go out to [a boy's home], it ain't a good idea. You'll end up hurting yourself more or hurting someone else. So, I'd rather hurt myself than someone else, you know that kind of way. So, I would have been about say fifteen, sixteen. ... At that time, that is when I started using heroin intravenously. That's when I started really using heroin intravenously.

I: Do you think in terms of starting that it was more to do with just the fact that you were homeless and had nowhere to live.

R: Well, it was everything. First of all, no stable accommodation, no cash, hungry, low self-image in yourself, you know, all these things contribute to the fact and I just went absolutely insane like. I wasn't the only one. There were a good few of us around, you know.

At the time of the interview, Barry was no longer engaged in sex working and was carving out a new life for himself, he was living independently and was no longer using drugs or alcohol; he was making substantial efforts to live a healthy life with a HIV diagnosis. He commenced alcohol and illicit drug use at the age of 12.

R: I found myself being abused from the age, the very early age of seven up to 14. I started getting into alcohol, drug taking, so I found with the alcohol, the drug taking that it was much easier to go out and sell myself, cos I was already after being abused and had no value on meself. ...Other male prostitutes, would have introduced me to, there was a group of 12 of us, now, there is only 3 of us left alive out of the group, there was 2 actually murdered there, in the field of prostitution, a lot of them died, HIV related and myself, I was diagnosed as HIV in 1990, and that still wasn't me turning point, I was still addicted, I was still in prostitution, and still addicted at that time.

I: But would you think it is separate between, you weren't doing the prostitution in terms of the money for the drinking or the tablets? Were the two connected?

R: No, I was doing prostitution for the money, 'cause I was going off, literally going off where anything that would pay me, and in male prostitution, which is also on the female side, of when you are addicted, it is a whole different story, when you are on the game. Punters and clients are working on your vulnerability, say I am with a punter one night and he is giving me €50, he will see me the next night, and say he'll know I am that desperate, he will offer me a tenner (€10).

He discussed the difficulties for male sex workers in terms of their own low self-esteem, their addiction issues and the difficulties of negotiating condom use with clients.

R: Condoms! And it is still a big issue today, condoms can be introduced into prostitution but most prostitutes with addiction, if they are asked not to use it, they won't use it. It's not an issue on the game, that would be like: "We're addicts", mm people like myself having no value on myself, like "Fuck it, I want to die anyway", like "I don't like this life", "I don't like myself" "I don't even wanna be here", you know, you just have no value like, 'cause when I was diagnosed, before I was diagnosed HIV, I was diagnosed negative, and they told me, they said "You're clean", like, it's the tip of the iceberg with you, like you are going to come back positive". Three months later, then I came back positive then.

Colm was also sexually abused as a young boy of 12 by a twenty year old male neighbour; he started using heroin at the age of 15 and started sex working at 16 to make money to buy drugs. He had contracted HCV before the introduction of needle exchanges.

R: I tell you, the needle exchanges have really, really been fantastic, because they have changed. I'm telling you a lot of people would be infected with HIV or Hepatitis C only for them. Whoever got that brought in may God bless them, I'm telling you, because I'm Hepatitis C, 'cause I was unlucky because I was using well before they allowed that, pass that agreement, you know.

He was unsure of his HIV status: 'One time they told me I had it and one time they told me I hadn't got it, I don't know'. There were occasions in the past when he didn't use condoms, but now always does so.

I: Can I ask you now about safer sex? Were there times when you didn't use condoms?

R: There was times when I didn't.

I: And do you think that was just at the beginning, years ago?

R: That was years ago and a couple of times I didn't and I escaped.

I: And what were the circumstances around that? Did the punter ask you not to?

R: He gives you plenty of, gives you more money if you don't. But then, then, it's not my fault like I didn't know.

I: You know you said you still occasionally would do people? Would they know your status or would you know their status?

R: No, I always bally [use a prophylaxis] up, I always use condoms, always.

In addition to receiving opiate substitution treatment (90 mg methadone) he was also injecting a quarter gram of heroin twice a week and taking both prescribed and un-prescribed benzodiazepines.

Darragh commenced drug use at the age of 12: 'I started off smoking hash, and then taking a few tablets like Upjohns, Roache 5, and things like that and napps then, and start banging up napps'. Unlike the three other men who were gay he was heterosexual and was the father of two children. He was currently in opiate substitute treatment and was prescribed 190 milligrams of methadone, but in addition he was also buying tablets on the street: 'But I do buy tablets as well, like Roache, and Dalmaine, Zimovane and all that'. He had not contracted HIV but was HCV positive. He accessed needles in his local needle exchange and had devised a strategy for when he ran out of needles: 'If I run out, I would end up using one of the old ones that I had, or else I would try and buy a new one off someone else, like you know'.

He was currently sex working in well known places in Dublin city centre:

> R: *I'd be going to the Park from about four up to till half nine, ten. After that then you head into town like and you meet people coming out of the [X Pub]. Then you go into the [X city centre] buildings, find a little spot and do what you have to do, like.*
>
> I: *And how many times would you go to the Park?*
>
> R: *Most nights*
>
> I: *And how many clients would you see, how many clients would you see a night?*
>
> R: *In a night? It all depends, sometimes I would meet one client and he would give me €500, just for being with him for half an hour. And then sometimes I would meet a client and I would only get €70 or €80 off him. That's the way it goes, like.*
>
> I: *Would you have regular people?*
>
> R: *Ah yea, yea I have at the moment regular people that ring me. These are all barristers, and cops, top people, you know what I mean?*

If offered more money for sex without a condom, Darragh had a pragmatic and practical reason for agreeing to do so.

> I: *In terms of sexual health, do you bring condoms with you or would you bring condoms with you when you go to the Park?*
>
> R: *Mmm, no. They would say: "Ah no, I'm not into using them condoms", this, that and all, they make up an excuse like, they are not interested.*
>
> I: *Have you fucked anybody without a condom?*
>
> R: *I have, yea.*
>
> I: *And you can't charge more though for that, can you?*
>
> R: *You can, yea, they say I'll give you x amount if you do it without the condom, you do be saying to yourself, that extra few quid will save me coming up tomorrow like, you know what I mean?*

15. Discussion

The three categories of high risk behaviour (sex working, injecting drug use, men having sex with men) identified by the UNAIDS *Report on the Global AIDS Epidemic 2010* associated with the transmission of HIV are also the risk behaviours which emerged from the analysis of our data. These risks are similar in low, middle-income and higher income countries. Engaging in unsafe injecting (and sexual) practices facilitates the spread of the HIV and HCV viruses [25, 26]. For the participants in this study, blood borne viral infections (HIV, HCV) were transmitted as a result of accidents (sharing works, having a friend administer the injection, unwittingly using another's works, re-using old syringes), and of ignorance of the consequences of injecting drug use. Although some respondents were aware of the dangers of using another's injecting equipment, their judgement was impaired due to: being 'strung out' (suffering withdrawal symptoms), to administering the injection in a rushed unsterile environment, and to the distractions and confusion that can occur when injecting in the company of friends/drug buddies and allowing friends to administer the injection to them.

In a systematic review and meta-analysis of interventions to prevent Hepatitis C virus infection in injecting drug users, it was found that a complex of interventions worked best to reduce the incidence. For example combining counselling with strategies such as -- enabling the injector to maintain control over the injection process by not injecting in chaotic and rushed settings; maintenance in opiate substitution treatment of ≥ than 60 mg a day; and using sterile syringes obtained from a syringe exchange program [27]. In our study, most of the participants were accessing some of the elements in such a treatment complex. However, their attempts to reduce their risks were exacerbated by the fact that many were homeless and spent much time on the streets and were likely to inject in public places and spaces which lacked the necessary hygiene. Only three of the seven who reported being HIV positive were receiving anti retroviral treatment; two others were unsure of their HIV status. They are a high risk group in terms of passing on the virus to others. Other research has found that sex workers who are injecting drug users are associated with poorer engagement with Opioid Agonist Treatment and retention in treatment[28]. Other jurisdictions[24] in Europe have been successful in reducing the rates of new infections among people who inject drugs: for example in Switzerland and in the Netherlands, HIV infections have almost been eliminated (at most 5% of new infections in 2007 and 2008 respectively) amongst those who engage in 'social' drug use, involving several people using the same contaminated injecting equipment. Whereas in Ireland, the rate of new infections for intravenous drug users accounted for 7.9% of all newly diagnosed cases in 2009. And in this small study the rate of HIV infection among the 35 people interviewed was 21 per cent.

For sex workers and their clients, unprotected sex increases the risk of contracting and transmitting a range of sexually transmitted infections (STIs), including HIV [29] and HCV infection [30]. In this study, sex workers were aware of the importance of protected sex and were generally proactive in the use of condoms with clients. Offers of increased money for sex without a condom weakened their resolve. This suggests that it is clients rather than sex workers who are more prepared to take the risk of contracting HIV. The power dynamics and the inequalities in physical strength between a sex worker and a customer can rob the sex worker of the opportunity to negotiate condom use [31].Gender violence against women and rape also led to the transmission of the HIV virus. Rape was a common experience for the sex working men and women. Enhanced policing practices could help to reduce the possibilities of sex workers being raped, and therefore of contracting HIV through rape. The latest Home Office Review of Effective Practice document and the new ACPO (Association of Chief Police Officers) Strategy & Operational Guidance for Policing Prostitution and Sexual Exploitation [32] mention's the partnership work in Merseyside of the UK Network of Sex Work Projects. It endorses taking a harm reduction approach to prostitution by introducing schemes such as the 'Ugly Mugs' scheme which can help to improve safety by allowing sex workers to report incidents of violence, which in turn can enable information about dangerous individuals to be disseminated to other sex workers or be used to report a crime to the police for investigation.

In this study, the male interviewees, because they were men who have paid sex with other men, constitute a high risk group for transmitting blood borne viral infections, particularly if they are using used syringes, and are not practicing safe sex.

16. Conclusion

Despite the existence of harm reduction interventions such as opiate substitution treatment, needle exchanges for drug users who engage in sex working, this population remain a high-risk group for contracting blood borne viral infections and death. In Ireland, some injecting drug users and other young people are still taking risks as exemplified in the recent surveillance statistics[11]. The introduction of safe injecting spaces and places might enable intravenous drug users to inject in more hygienic and safer settings thereby reducing the risk of transmission. Health messages displayed in public places might inform the intravenous drug users of the harmful consequences of unhygienic injecting practices and sharing equipment and may therefore increase their awareness of the inherent risks. Marginalized, vulnerable young people such as those leaving residential care in the justice or social welfare systems need to be targeted and informed of the dangers of illicit drug use and sex work. Health messages should also target customers and potential customers of sex workers, their insistence on not wearing a condom during sexual intercourse is putting them and whoever else they are having sex with at risk.

A change in how drug use and addiction is perceived could result in a change in the risk environment in Ireland. For example, in Portugal [33], since heroin use has been decriminalised, public perceptions have changed from viewing opiate users as criminals and addicts to viewing then as sick people in need of treatment. In Switzerland and the Netherlands successful harm reduction interventions have reduced the rates of new infections among people who inject drugs

Changes to the risk environment in Ireland in terms of policy, perception and policing could lead to the creation of an enabling environment for injecting drug using sex workers so that changes in individual behaviour could be brought about by enhanced structural interventions [34]. This approach advocates all forms of social interventions (improved education, greater needle exchange coverage, enhanced condom provision) which are extra-individual – in other words interventions that change the context within which risks are produced and reproduced [12].

Author details

Teresa Whitaker[*, **]

Hallows College, Dublin, Ireland

---

* Corresponding Author

** The authors declared no conflicts of interest with respect to the authorship and/or publication of this article.

Paul Ryan
Department of Sociology, NUI Maynooth, Co. Kildare, Ireland

Gemma Cox
Young Ballymun, Dublin, Ireland

Acknowledgement

The authors gratefully acknowledge the courage of the sex workers who participated in the research notwithstanding the stigma attached to sex work and drug use in Irish society.

The opinions expressed in this article are those of the authors and do not necessarily reflect the views of the National Advisory Committee on Drugs; appreciation is expressed to the Committee for their permission to use the data.

The authors disclosed receipt of the following financial support for the research and/or authorship of this article: The National Advisory Committee on Drugs.

17. References

[1] Cox, G. and Whitaker, T. (2009) *Drug use, sex work and the risk environment in Dublin.*, Dublin: National Advisory Committee on Drugs.

[2] Department of Tourism Sport and Recreation (2000) *Building on Experience*. Dublin: Stationery Office.

[3] World Health Organization (2008) *Progress on Implementing the Dublin Declaration on Partnership to fight HIV/AIDS in Europe and Central Asia.* http://www.euro.who.int/Document/SHA/Dublin_Dec_Report.pdf.Accessed 2008 Aug 21.

[4] World Health Organization (2001) *STI/HIV Sex Work in Asia*. Regional Office for the Western Pacific.http://www.wpro.who.int/NR/rdonlyres/D01A4265-A142-4E19-99AE-6CC7E44F995C/0/Sex_Work_in_Asia_July2001.pdf Accessed 2008 Oct 15.

[5] World Health Organization (2005) *Toolkit for Targeted HIV/AIDS Prevention and Care in Sex Work Settings*. Geneva: World Health Organization.

[6] UNAIDS (2002) *Sex work and HIV/AIDS UNAIDS Technical Update UNAIDS Best Practice Collection*. 2002, Geneva: UNAIDS.

[7] UNAIDS (2010) *Global Report UNAIDS REPORT ON THE GLOBAL AIDS EPIDEMIC 2010*, in *Joint United Nations Programme on HIV/AIDS (UNAIDS)*. 2010, Geneva:United Nations. http://www.unaids.org/en/media/unaids/contentassets/documents/unaidspublication/2011/20111215_Report-UNAIDS-Advisory-group-HIV-Sex-Work_en.pdf. Accessed 2012 Apr 10.

[8] Department of Health and Children (2010) *Commitment on HIV and AIDS Ireland 2009*. Dublin: Department of Health and Children, Irish Aid, Department of Foreign Affairs.

[9] National Aids Strategy Committee (2008) *HIV and AIDS Prevention Plan 2008-2012 Mid Term Review.* http://www.drugsandalcohol.ie/15513/1/HIV_AIDS_education_and_prevention_plan_08-12.pdf. Accessed 2012 Apr 9.

[10] Safetynet (2010) http://www.chrysalisdrugproject.org/services/womens_mobile_health_clinic. Accessed 2012 Apr 9.

[11] Health Protection Surveillance Centre (2011) *STIs/HIVandAIDS/SurveillanceReports.* http://www.hpsc.ie/hpsc/A-Z/HIVSTIs/HIVandAIDS/SurveillanceReports/File,13068,en.pdf. Accessed 2012 Apr 9.

[12] Rhodes, T. and Simic, M. (2005) *Transition and the HIV risk environment.* BMJ, 331: p. 220-223.

[13] Whitaker, T., Ryan, P. and Cox, G. (2011) *Stigmatization among drug-using sex workers accessing support services in Dublin.* Qualitative Health Research, 21(8): p. 1086-1100.

[14] Cusick, L., (2006) *Widening the harm reduction agenda: From drug use to sex work.* International Journal of Drug Policy, 17(1): p. 3-11.

[15] Plumridge, L. and Abel, G. (2001) *A 'segmented' sex industry in New Zealand: Sexual and personal safety of female sex workers.* Australian and New Zealand Journal of Public Health,. 25: p. 78-83.

[16] Cusick, L., Martin, A. and May,T. (2003) *Vulnerability and involvement in drug use and sex work*, London: The Research, Development and Statistics Directorate, Home Office Research Study 268:

[17] Government of Ireland. (1993) *Criminal Law (Sexual Offences) Act, 1993, No. 20.* http://www.irishstatutebook.ie/1993/en/act/pub/0020/index.html.Accessed 2008 Aug 25.

[18] Connolly, J., Foran, S., Donovan, A. M., Carew, A. M.,Long, J. (2008) *Crack cocaine in the Dublin region: an evidence base for a Dublin crack cocaine strategy.*, Dublin: Health Research Board Series 6.

[19] Moore, G., McCarthy, P., MacNeela, P., MacGabhann, L., Philbin, M., Proudfoot, D.,(2004), *A review of harm reduction approaches in Ireland and evidence from the international literature.*, Dublin: National Advisory Committee on Drugs.

[20] European Monitoring Centre for Drugs and Drug Addiction (2011) *The State of the Drugs Problem in Europe.* http://www.emcdda.europa.eu/publications/annual-report/2011 Accessed 2012 Apr 9.

[21] Health Service Executive (2011) *The introduction of the Opioid Treatment Protocol.* http://www.drugs.ie/pdfs/2010/Opioid_Treatment_Protocol.pdf. Accessed 2012 Apr 9.

[22] O'Connell, B., (2012) *Is Ireland failing its heroin addicts?*, in *The Irish Times*.Dublin: The Irish Times.

[23] Health Research Board (2011) *Drug related deaths and deaths among drug users in Ireland. Revised 2009 figures from the National drug-related deaths index.* www.drugsandalcohol.ie/16365 Accessed 2012 Apr 9.

[24] UNAIDS, (2011) *The Report of the UNAIDS Advisory Group on HIV and Sex Work.* Geneva: UNAIDS.

[25] Smyth, B., Barry, J. and Keenan, E. (2005) *Irish injecting drug users and hepatitis C: the importance of the social context of injecting*. International Journal of Epidemiology, 2005. 90: p. 837-841.

[26] ACMD, *The primary prevention of hepatitis C among injecting drug users*. 2009, London: Home Office.

[27] Hagan, H. Pouget, E. R., and Des Jarlais, D. C. (2011) *A systematic review and Meta-analysis of interventions to prevent Hepatitis C virus infection in people who inject drugs*. The American Journal of Infectious diseases of America, 204: p. 74-83.

[28] Marchand, K., Oviedo-Joekes, E., Guh, D. Marsh, D. C., Brissete, S. Schechter, M. T., (2012) *Sex work involvement among women with long-term opioid drug dependence who enter opioid agonist treatment*. Harm Reduction Journal, 9(8).

[29] Darrow, W. J., Boles, and Cohen, J. (1991) *HIV Seroprevalence trends in female prostitutes, United States: 1986-1990*. Florence: Italy.

[30] Harcourt, C., van Beek, I., Heslop, J., McMahon, M., Donovan, B., (2001)*The health and welfare needs of female and transgender street sex workers in New South Wales*. Australian & New Zealand Journal of Public Health, 25: p. 84-89.

[31] Shannon, K. Strathdee, S., Shoveller, J., Rusch, M., Kerr, T., Tyndall, M., (2009) *Structural and environmental barriers to condom use negotiation with clients among female sex workers: Implications for HIV-prevention strategies and policy*. American Journal of Public Health, 99(4): p. 1-7.

[32] Association of Chief Police Officers (2011) *ACPO strategy for Policing Prostitution and Sexual Exploitation*. http://www.acpo.police.uk/documents/crime/2011/20111102%20CBA%20Policing%20Prostitution%20and%20%20Sexual%20Exploitation%20Strategy_Website_October%202011.pdf. Accessed 2012 Apr 9.

[33] Global Commission (2011) *War on drugs Report of the Global Commission on drug policy*. http://www.globalcommissionondrugs.org/reports/ Accessed 2012 Apr 9.

[34] Des Jarlais, D., (2000) *Structural interventions to reduce HIV transmission among injecting drug users*. AIDS, 14 (Supplement 1): p. 541-546.

Section 4

Immunodeficiency – HIV, Feline Model

Chapter 15

Feline Immunodeficiency

Fabiana Alves and Jenner Karlisson Pimenta dos Reis

Additional information is available at the end of the chapter

1. Introduction

Classic infectious causes of immunodeficiency in felines are the immunodeficiency by retroviruses, including feline immunodeficiency virus (FIV) and feline leukemia virus (FeLV). Immunodeficiency caused by these infectious agents may result from disruption of normal host barriers or deregulation of cellular immunity.

The feline immunodeficiency virus and the feline leukemia virus are detected worldwide and are among the most common infectious diseases of domestic cats, others small felids and wild cats, and causes immunodeficiency, with increased risk for opportunistic infections, neurologic diseases, and tumors.

Feline immunodeficiency virus and feline leukemia virus are retrovirus, but they differ in their potential to cause disease. FIV is classified as a *Lentivirus* and, FeLV as a *Gamaretrovirus*. The high incidence of FIV and FeLV is associated with density of cat population.

FIV causes immune dysfunctions in cats similar to those observed in people infected with human immunodeficiency virus (HIV). Diseases associated with FeLV and FIV may affect some organ, and may cause among other disorders, lymphoma, blood dyscrasias, alterations in the function of central nervous system, and secondary and opportunistic infections, with a significant number of opportunistic pathogens of viral, bacterial, protozoal, and fungal origin. Therefore, infected animals may play a role in transmission of various pathogens to human beings.

Risk groups for infection with FIV and FeLV are different: FIV is mainly associated with males, free access to streets and bites inflicted during fights for territory, therefore, the risk of FIV transmission is low in socially well-adapted cats, while FeLV infection is associated with social contacts and thus the FeLV infection is found almost equally between males and females, at a rate slightly elevate in male cats.

The diagnosis of FIV and FeLV can not be done based solely on clinical signs, but should be based on the demonstration of anti-FIV and FeLV antigen in the serum of infected animals.

FeLV and FIV do not survive for long outside the host and are easily inactivated by disinfectants, heating and drying. As prophylaxis against infection of FIV and FeLV is recommended castration to reduce aggression and lessen the bite. The rapid and accurate diagnosis of any secondary diseases is essential. In shelters, infected cats should be housed individually to prevent infection. All animals should be tested before being placed in shelters and breeding. Vaccines are available for both viruses; however, identification and segregation of infected cats remains the cornerstone for preventing new infections.

Studies and research about these viruses are continuously necessary to define prophylactic, management, and therapeutic measures for stray, feral and owned cats.

2. Feline immunodeficiency virus

The first isolation of feline immunodeficiency virus (FIV) has been described by Pedersen, 1987 in the city of Petaluma, USA. FIV is an important lentivirus that causes immune disorders in both domestic and nondomestic cats.

Like other retroviruses the FIV containing accessory genes in addition to *gag, pol* and *env*. The FIV *gag, pol* and *env* genes encode the capsid protein p24; protease, integrase, and reverse transcriptase proteins; the viral glycoprotein (gp120) and the transmembrane protein (gp41), respectively. Both gag and pol are relatively conserved between strains (Olmsted et al., 1989; Kenyon & Lever, 2011; McDonnel et al., 2012).

Species-specific strains of FIV circulate in many feline populations. Five genetically distinct subtypes or clades of FIV have been described: A, B, C, D and E, with considerable sequence diversity in the *env* gene. Studies have shown that is possible to use the env nucleotide sequence and the p17-p24 region of the gag gene for subtypes indentification but, once gag gene has a retention rate higher than the env gene, it is considered a good candidate for phylogenetic studies (Sodora et al., 1994; Kurosawa et al., 1999; Hosie et al., 2009; Kenyon & Lever, 2011).

2.1. Epidemiology and transmission

The seroprevalence of FIV is highly variable between geographic locations. Epidemiological studies show that FIV transmission is influenced by behavior: cats with free access to the streets, sick cats, and males are more susceptible to infection with FIV (Courchamp & Pontier, 1994; Sellon and Hatmann, 2006).

Feline immunodeficiency virus can be transmitted primarily by inoculation of virus present in saliva or blood, presumably by bite and fight wounds. Male cats with free access to streets are more susceptible to infection because males are territorialist, other ways such as via mucosal exposure, blood transfer, during mating, and vertically during prenatal and postnatal exposure, can also be responsible for transmission. In natural infections, the efficacy of colostral immunity is not known (Sellon & Hartmann, 2006; Medeiros et al., 2012).

2.2. Pathogenesis, immunity and clinical symptoms

FIV has a tropism for T cells, macrophages, dendritic cells and central nervous system cells. The major targets for FIV infection are activated CD4+ T lymphocytes (Fig. 1). These cells typically function as T helper cells, which have a central role in immune functions, facilitating the development of humoral and cell-mediated immunity (Fig. 1) (Sellon and Hartmann, 2006; Hosie et al., 2009; Simões et al., 2012) . FIV does not use CD4 as a primary *binding* receptor, its gp120 glycoprotein binds to the CD134 (OX40) a member of the tumor necrosis factor receptor (TNFR)/nerve growth factor receptor family of molecules as the binding receptor in conjunction with the chemokine receptor CXCR4 as a cofactor for infection (Yuan et al., 2003; de Parseval et al., 2005; Willett et al., 2006b; Elder et al., 2010). The CD134 co-stimulatory pathway has been shown to be critical for T, B and antigen-presenting cell (APC) cell activation. Studies have shown that antigen stimulation of infected B-cells is increased compared with non-infected cells. FIV-infection in cats also results in a sustained polyclonal activation of B-cells with the production of antibodies to a variety of non-viral antigens (Yuan et al., 2003; Willett et al., 2006b).

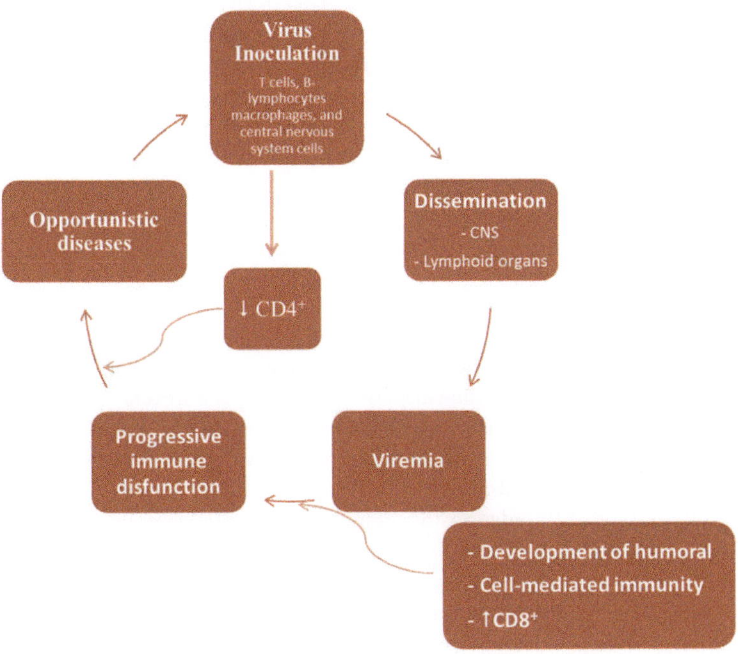

Figure 1. Diagram illustrating the stages of the pathogenesis of FIV. Modified from Sellon and Hartmann, 2006.

As for HIV, it has been classified some stages for FIV infection (Table 1 and Fig. 2 and 3): clinical symptoms during initial stages (acute phase) of infection include fever, leucopenia, gingivitis, lethargy, signs of enteritis, stomatitis, dermatitis, conjunctivitis, respiratory tract disease, neutropenia, and generalized lymphadenopathy (Sellon e Hartmann, 2006; Gunn-Moore & Reed, 2011; Hartmann, 1998; Hartamann, 2011; O'Brien et al., 2012). The progression of disease occurs in a manner similar to the HIV-1 infection in humans. In the first few days after infection, FIV replicates in dendritic cells, macrophages and CD4+ T lymphocytes, within 2 weeks appears in the plasma. FIV-specific CD8+ cytotoxic T cells are detected in the blood within one week of infection. The duration of the following asymptomatic phase varies but usually lasts many years, viral replication is controlled by the immune response, but there is a progressive decline in CD4+ T lymphocyte numbers, resulting in a decreased $CD4^{+}/CD8^{+}$ T lymphocyte ratio (Fig. 1) (Hartmann, 1998; Sellon e Hartmann, 2006; Gunn-Moore & Reed, 2011; Hartamann, 2011). The most infected cats exhibit an increase in CD8+ T cells along with a strong humoral antibody response which allows them to control this initial phase of the infection (Elder et al., 2010). After 2-4 weeks after infection, antibodies are detectable in plasma for FIV. Antibodies recognizing *env* related proteins appear earlier than those against the *gag* protein p24. Factors that influence the length of the asymptomatic stage include the pathogenicity of the infecting strain (also depending on the FIV subtype), exposure to secondary pathogens, and the age of the cat at the time of infection. In the last, symptomatic stage (FAIDS phase) of infection, clinical signs are a reflection of opportunistic infections, skin infections such as demodicosis and pediculosis, neoplasia such as B cell lymphosarcoma and squamous cell carcinoma, myelosuppression, and neurologic disease, similar to those observed in people infected with human immunodeficiency virus (HIV) (Hartmann, 1998; Sellon e Hartmann, 2006; Elder et al., 2010; Gunn-Moore & Reed, 2011; Hartamann, 2011; Korman et al., 2012; Sobrinho et al., 2012). The chronic gingivostomatitis is the most common clinical sign in infected cats and significantly degrade the quality of life of animals

Phases	Clinical sings	Duration
Acute Unspecific signs	Neutropenia, Fever, lethargy, peripheral, lymphadenopathy, weight loss	Weeks-months
Asymptomatic	No clinical signs, but there is a progressive decline in CD4+ T lymphocyte numbers	Years
Unspecific clinical signs	Apathy, weight loss, lymphadenopathy, fever, anorexia, depression, chronic gingivostomatitis (difficulty eating), chronic rhinitis, lymph adenopathy, immune-mediated glomerulo nephritis, leucopenia, bahvioral abnormalities	Several months
FAIDS	Above symptoms more opportunistic infections, clinical symptoms of immunodeficiency, neoplasia, neurological abnormalities and seizures.	Several months

Table 1. Stages of clinical sings of FIV infection.

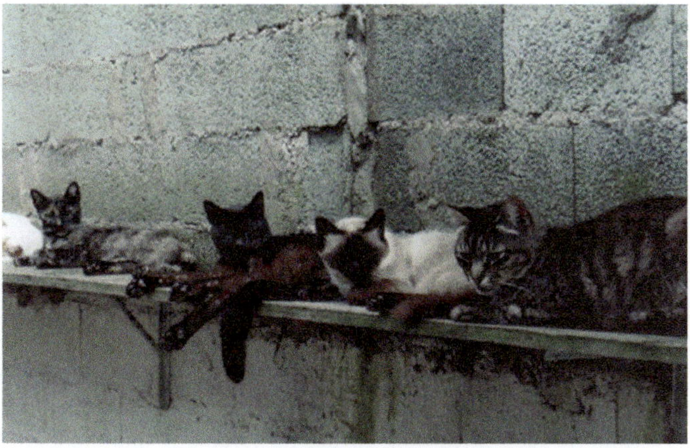

Figure 2. FIV infected cats. (Courtesy Bruno Teixeira, Universidade São Paulo, USP).

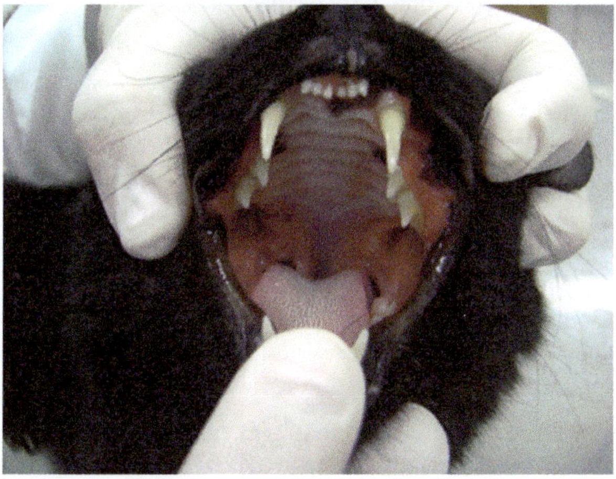

Figure 3. Stomatitis and gingivitis. (Courtesy Bruno Teixeira, Universidade São Paulo, USP).

Pathologic abnormalities described in FIV positive cats with alterations in the morphology of lymph node: hyperplastic during acute phase, follicular involution in the terminal phase of infection; thymus: cortical involution, atrophy, lymphoid follicular hyperplasia and germinal center formation; intestinal tract: villous blunting, pyogranulomatous colitis, lymphoplasmacytic stomatitis; liver: periportal hepatitis; bone marrow: dysplastic changes, granulocytic hyperplasia and the formation of marrow lymphoid aggregates; kidney: tubulointerstitial infiltrates, glomerulosclerosis; central nervous system: Perivascular cuffing, gliosis, myelitis, loss and reorganization of neurons, axonal sprouting, vacuolar myelinopathy; lung: interstitial pneumonitis, alveolitis; skeletal muscle: lymphocytic myositis, myofiber necrosis, perivascular cuffing; reproductive failure occurs in FIV infected cats (Sellon e Hartmann, 2006; Gunn-Moore & Reed, 2011; Hartmann, 2011).

2.3. Diagnosis and management of FIV-infected cats

The methods used currently for detection of FIV infection in domestic cats include virus isolation, immunological tests for detection of specific antibodies and molecular tests for detection of viral genomic sequences, associated with the clinical diagnosis. Virus isolation is a reliable diagnostic method but is laborious and not used routinely.

The preferred initial tests are ELISA or immunochromatographic test, which detect antibodies recognizing viral structural proteins (such as the capsid protein p24 and a gp41 peptide) and offer the advantage of speed and convenience. However, when the results are inconclusive by these tests a more specific test should be used, such as the Western blot (Hosie et al., 2009). The PCR can have doubtful results due to the great genetic variability of FIV, use of specific primers only for one subtype, low viral load during a long period of infection, and inadequate preparation of PCR components. The specificity and sensitivity of PCR may vary from 40-100% according to the methodology and standardization of the laboratory (House & Jarret, 1990; Hartmann et al., 2007; Hosie et al., 2009). There is also a technique of lymphocytes, for the visualization of $CD4^{+}/CD8^{+}$, however, due to the complexity of these tests are not used routinely.

The cats positive for FIV should not be euthanized based only on a positive test result for FIV. These animals have a long life as large as that of uninfected cats, however, should be subject to regular veterinary (at least every 6 months) queries including monitoring biochemistry, hematological, and weight routine, however, the euthanasia should be considered when the clinical problems relate to an advanced stage of FIV infection leading the animal to a poor living conditions.

However, it is important to isolate the animal infected with FIV from others non-infected, and maintain a good state of health of the animal infected, because other conditions can lead to the progression of immune deficiency. Positive cats should be neutered to reduce aggressive and laughter of contamination during fighting and copulation.

Vaccination is a controversial subject. Vaccines with inactivated viruses are available in the U.S.A, Australia, New Zealandand and Japan. These vaccines induce a rapid humoral response with antibodies indistinguishable from natural infection. However, there are several studies aimed at differential tests to indentify natural FIV infected animals from those vaccinated ones.

Early diagnosis is very important because it will enable early treatment of disease. There are treatments with corticosteroids and other immunosuppressive drugs in animals with chronic stomatitis, however, they cause many side effects. The Filgastrim (granulocyte colony-stimulation factor), a recombinant human cytokine (rHuG-CSF), has been used in cats with profound neutropenia, to increase the neutrophil count, however, can also increase the viral load. The recombinant human erythropoietin is also used successfully in cats with non-regenerative anemia, administration elevates blood cells, without increasing the viral load. Treatment with insulin-like growth factor-1 recombinant human induces thymic growth and stimulates T cell function, resulting in a significant increase in thymus size and thymic cortical regeneration, replenishing the peripheral T cell pool in experimentally FIV-infected cats (Hosie et al., 2009; Mohammadi & Bienzle, 2012).

Most of the antiviral drug for FIV is licensed for the treatment of HIV infections in humans, with AZT (3′-azido-2′,3′-dideoxythymidine), however, many human antiviral, are ineffective or toxic to cats. AZT (3′-azido-2′,3′-dideoxythymidine) is a nucleoside analogue (thymidine derivative) that blocks the retroviral reverse transcriptase and inhibits the replication of FIV in vivo and in vitro. As with HIV, FIV resistance may arise after 6 months of treatment (Hosie et al., 2009; Doménech et al., 2011; Mohammadi & Bienzle, 2012).

Some studies have shown promising results with the use of recombinant interferon for the treatment of FIV, increasing the survival of infected animals. Immunomodulators and interferon inducers are most utilized in infected animals, but there are controversies regarding the use, for nonspecific stimulation of the immune system, can also assist in an increase in viral load.

3. Human immunodeficiency virus type 1 (HIV-1) x Feline immunodeficiency virus (FIV)

Like the HIV, FIV belongs to the genus *Lentivirus* of the Retroviridae family. Since the discovery of human immunodeficiency virus type 1 (HIV-1) in 1982 there is an urgent need for animal models to study the pathogenesis of HIV-1 infection and possibilities for interventional strategies (Elder et al., 2008). FIV was descript in 1987, and since then, FIV has been proposed as a model for HIV studies, because, among non-primate vertebrates, FIV infection in the cat may be the closest model of HIV infection and acquired immunodeficiency syndrome (AIDS).

FIV is phylogenetically (though not antigenically) related to HIV-1. FIV and HIV share many features in their genomes in comprising three major open reading frames (ORF), gag, pol and env, especially in the pol gene and FIV also has a very similar life cycle to that of HIV (Table 2) (Savarino et al., 2007; Elder et al., 2008; Elder et al., 2010).

	FIV	**HIV**
Viral genes encoded		
Gag,Pol,Env,LTRs	Yes	Yes
Vif	Yes	Yes
Ver	Yes	Yes
Tat	No	Yes
Vpr	No	Yes
Vpu	No	Yes
OrfA	Yes	No
DU	Yes	No
Nef	No	Yes

Table 2. Comparative viral genes encoded. Modified from Elder et al., 2010.

The similarities and discrepancies in the physiopathology of feline and human viruses in their respective natural hosts presents striking analogies, and several intriguing differences (Tables 3 and 4). FIV and HIV share a common pattern on clinical signs, having initially a nonspecific acute phase, followed by an asymptomatic phase and a phase in which the immune system is compromised and the animal is subjected to secondary infections (Sellon e Hartmann, 2006; Gunn-Moore & Reed, 2011; Hartmann, 1998; Hartamann, 2011; Magden et al., 2011; O'Brien et al., 2012).

The dynamics of infection by FIV and HIV in their natural hosts are very similar, like HIV, FIV can be transmitted via mucosal exposure, blood transfer, and vertically via prenatal and postnatal routes, but FIV is principally transmitted through biting, while natural transmission of HIV occurs mainly via mucosal routes.

The development of disease and clinical signs are also similar in human and cat (Fig. 1 and Table 3), both virus preferentially infects CD4 + T cells, while the cell surface receptors CD4 and CD134 are used for HIV and FIV, respectively, differ: the SU glycoprotein of FIV initially binds to CD134, triggering the conformational changes in SU that allow subsequent interaction between SU and the receptor CXCR4 (Grant et al., 2009). While some viruses arising in the later stages of HIV infections are able to use CXCR4, most natural isolates of HIV use a different chemokine receptor, CCR5. Nevertheless, since CCR5 and CD134 in humans and cats, respectively, are predominantly expressed on CD4+ T cells (Table 4) (Willet et al., 2006a; Grant et al., 2009; Elder et al., 2010).

	FIV	**HIV**
Oral lesions	Yes	Yes
Lymphadenopathy	Yes	Yes
Neutropenia	Yes	Yes
CD4 T cell depletion	Yes	Yes
Hypergammaglobulinemia	Yes	Yes
Wasting, diahrrea	Yes	Yes
Secondary infections	Yes	Yes
CNS lesions	Yes	Yes
Neoplasia	Yes	Yes

Table 3. Comparative disease symptoms. Modified from Elder et al., 2010.

Host immune response against FIV in domestic cats is very similar to those induced in HIV-infected patients. Both viruses cause dysfunction of the CD4+ lymphocyte early in infection, although FIV also infects the CD8+ subset, B lymphocytes and macrophages and ultimately cause immune system collapse. Epitopes recognized by humoral and cytotoxic cellular immune responses have been described in both *Env* and *Gag* genes. Some studies suggest that progression to AIDS may be associated with a TH2-type response, while resistance may be higher in individuals with a strong THI-type response.

The evaluation of vaccine strategies in animal models is essential to instruct development of a vaccine against HIV. Currently, there are studies using transgenic cats expressing HIV proteins, serving as valuable models to study the pathophysiology of HIV.A vaccine against FIV, whose development has been the object of considerable international research effort, has intrinsic value as well as the potential to provide a powerful proof of concept in vaccination against human AIDS (Klonjkowski et al., 2009).

	FIV	HIV
Transmission		
Blood contact	Yes	Yes
Mucosal contact	Yes	Yes
Vertically via prenatal	Yes	Yes
Postnatal routes	Yes	Yes
Target cell		
CD4+ T cell	Yes	Yes
Macrophage	Yes	Yes
Dentritic cell	Yes	Yes
Subset B cells	Yes	?
Microglia	Yes	Yes
Receptors utilized		
CD4	No	Yes
CD134	Yes	No
CXCR4	Yes	Yes
CCR5	No	Yes

Table 4. Comparative properties of FIV and HIV. Modified from Elder et al., 2010.

4. Feline leukemia virus

Feline leukemia virus has been reported mainly in domestic cats and, was first described in 1964 by William Jarret and co-workers. It is considered more pathogenic than FIV and FeLV infection has higher impact on mortality, because causes more severe immunosuppression than that caused by FIV infection (Hartmann, 2006; Lutz et al., 2009).

The FeLV genome contains envelope (*env*), polymerase (*pol*) e group specific antigen (*gag*) genes that encode for the surface (SU) protein glycoprotein gp70 and the transmembrane (TM) protein p15E; reverse transcriptase, protease and integrase; internal virion proteins, including p15c, p12, p27 and p10; respectively. The p27, which is used for clinical detection of FeLV and gp70 defines the virus subgroup (Hartmann, 2006; Lutz et al., 2009).

Although it has not been described serotypes for FeLV virus isolates have variants or subgroups (FeLV-A, FeLV-B, FeLV-C and FeLV-T). These subgroups are distinguished by the nucleotide sequence of the *env* gene and, antigenically they are closely related. Variations in protein SU sequences would be responsible for use by the virus of different cell receptors, resulting in differences in tropism including bone marrow, salivary glands and respiratory epithelium, and pathogenicity of field isolates (Neil et al., 1991; Roy-Burman et al., 1995). Subtype A is more disseminated, it is involved in all clinical infections and is related to immunodeficiency. Only FeLV A is contagious and passed horizontally from cat to cat in nature. The host cell receptor used by FeLV is *Feline highaffinity thiamine transporter 1* (feTHTR1), found in absorption tissues and small intestine besides liver and kidneys, and also in cells of the lymphoid system. This wide distribution is consistent with the fact that the FeLV-A is found in a variety of tissues and cells and this subgroup can cause lymphomas, but usually causes injury moderate in the absence of other subgroups. Subtype B originates from recombination of FeLV-A is primarily associated with tumors. Subtype C considered the most pathogenic subgroup, emerges from mutations in the *env* gene of subtype A and is mainly associated with non-regenerative anemia. Subtype T was originally isolated from a cat with FeLV induced immunodeficiency (FAIDS). This subgroup arises from mutations in the SU gene sequence of the FeLV-A with approximately 96% similarity. It is defined by its T lymphotropism. This subgroup requires a membrane-spanning receptor molecule (PIT1) and a co-receptor protein (FeLIX) to infect T lymphocytes and causes usually severe immunosuppression. In fact, all naturally infected cats carry FeLV A either alone or in combination with FeLV B, FeLV C, or both (Neil et al., 1991; Roy-Burman et al., 1995; Hartamann, 2006; Lutz et al., 2009).

4.1. Epidemiology and transmission

The feline leukemia virus has a worldwide distribution. FeLV is contagious and spreads through close contact between viral shedding, but the prevalence of infection varies greatly depending on their age, health, environment, density of animals and lifestyle (Hard et al., 1976; Grant et al., 1980). The kittens are more susceptible, since the resistance develops with age. Because of advances in the diagnosis of disease and vaccination the prevalence of FeLV has dropped substantially in the last two decades. In Shelters and places where there is a high density of animals, it is advisable to proceed diagnosis of all animals. Infected animals should be euthanized or isolated from not infected animals.

FeLV is transmitted mainly by oronasal contact, through saliva, urine, feces, ingestion of contaminated food and water and also through bites. Transmission can also take place from an infected mother cat to her kittens, either before they are born or while they are nursing. Older cats are more resistant to FeLV infection, but can be infected by high viral doses (Lutz et al., 2009).

4.2. Pathogenesis, immunity and clinical symptoms

FeLV is present in the blood during two different stages of infection: primary viremia, an early stage of virus infection. During early stage some cats are able to mount an effective immune response, eliminate the virus from the bloodstream. The second stage is characterized by persistent infection of the bone marrow and other tissues (Table 5) (Hard et al., 1976; Hartmann, 2006; Fugino et al., 2008). If FeLV infection progresses to this stage it has passed a point of no return: the overwhelming majority of cats with secondary viremia will be infected for the remainder of their lives. The pathogenesis of FeLV is different in each cat and depends on immune status and age, but can be classified into six stages (Table 6) (Hard et al., 1976; Charreyre & Pedersen, 1991; Hartmann, 2006; Fugino et al., 2008; Lutz, 2009).

Classification of evolution of the disease	Classification of infected animals	Response immune	Days after infection	Healthy cat
Regressive infection extinct	Transient viremia	Efficient - virus neutralization	Days	FeLV negative - Animal resistant future infections for a period of time
Progressive	Persistent viremia	Failure to develop an immune response effective	3 weeks	FeLV positive
Regressive	Latent infection	Body inactive the virus, but not neutralizes	3-13 weeks	FeLV negative (complete elimation) FeLV positive (continued viremia)
Atypical		Complete virus is sequestered in the epithelial tissue, replicates itself, but leaves the cells	3-13 weeks	FeLV positve

Table 5. Immune responses following infection. Modified from Hartmann, 2006.

Clinical signs associated with FeLV infection are variable (Fig. 4). It has seen tumors in infected cats once FeLV is a major oncogene that causes different kind of tumors, most commonly malignant lymphoma and leukemia and other hematopoietic tumors. It also induces thymic atrophy and depletion of lymph node paracortical zones following infection Besides that it has been found immunosuppression with poor response to T-cell mitogens, reduced immunoglobulin production; hematologic disorders like lymphopenia and neutropenia; immune-mediated diseases; neuropathy; reproductive disorders; fading kitten syndrome and opportunistic infections. The lymphopenia may be characterized by preferential loss of $CD4^+/CD8^+$ ratio and losses of helper cells and cytotoxic supressor cells and primary and secondary humoral antibody responses are delayed and decreased (Hartmann, 2006; Lutz et al., 2009; Hartmann, 2011).

FeLV infected cats having concurrent protozoal, bacterial, viral, and fungal infections, most commonly bartonellosis, respiratory infections and coccidiosis (Wolf-Jäckel et al., 2012; Sobrinho et al., 2012). Diseases such as hemolytic anemia, glomerulonephritis, chronic enteritis with intestinal epithelial cell degeneration and necrosis of the crypts, liver disease, reabsorption fetal, abortion, stillbirth, lymphadenopathy, polyarthritis and neurological diseases such as peripheral neuropathies, may be related to FeLV infection (Hartmann, 2006; Lutz et al., 2009; Hartmann, 2011).

Stages	Replication region	Pathogenesis	Days post infection
I	Oropharynx and lymph nodes	Infects lymphocytes, which travel to the bone marrow	2- 12 days
II	Lymphocytes and monocytes	Immune suppression, thymic atrophy, lymphopenia, neutropenia, neutrophil function abnormalities, loss of $CD4^+$ cells and $CD8^+$ lymphocytes	2- 12 days
III	Systemic lymphoid centers	Immune suppression	2- 12 days
IV	Bone marrow cells and epithelial cell	Anaemia and lymphoma	2- 6 weeks
V	Bone marrow stem cells	Myelossuppression and leukemia	4- 6 weeks
VI	Viremia medullary epithelial and lymphoid	Thrombocytopenia and neutropenia	4- 6 weeks

Table 6. Stages of replication of the virus of feline leukemia (FeLV).

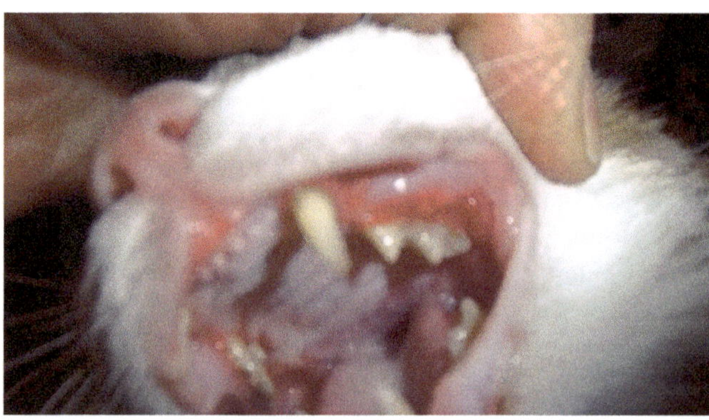

Figure 4. Gingivitis. (Courtesy Marcia Moller Nogueira).

The feline oncovirus associated-membrane antigens (FOCMA) may be associated with immunodeficiency that occurs because of depletion of lymphoid cells infected, probably due to antibody-mediated cytotoxic. Leukemia and anemia are induced by the transformation of stem cells, myeloid and lymphoid lineages, induced by infection with FeLV (Hard et al., 1976; Lutz et al., 2009; Hartmann, 2011).

4.3. Diagnosis and management of FeLV-infected cats

The correct and early diagnosis is important for prevention and control of FeLV infection Diagnostic tests detect antigens and, cats of any age should be tested. For the diagnosis of FeLV, virus isolation is not widely used, because it is difficult, time consuming to perform and requires special facilities, though viral antigens could be detected in peripheral blood cells, this method has been considered as the ultimate diagnostic criterion. Most often, the diagnosis of infection is done based on clinical history and detection of antigens, the FeLV core protein (p27), in leukocytes, plasma, serum or saliva of suspected animals (Barr, 1998; Hartmann, 2006). The direct immunofluorescence assay in blood smears, is the most commonly used diagnostic methods for detection of the virus, targeting mainly proteins p27 and p55 that are present in infected leukocytes (Hard, 1991). Tests such as ELISA and immunochromatography for the p27 protein have high sensitivity and specificity and are preferred used because they are less laborious, however, when doubtful results occurs it should be confirmed by direct immunofluorescence (Table 7) (Hard, 1991, Hartmann et al., 2007; Lutz et al., 2009). PCR is being used currently for detection of viral nucleic acid (RNA or proviral DNA) and is highly strain specific. PCR positive for FeLV proviral DNA indicates the presence of exogenous but not necessarily can be used as a diagnosis for viremia (Gomes-Keller et al., 2006). In these cases the RT-PCR detects the presence of viral RNA and informs the development of viremia in infected animals, but current reagents and testing protocols should be well standardized. As a retrovirus, mutations in FeLV occur naturally and may react negatively with a specific PCR.

It is necessary a good classification of the stage (Table 6) of the disease to obtain an accurate diagnosis. In phases I-III only ELISA can detect viral antigens for FeLV, and in the stages IV-VI can be detected by ELISA, immunofluorescence and PCR. The combination of testing determines the FeLV infection status of most cats. Recommend annual retesting after any discordant test result until agreement. A positive test doubtful a healthy animal, it should be done further confirmatory tests such as direct immunofluorescence and PCR for provirus (Gomes-Keller et al., 2006; Hartmann, 2006; Lutz et al., 2009).

For an accurate diagnosis, it is also necessary to evaluate the age and lifestyle of the animal (Table 7): Negative animals under 12 weeks who had contact with sick birds or other animals should be retested within 4-6 weeks; positive results indicate that at this age the animals are infected. Negative animals with more than 12 weeks who had contact with sick birds or other animals should be retested within 6-8 weeks; positive results at this age should be classified as follows: sick animals (positive), healthy animals, retesting within 6-8 weeks.

The early and precise diagnosis is needed to enable rapid intervention. FeLV-infected cats should be isolated from uninfected ones. It is also recemmented that they could be examined by the vet regularly (every 6 months), doing biochemical tests, complete blood count and urinalysis. Infected animals should be sterilized to minimize the transmission. The living environment should be cleaned periodically, because FeLV is sensitive to any type of disinfectant.

Age	Result of the diagnosis	Lifestyle of the animal	Interpretation	Measure
Less than 12 weeks	Negative	Kept contact with other animals and /or sick animals	Re-test after 4-6 weeks	The result of the last test will be conclusive
		Not kept contact with other animals and / or sick animals	Uninfected	
	Positive	Even that has ingested colostrum positive for FeLV	Infected	Isolation of animal and clinical control every six months.
More than 12 weeks	Negative	Animal exposed to sick or diseased animals	Re-test after 6-8 weeks	The result of the last test will be conclusive
		Animal no manifestations	Uninfected	
	Positive	Sick animal	Infected	
		Animal health	Re-test after 6-8 weeks	The result of the last test will be conclusive

Table 7. Interpretation of results obtained by ELISA and direct immunofluorescence. Modified from Hartmann, 2006.

As immunomodulatory therapy are used to good clinical improvement, but are still under study. Antivirals such as AZT that acts effectively against FeLV replication in vitro and in vivo reducing the viral load, improving the immune response and clinical condition of the animal (Cotter, 1991; Hartmann, 2006; Lutz et al., 2009). Infected animals should be treated for other infections promptly to prevent an impaired immune system and should be vaccinated regularly against other pathogens like rabies virus, feline panleukopenia, rhinotracheitis, calicevirose, chlamydiosis and other (Cotter, 1991; McCaw, 1995, Lutz et al., 2009). Corticosteroids should be avoided, but if stomatitis or gingivitis occurs they can be used to facilitate the intake of food. In cats with anemia, blood transfusions may be useful and leukopenia can be treated with colony-stimulating factors (Cotter, 1991; McCaw, 1995, Lutz et al., 2009).

All animals should be tested for FeLV and thereafter be vaccinated at the age of 8-9 weeks and again at 12 weeks with annual boosters. Older animals are less susceptible to infection and can be vaccinated at intervals of 2-3 years. Vaccines prepared with inactivated whole virus obtained from cell cultures are available commercially, as well as vaccines containing recombinant viral proteins expressed in heterologous systems. No FeLV vaccine provides 100% efficacy of protection for FeLV and none prevents infection, but vaccination offers good prevention of fatal cases. The immunization of animals with inactivated vaccines may result in a reduction of 70% incidence of the disease. FeLV immunization should be part of the routine vaccination programmed for pet cats. However, the most effective way to prevent the spread of infection is testing for FeLV and preventing exposure of healthy cats to FeLV infected cats (Cotter, 1991; McCaw, 1995, Hartmann, 2006; Lutz et al., 2009).

Author details

Fabiana Alves and Jenner Karlisson Pimenta dos Reis
Universidade Federal de Minas Gerais, Brazil

5. References

Barr, F. (1998). Feline Leukemia Virus. *J. Small Anim. Pract.* 39(1):41-43.

Charreyre, C., Pedersen, N. C. (1991). Study of feline leukemia virus immunity. *J. Am. Vet. Med. Assoc.* 199(10):1316-24.

Cotter, S. M. (1991). Management of healthy feline leukemia virus-positive cats. *J. Am. Vet. Med. Assoc.* 199(10):1470-3.

Courchamp, F., Pontier, D. (1994). Feline immunodeficiency virus: an epidemiological review. *C. R. Acad. Sci. III.* 317(12):1123-34.

de Parseval, A., Chatterji, U., Morris, G., Sun, P., Olson, A. J. & Elder, J. H. (2005). Structural mapping of CD134 residues critical for interaction with feline immunodeficiency virus. *Nat. Struct. Mol. Biol.* 12(1):60-6.

Doménech, A., Miró, G., Collado, V. M., Ballesteros, N., Sanjosé, L., Escolar, E., Martin, S. & Gomez-Lucia E. (2011). Use of recombinant interferon omega in feline retrovirosis: from theory to practice. *Vet. Immunol. Immunopathol.* 143(3-4):301-6.

Elder, J. H., Sundstrom, M., de Rozieres, S., de Parseval A., Grant, C. K., Lin Y. C. (2008). Molecular mechanisms of FIV infection. *Vet. Immunol. Immunopathol.* 15;123(1-2):3-13.

Elder, J. H., Lin, Y. C., Fink, E. & Grant, C. K. (2010). Feline immunodeficiency virus (FIV) as a model for study of lentivirus infections: parallels with HIV. *Curr.* HIV *Res.* 8(1):73-80.

Fujino, Y., Ohno, K., Tsujimoto, H. (2008). Molecular pathogenesis of feline leukemia virus-induced malignancies: insertional mutagenesis. *Vet. Immunol. Immunopathol.* 123(1-2):138-43.

Gomes-Keller, M. A., Gönczi, E., Tandon, R., Riondato, F., Hofmann-Lehmann, R., Meli, M. L., Lutz, H. (2006). Detection of feline leukemia virus RNA in saliva from naturally infected cats and correlation of PCR results with those of current diagnostic methods. *J. Clin. Microbiol.* 44(3):916-22.

Grant, C. K., Essex, M., Gardner, M. B., Hardy, W. D. Jr. (1980). Natural feline leukemia virus infection and the immune response of cats of different ages. *Cancer Res.* 40(3):823-9.

Grant, C. K., Fink, E. A., Sundstrom, M., Torbett, B. E., Elder, J. H. (2009). Improved health and survival of FIV-infected cats is associated with the presence of autoantibodies to the primary receptor, CD134. *Proc. Natl. Acad. Sci. U S A.* 24;106(47):19980-5.

Gunn-Moore, D. A. & Reed, N. (2011). CNS disease in the cat: Current knowledge of infectious causes. *J. Feline Med. Surg.* 13(11):824-36.

Hardy, W. D. Jr., Hess, P. W., MacEwen, E. G., McClelland, A. J., Zuckerman, E. E., Essex, M., Cotter, S. M., Jarrett, O. (1976). Biology of feline leukemia virus in the natural environment. *Cancer Res.* 36(2 pt 2):582-8.

Hardy, W. D. Jr. (1991). General principles of retrovirus immunodetection tests. *J. Am. Vet. Med. Assoc.* 199(10):1282-7.

Hartmann, K. (1998). Feline immunodeficiency virus infection: an overview. *Vet. J.* 155(2):123-37.

Hartmann, K. (2006). Feline Leukemia Virus infection. Greene, C. E. In: *Infectious diseases of the dog and cat*. 3ª ed. Elsevier, p. 105-131.

Hartmann, K. (2011). Clinical aspects of feline immunodeficiency and feline leukemia virus infection. *Vet. Immunol. Immunopathol.* 143(3-4):190-201.

Hartmann, K., Griessmayr, P., Schulz, B., Greene, C. E., Vidyashankar, A. N., Jarrett, O. & Egberink, H. F. (2007). Quality of different in-clinic test systems for feline immunodeficiency virus and feline leukaemia virus infection. *J. Fel. Med. Surg.*, v. 9, n. 6, p. 439-45.

Hosie, M. J. & Jarrett, O. (1990). Serological responses of cats to feline immunodeficiency virus. *AIDS.* 4(3):215-20.

Hosie, M. J., Addie, D., Belák, S., Boucraut-Baralon, C., Egberink, H., Frymus, T., Gruffydd-Jones, T., Hartmann, K., Lloret, A., Lutz, H., Marsilio, F., Pennisi, M. G., Radford, A. D., Thiry, E., Truyen, U. & Horzinek, M. C. (2009). Feline immunodeficiency. ABCD guidelines on prevention and management. *J.* Feline *Med. Surg.* 11(7):575-84.

Kenyon, J. C., Lever, A.M. (2011). The molecular biology of feline immunodeficiency virus (FIV). *Viruses.* 3(11):2192-213.

Klonjkowski, B., Klein, D., Galea, S., Gavard, F., Monteil, M., Duarte, L., Fournier, A., Sayon, S., Górna, K., Ertl, R., Cordonnier, N., Sonigo, P., Eloit, M., Richardson, J. (2009). Gag-specific immune enhancement of lentiviral infection after vaccination with an adenoviral vector in an animal model of AIDS. *Vaccine.* 5;27(6):928-39.

Korman, R. M., Cerón, J. J., Knowles, T. G., Barke,r E. N., Eckersall, P. D., Tasker, S. (2012). Acute phase response to Mycoplasma haemofelis and 'Candidatus Mycoplasma haemominutum' infection in FIV-infected and non-FIV-infected cats. *Vet. J. in press.*

Kurosawa, K., Ikeda, Y., Miyazawa, T., Izumiya, Y., Nishimura, Y., Nakamura, K., Sato, E., Mikami, T., Kai, C., Takahashi, E. (1999). Development of restriction fragment-length polymorphism method to differentiate five subtypes of feline immunodeficiency virus. Microbiol Immunol. 43(8):817-20.

Lutz, H., Addie, D., Belák, S., Boucraut-Baralon, C., Egberink, H., Frymus, T., Gruffydd-Jones, T., Hartmann, K., Hosie, M. J., Lloret, A., Marsilio, F., Pennisi, M. G., Radford, A. D., Thiry, E., Truyen, U. & Horzinek, M. C. (2009). Feline leukaemia. ABCD guidelines on prevention and management. *J.* Feline *Med. Surg.* 11(7):565-74.

Magden, E., Quackenbush, S. L. & VandeWoude, S. (2011). FIV associated neoplasms--a mini-review. *Vet. Immunol. Immunopathol.* 143(3-4):227-34.

McCaw D. (1995). Caring for the retrovirus infected cat. *Semin. Vet. Med. Surg. (Small Anim.).* 10(4):216-219.

McDonnel, S. J., Sparger, E. E., Luciw, P. A., Murphy, B. G. (2012). Transcriptional Regulation of Latent Feline Immunodeficiency Virus in Peripheral CD4+ T-lymphocytes. *Viruses.* 4(5):878-88.

Medeiros, S. O., Martins, A. N., Dias, C. G., Tanuri, A., Brindeiro, R.D. (2012). Natural transmission of feline immunodeficiency virus from infected queen to kitten. *Virol. J.* 25;9(1):99.

Mohammadi, H., Bienzle, D. (2012). Pharmacological Inhibition of Feline Immunodeficiency Virus (FIV). *Viruses.* 4(5):708-24. Epub 2012 Apr 27.

Neil, J. C., Fulton, R., Rigby, M., Stewart, M. (1991). Feline leukaemia virus: generation of pathogenic and oncogenic variants. *Curr. Top. Microbiol. Immunol.* 171:67-93.

O'Brien, S. J., Troyer, J. L., Brown, M. A., Johnson, W. E., Antunes, A., Roelke, M. E., Pecon-Slattery, J. (2012). Emerging viruses in the Felidae: shifting paradigms. *Viruses.* 4(2):236-57.

Olmsted, R. A., Hirsch, V. M., Purcell, R. H., Johnson, P. R. (1989). Nucleotide sequence analysis of feline immunodeficiency virus: genome organization and relationship to other lentiviruses. *Proc. Natl. Acad. Sci. U S A.* 86(20):8088-92.

Pedersen, N. C., Ho, E.W., Brown, M. L., Yamamoto, J. K. (1987). Isolation of a T-lymphotropic virus from domestic cats with an immunodeficiency-like syndrome. *Science.* 235(4790):790-3.

Roy-Burman, P. (1995). Endogenous env elements: partners in generation of pathogenic feline leukemia viruses. *Virus Genes.* 11(2-3):147-61.

Savarino, A., Pistello, M., D'Ostilio, D., Zabogli, E., Taglia, F., Mancini, F., Ferro, S., Matteucci, D., De Luca, L., Barreca, M. L., Ciervo, A., Chimirri, A., Ciccozzi, M., Bendinelli, M. (2007). Human immunodeficiency virus integrase inhibitors efficiently suppress feline immunodeficiency virus replication *in vitro* and provide a rationale to redesign antiretroviral treatment for feline AIDS. *Retrovirology.* 30;4:79.

Sellon, R. K. & Hartmann, K. (2006). Feline Immunodeficiency Virus infection. Greene, C. E. In: *Infectious diseases of the dog and cat.* 3ª ed. Elsevier, p. 131-142.

Simões, R. D., Howard, K. E., Dean, G. A. (2012). In Vivo Assessment of Natural Killer Cell Responses during Chronic Feline Immunodeficiency Virus Infection. *PLoS One.* 7(5):e37606.

Sobrinho, L. S., Rossi, C. N., Vides, J. P., Braga, E.T., Gomes, A. A., de Lima, V. M., Perri, S. H., Generoso, D., Langoni, H., Leutenegger, C., Biondo, A. W., Laurenti, M. D. & Marcondes, M. (2012). Coinfection of Leishmania chagasi with Toxoplasma gondii, Feline Immunodeficiency Virus (FIV) and Feline Leukemia Virus (FeLV) in cats from an endemic area of zoonotic visceral leishmaniasis. *Vet Parasitol, in press.*

Sodora, D. L., Shpaer, E. G., Kitchell, B. E., Dow, S. W., Hoover, E. A., Mullins, J. I. (1994). Identification of three feline immunodeficiency virus (FIV) env gene subtypes and comparison of the FIV and human immunodeficiency virus type 1 evolutionary patterns. *J Virol.* 68(4):2230-8.

Willett, B. J., McMonagle, E. L., Ridha, S., Hosie, M. J. (2006). Differential utilization of CD134 as a functional receptor by diverse strains of feline immunodeficiency virus. *J. Virol.* 80(7):3386-94a.

Willett, B. J., McMonagle, E. L., Bonci, F., Pistello, M. & Hosie, M. J. (2006). Mapping the domains of CD134 as a functional receptor for feline immunodeficiency virus. *J. Virol.* 80(15):7744-7b.

Wolf-Jäckel, G. A., Cattori, V., Geret, C. P., Novacco, M., Meli, M. L., Riond, B., Boretti, F. S., Lutz, H., Hofmann-Lehmann, R. (2012). Quantification of the humoral immune response and hemoplasma blood and tissue loads in cats coinfected with 'Candidatus Mycoplasma haemominutum' and feline leukemia virus. *Microb. Pathog.* 53(2):74-80.

Yuan, X., Salama, A. D., Dong, V., Schmitt, I., Najafian, N., Chandraker, A., Akiba, H., Yagita, H. & Sayegh, M. H. (2003). The role of the CD134-CD134 ligand costimulatory pathway in alloimmune responses in vivo. *J. Immunol.* 170(6):2949-55.

Chapter 16

Simian-Human Immunodeficiency Viruses and Their Impact on Non-Human Primate Models for AIDS

Lara E. Pereira, Priya Srinivasan and James M. Smith

Additional information is available at the end of the chapter

1. Introduction

Non-human primates (NHP) have been indispensable to the study of simian immunodeficiency (SIV)/human immunodeficiency (HIV) infection, pathogenesis, and the development of prophylactic and therapeutic interventions to prevent transmission and progression to disease. A number of SIV and chimeric simian-human immunodeficiency virus (SHIV) challenge stocks have significantly advanced the NHP model, making it possible to identify and better understand factors that influence virus transmission, acute infection, pathogenesis and the eventual progression to AIDS. The development of SHIV recombinant viruses, in particular, has been especially advantageous in that it provides a more relevant research tool for studying properties of HIV-1 infection in a NHP setting. These include HIV-1 envelope characteristics that affect transmission and pathogenesis. SHIV constructs also allow for the evaluation of the efficacy of anti-HIV microbicide formulations and vaccines that are directed against envelope and other critical virus components such as reverse transcriptase. While beneficial, the vast number of virologically-distinct challenge stocks and the growth of the NHP challenge model repertoire to now include rhesus, pigtail and cynomolgus macaques, have collectively introduced an increased level of complexity with regard to experimental design and data interpretation. Furthermore, some virus stocks have virological properties that limit applications in novel areas of drug discovery, prompting the development of new generation SHIV challenge stocks. The purpose of this chapter is to therefore summarize efforts that have been made to characterize both SIV/SHIV challenge stocks and NHP hosts, to highlight the development of new generation SHIV, and how these novel challenge stocks have advanced the SHIV NHP challenge model and anti-HIV drug and vaccine development.

2. Current NHP models: Overview of NHP species origin, susceptibility to infection and pathogenesis/disease course

2.1. Old World NHP natural hosts

As many as 40 NHP species have been identified to be naturally infected with SIV, with each species exhibiting distinct virus lineages that share a considerable degree of genetic identity. Epidemiological and phylogenetic analyses have established that the origin of the HIV-1 and HIV-2 strains is the result of cross-species transmission of the NHP lentivirus equivalents SIVcpz and SIVsm from Eastern/Central African chimpanzees and the West African sooty mangabey, respectively [1-8]. More recently, there was also evidence demonstrating cross-species transmission of a distinct SIV lineage from gorillas [9]. Due to cost and ethical reasons, the study of SIVcpz infection has been limited to small numbers of chimpanzees tracked in the wild or in captivity, with limited opportunities to monitor natural SIVcpz infections. Laboratory-adapted HIV-1 strains were initially tested in chimpanzees and were found to recapitulate some, but not all, aspects of pathogenesis observed in HIV-1 infected humans [10]. Changes in the environmental protection status of this species have led to a halt in invasive studies thereby limiting their research capacity. Experimental SIV infection of sooty mangabeys has also ceased due to their endangered status, but previously acquired samples and animals with existing SIV infections are permitted for study. Two other animal models of natural SIV infection that are available for experimental AIDS research include the African green monkey (AGM), and more recently, mandrills that are native to Gabon [11, 12]. Although initial studies were performed in AGM of African origin, the import of this NHP species to the Caribbean has facilitated their availability, making AGM of Caribbean origin the source of more recent SIV studies. The breadth of research in mandrills is not yet as extensive as that conducted in the other Old World NHP species, thus the majority of information on non-pathogenic SIV infections have been gained from studies in sooty mangabeys and AGM. Research on these natural NHP SIV hosts has collectively revealed what have come to be known as the hallmarks of SIV infection in Old World NHP natural hosts: attenuated anti-SIV immune responses and a typical lack of progression to an AIDS-like disease.

Natural hosts of SIV generally exhibit elevated acute innate and adaptive immune responses in the early phase of infection, followed by a downregulation of Type I interferon responses during the chronic phase of infection [13, 14]. In addition, while humoral immune responses are mounted during SIV infection, these are relatively minimal as demonstrated by the detection of low neutralizing antibody titers in SIV-infected sooty mangabeys and AGM [15, 16]. This immunologic attenuation collectively contributes to limited T-cell apoptosis and maintenance of peripheral CD4+ T-cells even though viral loads comparable to those in pathogenic SIV infection are observed [17-19]. The precise mechanism that triggers the downregulated immune response is unclear, but is likely to involve a combination of proposed processes that include, (1) enhanced responses of immunosuppressive regulatory T-cells and IL-17 producing Th17 cells (2) a robust early innate immune response that is swiftly constrained, and (3) controlled regulation of cellular factors or receptors associated with activation, apoptosis, or virus binding [20-32]. Furthermore, in contrast to the massive immune depletion that occurs in the gastrointestinal (GI) tract of non-natural hosts of SIV or HIV infection, natural NHP SIV hosts maintain GI epithelial integrity and exhibit a lack of microbial translocation that may in part account for minimal systemic immune activation [33, 34]. Limiting the pool and/or proliferative capacity of target cells may also play a role in disease resistance, as demonstrated by studies in sooty mangabeys in which SIV replication was shown to be restricted to primarily short-lived activated CD4+ T-cells, which likely contributes to the preservation of central memory CD4+ T-cells [35, 36]. A population of double negative (CD4-CD8-) T-cells capable of producing Th1, Th2 and Th17 cytokines have also been identified in sooty mangabeys, and are thought to compensate for CD4+ T-cell helper functions in SIV-infected animals [37].

Although the vast body of evidence points toward a disease-resistant phenotype, a low level of AIDS-like mortalities have been described among natural NHP hosts of SIV. An increasing number of studies suggest that SIV-infected chimpanzees in particular do not necessarily follow the disease-resistant paradigm and can in fact develop AIDS-like symptoms that include depleted CD4+ T-cell counts, reduced fertility in females, low offspring survival rates and increased risk of death following infection [38]. A case of immunodeficiency was also observed in a sooty mangabey that had been naturally infected with SIV for nearly two decades [39]. Collectively, these reports suggest different incubation periods for the SIVcpz and SIVsm lineages and/or that the asymptomatic period in SIV-infected Old World NHP may be longer than what is typically noted for HIV-infected humans. These NHP models have therefore provided valuable insight into both host and virus factors that have co-evolved to result in this attenuated disease phenotype. The slow progression to AIDS-like symptoms, if at all, in these species share important parallels with HIV-1 infected individuals who are long-term non-progressors and with HIV-2 infected individuals who typically exhibit a less severe clinical course , thereby providing clues about protective immune correlates of HIV infection that will undoubtedly influence vaccine and therapeutic design. It has also become increasingly apparent that immune factors alone may not influence the course of disease, as targeted CD4+ T-cell, CD8+ T-cell or CD20+ B-cell in vivo depletion via cell-specific antibody infusion in sooty mangabeys or AGM had negligible effects on viremia and disease progression [40-42], adding an additional layer of complexity and also highlighting that the virus itself needs to be taken into account. Continued research on the intricate interplay between host and virus factors in natural NHP hosts will continue to shed light on mechanisms that may have applications for health preservation in individuals already living with HIV infection.

2.2 .Old World NHP non-natural hosts

While natural NHP hosts of SIV have afforded a wealth of information about non-pathogenic infections, current environmental and ethical laws alluded to above restrict the availability and/or experimental infection of some of these species thereby limiting studies involving SIV transmission and evaluation of early anti-SIV immune responses. Furthermore, the non-pathogenic status of these natural hosts is not applicable to studies that seek to develop and test new prophylactic and therapeutic tools aimed at preventing and/or treating HIV infections. Such research has however been greatly facilitated by the utilization of Old World NHP macaque species since virus isolates and derivatives of SIVsm and SIVagm readily infect these animals, resulting in a pathologic process that is strikingly similar to that observed in HIV-1 infected individuals who progress to AIDS. Also of note, baboons (*Papio cynocephalus*) are readily infected with HIV-2, and exhibit a disease course resembling the slow progression that is observed in chronic HIV-1 infection in humans [43]. Baboons have therefore proven to be useful in studies evaluating viral latency and clinical stages of the disease. However, due to a number of factors that include differences in the HIV lineages, animal resource availability, and the time to disease development, studies modeling HIV-1 infection and vaccine development have primarily involved macaque species. The degree of susceptibility to infection and severity of disease course is highly dependent on both the macaque species and the challenge virus. Infection of Rhesus macaques (*Macaca mulatta*) with SIVsm isolates and its derivatives, but not SIVagm, typically leads to simian AIDS [44, 45]. Pigtail macaques (*Macaca nemestrina*) succumb to AIDS-like symptoms after infection with SIVsm and SIVmac, with only certain strains of SIVagm, and with SIVl'hoest and SIVsun which are isolates of l'Hoest (*Cercopithecus lhoesti*) and Sun tailed monkeys (*Cercopithecus solatus*), respectively[45-47]. Cynomolgus macaques (*Macaca fascicularis*) are readily infected with SIVmac251, an isolate from a captive rhesus macaque thought to have been infected with SIV from sooty mangabeys, but this species exhibits diminished pathogenicity and lower viremia when compared to SIV infected rhesus macaques [48].

Thus, while there is a fairly broad repertoire of macaques as animal models for AIDS research, their distinct pathogenic outcomes and innate physiological and biological makeup have to be carefully accounted for prior to selection for experimental studies. There is healthy skepticism regarding the extent to which macaques can accurately reflect HIV pathogenesis and predict efficacy of vaccines or other prophylactic tools in humans, and this is especially highlighted by negative results of the vaccine clinical trials AIDSVAX and STEP [49]. However, NHP macaques continue to be the best available model that researchers can utilize to study in vivo host-virus interactions in a system that is similar to HIV infected individuals. Furthermore, macaque models can be utilized to conduct retrospective studies to recapitulate vaccine clinical trials that have been conducted in humans. The most recent Phase IIb vaccine clinical trial, RV144, demonstrated a modest level of protection (31.2%) with a prime-boost platform involving ALVAC HIV (vCP1521) and AIDSVAX B/E gp120 candidate vaccines, and a working group has been set up to identify correlates of protection conferred by this vaccination in macaques in order to compare and contrast degrees of protection and associated protective immune responses . Drawing parallels between macaque models and vaccine trial participants may inform the design of future clinical trials as well as guide the choice of NHP model for prospective pre-clinical studies. The nature of the challenge virus itself has to also be considered. Indeed, as reviewed below, virus stocks utilized in NHP research have grown past SIV to include chimeric SHIV strains as well as simian-tropic HIV-1 strains, to better reflect properties of HIV-1 specific transmission and associated immune responses, and to facilitate experimental studies on anti-retroviral treatments and anti-HIV vaccines in NHP models. The selection of a NHP model will also require careful thought of the scientific questions being evaluated, the impact of these studies on the design of clinical trials in humans, as well as the cost and availability associated with each macaque species. These considerations are detailed below and are summarized in Table 1.

Macaque model	**Pros**	**Cons**
Rhesus macaques (*Macaca mulatta*)	-intravenous, intra-rectal, intra-vaginal and penile-exposure models established (single high and repeat low dose challenge). - SIV/TB co-infection models. - Well characterized MHC allelic profiles in Indian origin macaques. -Model of choice for vaccine candidates.	-Supply of Indian rhesus macaques dependent on domestic breeding capacity. -Chinese rhesus macaques: Poorly characterized MHC allelic profiles, exhibit low viral loads and not suitable for vaccine studies. -Primarily seasonal breeders: shortage of female macaques, not suitable for comparative menstrual cycle-related SIV/SHIV studies.
Pigtail macaques (*Macaca nemestrina*)	-Vaginal ecology and physiology similar to women. -Well-characterized repeat low dose model of intravaginal virus challenge. -SIV/SHIV and STI co-infection models. -Shows promise as a macaque model utilizing modified HIV-1.	-SIVmac infections typically aggressive and not reflective of HIV-1 infection. -Limited breeding facilities in the US, expensive. -Less established as a model for testing vaccine candidates.
Cynomolgus macaques (*Macaca fascicularis*)	-Smaller in size, easier to handle. -Widely available. -Mauritian origin macaques exhibit high MHC allele homogeneity.	-Smaller size restricts volume and/or frequency of blood and specimen collections. -Exhibit low viral loads. Limited suitability for vaccine studies. -Repeat low dose model not optimized.

Table 1. Summary of advantages and disadvantages of current NHP models for AIDS.

2.3. Research applications and species-specific advantages of macaque models for AIDS

2.3.1. Rhesus macaques (Macaca mulatta)

Rhesus macaques have been extensively used in AIDS research, which was in part facilitated by their availability. These macaques are now less easily obtained in part due to demands for these animals in non-HIV areas of research. This species is highly susceptible to infection with a wide range of SIVmac and SHIV strains via intravenous, intrarectal and intravaginal routes of infection [50-52], and it is perhaps the best characterized NHP model of low dose penile exposure studies [53, 54]. Co-infection models involving SIV and tuberculosis have also been established in rhesus macaques [55]. SIV replicates to high levels in macaques of Indian origin. This can be advantageous in applications that involve stringent testing of vaccine and/or therapeutic efficacy that utilize viral load readouts as primary endpoints. However, the high levels of viremia and relatively rapid decline in CD4+ T-cells lead to simian AIDS in an average of 2-3 years, which is not reflective of the typical rate of pathogenesis in HIV-1 infected humans who tend to develop AIDS over a longer period of 10 years. The comparatively faster disease course in rhesus macaques may underestimate the efficacy of prophylactic or therapeutic interventions in preclinical studies. Nonetheless, this NHP model still has wide applications in vaccine studies since experimental and disease outcomes can be determined in a shorter time frame. Furthermore, certain HIV-1 infected individuals do exhibit rapid disease progression (2-5 years) [56] and thus SIV-infected rhesus macaques could serve useful in this context as well. In humans rapid progression to AIDS and death in individuals homozygous at one or more loci (A, B, and C) and the association of rapid development of AIDS and the presence of HLA class I alleles B*35 and Cw*04 was demonstrated previously [57]. Genes of MHC class I alleles such as HLA B*5701, HLA C and the specific combination of KIR3DS1 with HLA-B alleles that encode molecules with isoleucine at position 80 (HLA-B Bw480I) were associated with an efficient immune control of the kinetics on AIDS progression [58]. Variant genotypes of the chemokine receptors of HIV CCR2 (CCR2-64I) and CCR5 (CCR5-Δ32) in the homozygous or heterozygous states have been implicated in combating the progression of AIDS [59].

The lower viral load and slower decline in CD4+ T-cells observed in most HIV-1 infected individuals is recapitulated better by SIVmac infection in rhesus macaques of Chinese origin[60]. However, there is limited genotypic information on Chinese rhesus macaques [61, 62], with major histocompatibility (MHC) Class I alleles and relevant SIV epitopes being more extensively characterized in Indian macaques [63-66]. MHC class I-restricted CD8+ T-cell responses are a critical component of adaptive immunity that contributes to HIV-1 and SIV control. MHC-typing can be especially informative when selecting cohorts for studies that may require exclusion of animals expressing protective alleles known to confer disease resistance. Paradoxically, the advances in genotyping rhesus macaques have contributed to high levels of demand for animals with specific protective alleles such as Mamu-A*01, driving up their cost and limiting their availability. Homologues of the MHC class I alleles HLA-A and HLA-B exist in rhesus macaques. The high frequency of MHC class I (Mamu-

A*01) in rhesus macaques of Indian origin resulting in the restriction of epitopes in different regions of SIV has been reported [67]. Mamu-A*01 positive rhesus macaques naturally restrict SIVmac251 replication and significantly contain viremia following intrarectal challenge. Significant preservation of absolute CD4 counts but the absence of viremic control was observed in Mamu-A*01 positive macaques upon intravenous infection with SIVmac251 or SIVsmE660 [68]. The ability of Mamu-A*01 positive macaques to restrict SIVmac251 replication at peak and set-point following intravenous challenge was demonstrated recently [69].

Elite controllers or long-term non-progressors have a high frequency of HLA-B27 and HLA-B57. The presence of homologues in rhesus macaques of the above HLA alleles led to the identification of Mamu-B*08 in a high frequency (38%) in a group of macaques defined as elite controllers (geometric mean of chronic phase of plasma viremia is below 1000 copies/mL). The association of MHC class I alleles Mamu-B*17 and Mamu B*29 and Mamu-A*01 with several fold reduction in chronic-phase plasma viral load was established in a group of 181 rhesus macaques infected with SIVmac239 [70].

Although the genotype of rhesus macaques has been well characterized, this species has limitations in studies involving SIV/SHIV infection and the reproductive cycle. Rhesus macaques are seasonal breeders [71], with female macaques exhibiting irregular menstrual cycles during non-breeding periods. These reproductive patterns put further restrictions on the general availability of female macaques and their applications in SIV/SHIV studies involving the role of the female reproductive tract and/or hormonal cycle on virus infection. Some researchers have circumvented the problem of irregular cycling by using Depo Provera, a progestin-based contraceptive, to thin the vaginal wall of rhesus macaques and to generate a prolonged luteal phase-like state that allows for consistent vaginal infections. An in depth description of this is provided below, in the section detailing Routes and Dose of Virus Inoculation.

2.3.2. *Pigtail macaques (Macaca nemestrina)*

In recent years, pigtail macaques have increasingly become an alternative NHP model for AIDS research. However, recent closures of several breeding facilities in the US have created logistical challenges for their acquisition and resultant increased cost. The benefit of this macaque model is that this species is readily infected with SIVmac, SIVagm, and SHIV strains [72]. SIVmac-infected pigtail macaques tend to progress rapidly to AIDS and can potentially develop thrombocytopenia [136] which is a common autoimmune disease that can also manifest in untreated HIV-1 infected individuals. Pigtail macaques in some breeding colonies may exhibit certain pre-existing immunologic conditions such as compromised mucosal integrity, increased microbial translocation and lower levels of naïve and central memory CD4+ T-cells,have been described [34, 73]. SIV/SHIV infected pigtail macaques also exhibit considerable variability in set point viral loads which is a trend that is noted in HIV-1 infected humans. This may be partially dependent on host genetics, which in part prompted the study of MHC Class I alleles in this macaque species (Mane). To date, 16

Mane-A and 22 Mane-B MHC Class I alleles have been identified, and further characterization of the frequency and distribution of at least 10 of these alleles was performed in pigtail macaques of Indonesian, North American, and Australian origin [74, 75]. New alleles continue to be identified as the genetic characterization of pigtail macaques progresses, and this is likely to increase their application in vaccine research.

Although pigtail macaques have not served as the primary NHP model for HIV vaccine studies, other similarities that are shared by this species and humans have encouraged their use in other areas of AIDS research. One of the main advantages of pigtail macaques is that the females exhibit continuous lunar menstrual cycles as do women [76], making this species particularly valuable for studies examining the impact of the menstrual cycle and accompanying changes in the vaginal environment on SIV/SHIV susceptibility. Research on the role of the female reproductive system in HIV acquisition and transmission is especially critical given recent findings that demonstrated a higher risk for women receiving the Depo Provera synthetic progesterone injection for the purpose of birth control [77]. Indeed, studies in pigtail macaques have demonstrated a similar increase in susceptibility to infection during the late luteal phase of the menstrual cycle when progesterone levels are high, which is when thinning of the vaginal epithelium, reduced local immunity and other factors conducive to virus infection occur [78]. Furthermore, pigtail macaques are a well-characterized model for repeated low dose SHIV challenge studies involving the intravaginal route [79] which are more reflective of infectious HIV doses that are mucosally transmitted in humans. In addition, a co-infection model has been developed using this species, allowing for the study of sexually transmitted infections in the context of SHIV infection [80].

An intriguing feature of pigtail macaques is that they are partly permissive to HIV-1 and HIV-2 infection although virus replication and persistence are transient in vivo [72]. Nonetheless, the implication that this macaque species could potentially serve as a primate model that utilizes HIV strains as the challenge virus is incredibly appealing given that current models depend on SIV or SHIV viruses that exhibit enough divergence from HIV-1 to impede their applications in certain preclinical studies. The discovery that pigtail macaques carry a variant form of the host restriction factor TRIM5alpha [81-83] that fails to inactivate incoming HIV particles has led to the design of new generation recombinant SHIVs (described below) that exploit this feature, opening doors for the application of this macaque species as a challenge model in studies evaluating a number of pre-exposure prophylaxis (PrEP) approaches targeting HIV-1.

2.3.3. *Cynomolgus macaques (Macaca fascicularis)*

Like pigtail macaques and humans, cynomolgus macaques also have monthly menstrual cycles. While high dose virus challenge is widely used in these macaques, they are less well characterized for the repeat low dose challenge model. Cynomolgus macaques are small and easier to handle than rhesus or pigtail macaques, but this can restrict peripheral blood sampling volumes and the frequency of other specimen collections. Perhaps one of the biggest advantages of this NHP species is that they are more widely available, with the Indian Ocean island, Mauritius, being its largest exporter. A caveat of cynomolgus macaques in AIDS research is that in order to establish a pathogenic SIV infection, a higher inoculation dose is required, at least when challenged mucosally, and the resulting viral loads are typically lower than levels observed in rhesus macaques, and are more similar to those noted in HIV-infected humans [84]. This can pose a problem for vaccine studies that depend on virus load reductions as end points. However, due to the natural geographical isolation of the Mauritian species, cynomolgus macaques exhibit a rather homogeneous genetic profile, with the majority of animals possessing the allele combination Mafa-B*430101, Mafa-B*440101 and Mafa-B*460101 [85, 86]. This degree of MHC identity can be immensely beneficial to vaccine studies that require evaluation of CD8+ T-cell immune responses to defined viral epitopes. Furthermore, the well characterized and limited diversity of MHC alleles in this macaque species allows for their application in studies to evaluate non-MHC correlates of protection. As with rhesus macaques, an SIV/tuberculosis model has also been established in cynomolgus macaques, with this species being particularly informative with regard to latent/reactivated tuberculosis [87].

3. SIV/SHIV challenge stocks

3.1. SIV strains utilized in AIDS research: Origins, phylogeny, characteristics and applications

To date, at least seven distinct lineages of the primate lentivirus SIV have been identified [5, 88-94], and these share up to 50% identity in Gag and Pol proteins, which are the most conserved and encode structural and enzymatic viral proteins, respectively. The genomic organization for SIV lineages is generally LTR-gag-pol-vif-vpr-tat-rev-env-nef-LTR, but some differences exist, with the vpu gene being unique to SIVcpz and HIV-1 and a number of strains from Cercopithecus monkeys . However, SIVsm, HIV-2 and SIVmac strains harbor a vpx gene upstream of vpr. Genes expressing Vpr or Vpu are absent in the all other SIV lineages that include SIVagm.

Sooty mangabey SIV is the origin of most virus challenge stocks for studies involving NHP non-natural hosts, although SIVagm.sab from the AGM species sabaeus has also been used to infect rhesus macaques in a number of studies. Commonly utilized SIV strains are listed in Table 2. The 'parent' SIVmac strains, SIVmac251 and SIVmac239, have been derived from rhesus macaques that are thought to have to been infected by SIV+ sooty mangabeys [95-98]. SIVmac251 is a swarm, containing different quasispecies, that was isolated from a lymphoma of an infected rhesus macaque. Further passage of this isolate through additional macaques yielded a clonal stock , SIVmac239. The SIVmac316 clone was generated in a similar manner following passage of SIVmac239 [99]. Several other isolates, either swarms or clones, were derived from the plasma or PBMC of sooty mangabeys that were passaged through rhesus macaques, or were expanded in cell lines in vitro. It is also important to note that several attenuated SIV strains, primarily from the SIVmac239 and SIVmac251 lineages, have been designed for the purposes of vaccine research. Live attenuated strains, that include SIV-Δvpr, SIVmac239Δnef, and SIVmac251Δnef, have been utilized to study protective effects against intravenous or mucosal challenge with heterologous or homologous virus stocks in rhesus macaques (reviewed in [100]). While the risk associated with a live attenuated HIV vaccine precludes use in humans, vaccine studies in macaques serve to provide an understanding of the basis of protection that is conferred by attenuated strains, by shedding light on immune memory mechanisms and virus targets that could be applied in HIV vaccine design.

Strain	**Source**	**Stock composition**	**References**
SIVsmE660	Passaged in rhesus macaques originally infected with SIVsmE038	Swarm	[236]
SIVsmE543 SIVsmE543-3	Passaged in rhesus macaques originally infected with SIVsmE038	Swarm -Clone	[112]
SIVmac251	Rhesus macaque isolate	Swarm	[95, 97, 98]
SIVmac239	Passaged in rhesus macaques infected with SIVmac251	Clone	[95, 96]
SIVmac316	Passaged in rhesus macaque infected with SIVmac239	Clone	[99]
SIVagm.sab92018	African green monkey plasma and PBMC isolate	Swarm	[12, 18]
SIVPBj14 SIVsmPBj6.6 SIVsmPBj6.9	Rhesus macaque isolate originally infected with SIVsm9	Swarm -Clone -Clone	[237, 238]
SIVmne SIVmneCl8 SIVmne170 SIVmne027	Pigtail macaque lymph node isolate	Swarm -Clone -Clone -Clone	[230, 231, 239-243]

Table 2. Commonly utilized SIV strains.

Although the SIVmac and SIVsm strains share common ancestry, differences in the source, number of animal passages and/or laboratory in vitro propagation techniques can confer distinct virological properties, such as replicative capacity and pathogenicity, to each challenge stock. The selection of a challenge stock for any study therefore requires careful consideration of these virus-specific characteristics. SIVmac239, being a molecular clone, allows for better experimental reproducibility, and the nature of escape mutations from CD8+ T-cell responses are well defined for this stock. However, a clonal virus stock is not representative of human exposures where a number of quasispecies exist per exposure. This issue can be circumvented by utilizing swarm virus stocks such as SIVmac251 and SIVsm strains. These viruses are typically more aggressive but can serve as stringent challenges in vaccine studies. However, as mentioned earlier, their high pathogenicity could also underestimate the efficacy of vaccines and other prophylactic interventions. Furthermore, lab-specific propagation techniques can affect swarm challenge stocks, such as SIVmac251, leading to variations in the composition of quasispecies within what should in theory be the same stock. It is unclear if these differences can significantly affect the infectivity and course of pathogenesis in macaques, but nonetheless highlights the importance of addressing the phylogeny of challenge stocks used in NHP experiments.

Phylogenetic analysis of challenge stocks has greatly advanced since the advent of single genome amplification (SGA) which accurately determines the number and nature of viral quasispecies during the stages of transmission, acute, and chronic infection . This technique has demonstrated that the majority of mucosal HIV-1 infections (60-90%) originate from a single virus variant [101, 102]. This phenomenon, termed the genetic bottleneck, does not necessarily apply to high-risk individuals, who are typically infected with a more heterogeneous population that also correlates with more rapid disease progression [103-105]. An in-depth understanding of lentiviral phylogeny can therefore contribute immensely to the design of preventative strategies aimed at viral variants that are transmitted and go on to establish infection. Importantly, the features of HIV-1 transmission and early diversification are mirrored in SIV-infected macaques. SGA analysis of swarm challenge stocks SIVmac251 or SIVsmE660, and isolated virus soon after intra-rectal or intravaginal inoculation of macaques have demonstrated the presence of low diversity env sequence lineages that share a high level of genetic identity to the env spectrum in the challenge stock [53, 106, 107]. Indeed, it was found that a limited number of transmitted variants (1-10 species) establish infection, thus offering strong support for and confirmation of the observed patterns of HIV-1 transmission. Studies have also been performed on SIV evolution in the male genital tract of rhesus macaques, with results demonstrating similar virus sequence distribution in the blood and semen at peak viral load, while a compartmentalization of quasispecies begins to develop after set point [108]. Thus, SIV phylogenetic studies of challenge stocks and transmitted strains combined with knowledge of the dose and timing of transmission allows for more defined evaluation of virus evolution. In addition to shedding light on virus factors influencing transmission, analysis of SIV by SGA, or other next generation sequencing methods, can help identify variant-specific cellular or humoral responses generated by the host at early and late stages of infection.

Some SIV strains, such as SIVmac251, SIVmac239, and SIVsmE543-3, can be resistant to neutralizing antibodies, restricting their application in vaccine studies designed to elicit humoral immune responses [84, 109-114]. In contrast, SIVmac316 is sensitive to antibody neutralization while others, that include SIVsmE660, demonstrate variable sensitivity [109, 110]. Furthermore, while neutralizing antibodies may be produced in response to some of these viruses following infection, successful control of viral replication is still not achieved. Given these variations, evaluation of neutralizing antibody responses typically involve a tiered approach, and patterns of sensitivity are defined for viruses based on whether there is very high (Tier 1A), above average (Tier 1B), moderate (Tier 2), or low (Tier 3) sensitivity to antibody-mediated neutralization [115, 116]. Although levels of elicited humoral immune responses are inconsistent among the various challenge stocks, a close evaluation of these differences can help delineate molecular determinants of neutralization.

A unique characteristic of SIV strains is that CCR5 is the primary co-receptor of choice, with few utilizing CXCR4, and this CCR5-specificity is reflective of the majority of HIV-1 strains. Furthermore, a number of alternate co-receptors have also been identified for SIV, including GPR15, STRL-33, GPR-1, ChemR23 and CCR8 [117, 118]. The affinity for one or more of these co-receptors varies for each challenge stock. In addition to co-receptor usage patterns, several of the commonly utilized SIV strains, such as SIVmac251 and SIVmac316, are M-tropic, and SIV-infected macaques switch from M-tropism (macrophages, memory or activated CD4+ T-cells) to dual or T-tropism (naïve/resting and memory T-cells) during infection, as do many HIV-infected individuals [119].

Given that the cellular tropism of SIV strains affects cell populations other than CD4+ T-lymphocytes, such as macrophages and dendritic cells, NHP macaques are also utilized to address other aspects of SIV pathogenesis. HIV-1 infection in humans has been shown to cause complications that include encephalopathy, neurological diseases, interstitial pneumonia, and nephropathies [120]. Some of these pathologies have been successfully modeled in SIV-infected rhesus and pigtail macaques, and studies have focused on elucidating viral determinants of macrophage tropism, since the infection of this cell population was observed in perivascular, meningeal and microglial cells, and in alveolar macrophages, which contribute to neurological diseases and interstitial pneumonia, respectively [121]. However, macrophage tropism alone is not sufficient to cause these diseases, and these pathologies only manifest in a fraction of SIV-infected macaques or HIV-infected humans. Efforts to determine host and virus factors that influence the development of these diseases are ongoing.

While SIV strains have a wide range of applications in NHP macaque models of AIDS, the genetic, structural and antigenic differences between SIV and HIV-1, particularly in the virus envelope (Env), pose limitations in areas addressing cellular tropism or co-receptor affinity, antibody neutralization, and immune-driven evolution and adaptation of Env. These differences in Env and other viral components can restrict the utility of SIV challenge models when evaluating Env-based vaccine strategies, or when testing methods of PrEP that employ entry inhibitors and/or post-entry inhibitors. To circumvent this issue, chimeric simian/human immunodeficiency viruses have been developed to create challenge stocks that better mimic the infectivity and pathogenic properties of HIV-1 in a macaque model setting.

3.2. SHIV challenge stocks

3.2.1. Strains, transmissibility, and in vivo virological characteristics

The similarity in the genetic organization and composition of HIV-1 and SIV make it possible to construct replication-competent recombinant viruses that exhibit properties of both lineages. The genetic backbone of the majority of SHIV strains is SIVmac239. These viruses have been engineered to contain not only HIV-1 env, but also genes encoding Tat, Rev, Vpu, Vpr, Nef, integrase and/or reverse transcriptase. Initial SHIV constructs were found to have attenuated pathogenesis in macaques compared to parental SIVmac strains. However, the isolation of variants obtained from serial passage and in vivo adaptation in macaques yielded challenge stocks that variably increased their pathogenicity. The dual-tropic chimera SHIV89.6 that was originally developed by Reimann et al, contains the env gene from cytopathic primary patient isolate HIV-1 89.6, and although CD4+ T-cell loss and some degree of persistent infection was observed following intravenous inoculation in rhesus macaques, no disease developed [84]. In contrast, serial transfusion of peripheral blood from a rhesus macaque infected with SHIV89.6 yielded more pathogenic variants, SHIV89.6P (isolated from PBMC, LN and spleen) and SHIV89.6PD (plasma-derived), that had primarily CXCR4-tropism and resulted in higher viral loads and CD4+ T-cell decline, as well as simian AIDS [84, 122]. This SHIV construct and its derivatives have since been utilized to decipher host and virus factors influencing transmission and early T-cell and antibody responses following intravenous and intravaginal inoculation in macaques, and have also been applied in a number of pre-clinical vaccine trials. However, the suitability of HIV89.6P as a challenge virus in rhesus macaque models, particularly when evaluating vaccine candidates, has been called into question given their CXCR4-tropism. The affinity for the CXCR4 co-receptor allows for infection of naïve CD4+ T-cells which has a major impact on the kinetics of CD4+ T-cell depletion, resulting in rates of lymphopenia that are not reflective of that caused by HIV-1 and most SIV strains that are CCR5-tropic.

Another CXCR4-specific construct, SHIVSF33, which encodes Env from the patient PBMC isolate HIV-1SF33, exhibited similar properties in that the original molecular clone was minimally virulent, with in vivo adaptation in rhesus macaques cells yielding a more pathogenic isolate termed SHIVSF33A [123, 124]. This virus stock resulted in productive infections in rhesus macaques via both intravenous and intravaginal routes of challenge. The increased virulence of these SHIV derivatives were mapped to distinct amino acid changes throughout Env. Indeed, certain CXCR4-tropic constructs, such as SHIVku-1 which is a pathogenic variant derived by sequential passage of SHIV-4 (Table 2) in pigtail macaques leads to CD4+ T-cell depletion within 4 weeks of infection and simian AIDS in as early as 8 months [125]. However, this particular construct and its rhesus macaque-passaged counterpart SHIVku-2, lead to productive infection in the central nervous system and glomerulosclerosis of the kidney [126, 127], and so have applications in modeling neuropathogenesis and renal diseases that manifest in some HIV-1 infected individuals.

Thus, despite the drawbacks of utilizing CXCR4-tropic SHIV in vaccine studies, these chimeric constructs are still highly relevant in other areas of AIDS research. For instance, the infection of cynomolgus macaques and rhesus macaques of Chinese origin with SHIV89.6 results in a robust acute immune response, lower viremia, slower decline in CD4+ T-cells, and general maintenance of virus-specific immune responses and prolonged survival [84], similar to the scenario in HIV-1 infected humans. The early robust cell-mediated responses to SHIV89.6P infection and subsequent reduction in viral replication offer clues about immune correlates of protection and help determine prophylactic or therapeutic interventions aimed at inducing strong immune responses during the acute infection period. Furthermore, the transmission of SHIV89.6P, SHIVSF33 and SHIVku-1 constructs via the vaginal route in macaques demonstrate that CXCR4-utilizing virus strains can successfully cross the cervicovaginal mucosa to result in persistent viremia, CD4+ T-cell loss and simian AIDS [128-130]. Thus, although there is a higher prevalence of CCR5-tropic transmitted HIV-1 variants, these SHIV constructs can be utilized to address early T-tropic pathogenesis, as well as prophylactic and/or therapeutic strategies aimed at CXCR4 HIV-1 variants.

SHIV CCR5-tropic chimeric viruses have been developed in recent years. One of the best characterized of these is SHIV162 [124]. Recombinant virus was generated by replacing the tat, rev and env genes of SIVmac239 with those of HIV-1SF162. Intravenous challenge of rhesus macaques with SHIV162 yielded lower viral loads than the parental SIVmac239 strain, and although viremia persisted for over a year, immunodeficiency did not develop in any of the animals under study. However, three sequential blood-bone marrow transfusions in naïve rhesus macaques resulted in pathogenic variants termed SHIV162P3 and SHIV162P4 [131], the former being isolated from lymph node mononuclear cells. Infection of macaques with these in vivo adapted strains leads to peak viral loads of 10^6-10^8 viral RNA copies/ml plasma, viral set points of 10^3-10^6 viral RNA copies/ml, a gradual CD4+ T-cell decline, severe weight loss, and opportunistic infections, which are reflective of HIV-1 infection in humans. Importantly, productive infection via intrarectal, intravaginal or intravenous routes can be consistently obtained in rhesus, pigtail and cynomolgus macaques, therefore making this virus chimera a useful tool in a wide range of studies that involve host-specific immune responses and/or prophylactic or treatment regimens targeting HIV-1 envelope protein.

Another clade B chimera that productively infects rhesus, pigtail and cynomolgus macaques is SHIV Ba-L, which expresses tat, rev, vpu and env genes from R5-tropic HIV-1 Ba-L [132]. However, HIV-1 Ba-L is a laboratory adapted strain which may not truly reflect virologic properties of primary isolates. Furthermore, virus persistence of SHIV Ba-L is comparatively shorter (42 weeks) than has been observed for SHIV162P3/P4. A dual R5- and X4-tropic Clade B chimera, SHIVDH12 replicates to high titers and causes immunodeficiency in pigtail macaques, while its derivative SHIVDH12R induces CD4+ T-cell loss in rhesus macaques [133]. However, mucosal transmission of this construct has not been described. Nonetheless, the utilization of these recombinant viruses, which encode HIV-1 subtype B Env, has collectively contributed greatly to our understanding of host and viral determinants influencing the transmission of an HIV-1 clade that is highly prevalent in North America and Europe. However, diverse HIV-1 genotypes exist due to the high genetic variability of this virus, leading to classification of distinct classes (Group M, N and O) and subtypes based on env or gag nucleotide sequence comparisons. Group M is the major class and consists of 9 subtypes (A-D, F-H, J and K) that collectively constitute greater than 90% of HIV infection cases across the globe. Clades A, C, and D are predominant subtypes in sub-Saharan Africa, with Clade C being prevalent also in India and China. CRF01_AE is widespread in Thailand and neighboring regions of Southeast Asia. Recombinants of HIV-1 have also been identified in areas with populations infected with two or more subtypes. Thus, SHIV constructs have been tailored to encode clade-specific Env proteins in order to develop virus and macaque models that better reflect HIV transmission that is local to these regions.

Strain & derivatives	**SIVmac components**	**HIV-1 components**	**Source HIV-1 Clade**	**Tropism**	**Reference**
$SHIV_{89.6}$ $SHIV_{89.6P}$ $SHIV_{89.6PD}$	*gag, pol, vif, vpx, vpr, nef*	*env, tat, vpu, rev* from 89.6/HXBc2	B	X4/R5X4	[122]
$SHIV_{SF33}$ $SHIV_{SF33A}$	*gag, pol, vif, vpx, vpr, nef*	*env, tat, rev, vpu* from SF33	B	X4	[124]
SHIV-4 $SHIV_{KU-1}$ $SHIV_{KU-2}$	*gag, pol, vif, vpx, vpr, nef*	*env, tat, rev, vpu* from HXBc2	B	X4	[229]
$SHIV_{162}$ $SHIV_{162P3}$ $SHIV_{162P4}$	*gag, pol, vif, vpx, vpr, nef*	*env, tat, rev, vpu* from SF162	B	R5	[124]
SHIV Ba-L	*gag, pol, vif, vpx, vpr, nef*	*env, tat, rev, vpu* from Ba-L	B	R5	[132]
$SHIV_{DH12}$ $SHIV_{DH12R}$	*gag, pol, vif, vpx*, 20% *vpr*	80% *vpr* from NL43 and DH12; *tat, rev, env, vpu, nef* from DH12	B	R5X4	[133, 232]
$SHIV_{1157i}$ $SHIV_{1157ip}$ $SHIV_{1157ipd3n4}$ $SHIV_{ipEL}$	*gag, pol, vif, vpx, vpr, nef*	*tat, rev, vpu* from HXBc2; *env* from 1157i isolate from Zambian infant	C	R5	[134-136]
$SHIV_{CHN19}$	*gag, pol, vif, vpx, vpr, nef*	*env, tat, vpr, vpu, rev* from CHN19	C	R5	[137]
SHIV-E-CAR SHIV-E-P4	*gag, pol, vif, vpx, vpr, nef*	*rev, tat* and *env* ectodomain from CAR-402; *rev, tat* and *env* TM domain from SF33	E	X4	[228]

Table 3. List of common SHIV recombinant viruses and their genetic composition.

The chimera SHIV-1157i is an infectious molecular clone that encodes Env from an R5 clade C HIV-1 strain that was isolated from a 6 month old Zambian infant born to an HIV+ mother. As can be expected, the in vivo passage of this recombinant virus in rhesus macaques yielded a pathogenic isolate, SHIV-1157ip, which induces simian AIDS but at a relatively slow rate [134]. A clonal derivative, SHIV-1157ipd3N4, was designed to contain an additional NF-KB site to accelerate viral replication and also contains the 3′ half of provirus isolated from the PBMC of a SHIV-1157ip infected rhesus macaque that progressed to simian AIDS [135]. This construct was found to exhibit a Tier 2 neutralization phenotype. A Tier 1 SHIV derivative, SHIV-1157ipEL, was generated to encompass both the neutralizing-sensitive Env from SHIV-1157ip and the increased replicative capacity of SHIV-1157ipd3N4 [136]. The passaged virus, SHIV-1157ipEL, retains its R5 tropism, is mucosally transmissible and induces a pathogenic profile that is consistent with HIV infection. SHIV strains with different sensitivities to neutralizing antibodies can also provide a tiered testing platform for humoral-based vaccine candidates. Another Clade C recombinant virus, SHIVCHN19, encodes Env from an HIV-1 isolate local to China [137]. The passaged virus exhibits viral loads of up to 10^9 vRNA/ml of plasma in pigtail macaques and persists for 28-31 weeks, but its pathogenicity in rhesus macaques requires further characterization. This and other SHIV constructs are summarized in Table 3.

The sizeable repertoire of studies involving SHIV recombinant viruses has revealed a number of characteristics about these chimeras. First, they are highly versatile and can be engineered to reflect viral envelope properties of a wide range of HIV-1 subtypes. Second, these viruses have varying levels of transmissibility, pathogenicity and host specificity, thereby providing investigators with options that can be tailored to fit their research interests and available resources. These SHIV constructs also successfully establish infections when applied in repeat low dose models. Finally, despite pathogenic effects in some macaques, SHIV viremia in many of these animals is typically controlled or is ultimately cleared due to either intrinsic replicative properties of the recombinant virus and/or early robust host cell-mediated responses or neutralizing antibodies. While this may limit their application in some studies, SHIV constructs are still tremendously useful for evaluating prophylactic strategies aimed at preventing mucosal virus transmission, and for examining viral evolution in the context of prophylactic or therapeutic regimens during the acute infection period. The inclusion of env from different HIV-1 subtypes in these recombinant viruses has shed light on envelope-related factors such as cellular tropism that influence transmission, as well as host immune defense mechanisms that are required to inhibit envelope-mediated entry and infection. However, the constantly evolving nature of HIV-1 env poses a challenge for certain existing prophylactic methods, prompting a focus on other virus components as potential drug targets. This has yielded a new generation of SHIV chimeras that allow for preclinical evaluation of a wide range and/or combination of antiviral drugs.

3.2.2. New generation SHIV recombinants

While the SHIV constructs designed thus far have contributed significantly to the field of NHP preclinical AIDS research, the genetic distance between these recombinant viruses and

HIV-1 is still substantial (up to 70%), which makes it difficult to definitively predict the efficacy of proof-of-concept studies in NHP models in downstream clinical trials. Furthermore, emerging drug resistance and/or drug toxicities underscore the need for alternate targets and novel anti-retroviral (ART) drugs. To facilitate these studies in NHP models, SHIV recombinant viruses encoding one or more HIV-1 genes in addition to env have therefore been developed and will be highlighted in this section.

Current HIV-1 treatment regimens involve nucleoside reverse transcriptase inhibitors (NRTIs) or non-nucleoside reverse transcriptase inhibitors (NNRTIs) either alone or in combination with other ARTs. The reverse transcriptase (RT) protein of HIV-1 shares approximately 60% identity with that of SIV. For this reason, NNRTIs, which exhibit high specificity for HIV-1 RT, do not effectively inhibit SIV or SHIV chimeras that contain SIV RT. To overcome this limitation, the construct RT-SHIVHXB2 in which the entire RT of SIVmac239 was replaced with RT from the HXB2 clone of HIV-1 IIIB, was designed [138, 139]. The initial construct exhibited a severe impairment in replicative capacity, but this was significantly improved by introducing a T to C substitution at position 8 of the SIV tRNA primer binding site. The resulting chimera has been shown to replicate to high levels (10^5-10^7 vRNA copies/ml) following intravenous or intra-rectal challenge in rhesus macaques, or intra-vaginal challenge in pigtail macaques both with and without Depo Provera treatment. In addition, RT-SHIVHXB2 also exhibited sensitivity to a number of NNRTIs (efavirenz, nevirapine and UC781) and NRTIs (tenofovir and emtricitabine) both in vitro and in vivo. Similar studies have been performed in pigtail macaques utilizing RT-SHIVmne, which contains HIV-1 RT in the genetic background of SIVmne, a pathogenic isolate from the lymph node of an infected pigtail macaque [140]. Importantly, plasma virus isolates from macaques infected with either RT-SHIVHXB2 or RT-SHIVmne, and treated with NRTIs/NNRTIs, contained genetic mutations known to confer drug resistance such as K65R (tenofovir), V108I (efavirenz,) and K103N and M184I (emtricitabine), making these chimeras useful tools for the preclinical evaluation of in vivo drug resistance [140-143].

Newer prevention and treatment strategies typically employ ART combinations that target two or more components of HIV-1. The utilization of RT and entry inhibitors, in particular, has gained momentum since this approach targets the virus at both early and post-entry stages of its life cycle, potentially increasing efficacy. This combined method has been difficult to model in macaques since the majority of SHIV constructs, containing either Env or RT from HIV-1, have limitations in evaluating certain combination drug strategies for prevention or treatment. To facilitate this line of study in NHP models an RT Env SHIV construct which used RT-SHIVHXB2 and SHIV162P3 as templates to generate a chimera containing both RT and Env from HIV-1was developed [144]. In vivo passaging in rhesus macaques yielded a virus stock that infects intravenously, intra-rectally or intra-vaginally (without Depo Provera treatment). Viral loads of 10^6-10^7 vRNA copies/ml are observed, with viremia being detected up to 20 weeks post-challenge [145]. Furthermore, this virus retains sensitivity to both RT and entry inhibitors that include the NNRTI dapivirine, the NRTI tenofovir, and the CCR5 antagonist maraviroc. In vitro testing of dual drug combinations indicated additive inhibitory effects on RT Env SHIV replication. Collectively, these studies open the door for further in vivo applications of this chimera in macaques and allow for the evaluation of dual drug combinations in prophylactic and treatment strategies.

In order to stay one step ahead of drug resistance mutations that develop, ARTs targeting components other than RT and Env have also been developed. These include a broad range of HIV protease inhibitors (PIs), fusion inhibitors and integrase inhibitors. The recombinant virus SHIV-pr, which contains the pol segment encoding protease from HIV-1 NL432, replicates to levels of 10^6-10^7 vRNA copies/ml following intravenous challenge in rhesus macaques, reaching a set point of approximately 10^5 copies/ml with infection persisting for up to 12 weeks [146]. Importantly, in vivo viral load was lowered to or below the detection limit when macaques were treated with a combination of the PIs lopinavir and ritonavir. However, further characterization of this virus stock in mucosal transmission applications and in other NHP models is required.

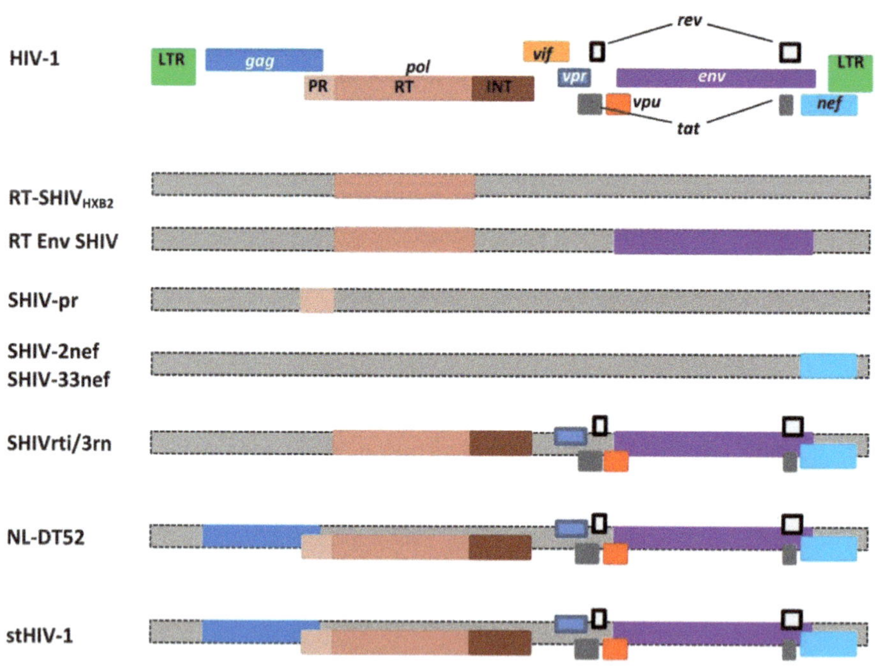

Figure 1. New generation SHIV constructs. The schematic illustrates HIV-1 genetic components in an SIV background (pale grey) for the various SHIV recombinants.

In recent years, scientists have worked toward generating recombinant SHIV constructs that are minimally divergent from HIV-1, such that they share greater than 90% genomic identity. This would undoubtedly expand the utility of these chimeric viruses and would also reduce the complexity of data interpretation when comparing prophylactic and treatment studies in NHP macaque models and human clinical trials. However, the creation of such chimeric viruses has proven to be difficult with the major reason being innate restriction factors of macaque cells that inhibit HIV-1 replication. In particular, TRIM5alpha and APOBEC3 proteins in rhesus macaque cells prevent HIV-1 infection, while the capsid and Vif protein sequences of HIV-1 enable it to overcome the human forms of TRIM5alpha and APOBEC3. Interestingly, pigtail macaques express TRIMCyp, which is a fusion protein of CypA and TRIM5, and does not inhibit HIV-1 transmission and replication [81-83]. However, HIV-1 replication is not sustained in vivo in these macaques. Some degree of persistent viremia was noted for two modified HIV-1 constructs, SHIVrti/3rn and NL-DT5R, in pigtail macaques. SHIVrti/3rn contains the reverse transcriptase and integrase-encoding regions of HIV-1 in addition to the 3' half genomic region of HIV-1, while NL-DT5R is an HIV-1 derivative that contains sequences encoding a 7 amino acid segment of capsid protein and the entire vif gene from SIV. Persistent replication of both these strains in pigtail macaques was attributed to replacement of HIV-1 vif with that from the HIV-2/SIVsm/SIVmac lineage. However, replication levels were low and plasma viremia was cleared by 5-12 weeks post-infection. In vivo treatment with a CD8+ T-cell-depleting antibody was also necessary to establish infection in some of the macaques. A promising study by Hatziioannou et al described the generation of simian-tropic (st) HIV-1 strains that not only persisted for greater than 20 weeks after intravenous inoculation, but also replicated at levels comparable to that in HIV-infected humans (10^5-10^6 vRNA copies/ml plasma) [147, 148]. Furthermore, the stHIV-1 strains demonstrated sensitivity to a wide range of RT and protease inhibitors in vitro, and the PrEP application of a tenofovir/emtricitabine/efavirenz triple drug combination in two naïve pigtail macaques demonstrated protection against a high dose intravenous challenge by stHIV-1. In depth characterization of the stHIV-1 model is still necessary, but results thus far show promise for its application in candidate vaccine studies and alternative PrEP research involving drug combinations. A limitation of the modified stHIV-1 constructs described above is that they encode a Clade B env that is primarily CXCR4-tropic and so do not model the dominant CCR5-mediated mode of transmission. More recently, a study by Humes and Overbaugh described the generation of HIVAQ23/SIVvif, which is a CCR5-tropic subtype A HIV-1 molecular clone encoding the vif gene from SIVmac239 [149]. Two adaptive mutations in Env were found to confer increased infectivity and replication in pigtail macaque cells in vitro. Thus, while further in vivo characterization of this modified HIV-1 construct is necessary, it is clear from the studies described above that the SHIV molecular virology field is making great strides in generating strains that not only maximally mimic transmitted HIV-1 strains but are also viable tools that can be implemented in vivo in NHP macaque models. Figure 1 summarizes the genomic content of the new generation SHIV/modified HIV-1 constructs.

3.2.3. Routes and dose of virus inoculation

Researchers have struggled for decades to mimic human HIV transmission and pathogenesis in animal models. A wide variety of combinations of NHP species, route and dose of infection, and recombinant viruses have been established over the last few decades. The specific combination to be used by an individual researcher is determined primarily by the research question being addressed. The varying degrees of resistance to different mucosal routes of infection with SIV or SHIV make the process even more complex. This is quite pronounced in vaginal transmission models. Unlike the rectum, the vaginal cavity has naturally evolved to resist and fight pathogens like bacteria and viruses and foreign material introduced via intercourse. The existence of multiple layers of the squamous epithelium in the vagina, innate immune factors, vaginal microflora, and mucus are some of the factors that occur in vivo to protect the female reproductive tract against sexually transmitted infections.

Earlier NHP models used supraphysiological doses that are far greater than the viral inoculum seen in human semen to demonstrate the efficacy of HIV therapeutics . Traditional methods of SIV/SHIV infection of macaques involve the administration of a single high dose of virus sufficient to infect all of the naïve controls. However, much lower doses of HIV exist in mucosal fluids of humans during sexual transmission. Thus these high dose inoculums may underestimate the degree of efficacy when evaluating HIV vaccines or antiretroviral drugs that are effective in preventing HIV infections at a physiologically relevant dose. Infection of macaques with lower intermediate doses of virus was therefore adopted. The intermediate dose in rhesus macaques generally includes the exogenous administration of Depo-Provera (a progestin-based contraceptive) to thin the vaginal epithelium and therefore increase the susceptibility to infection with SIV/SHIV [51, 150]. Although this model is reliable in obtaining consistent infection rates, it does not model HIV transmission in humans that are not on hormonal contraceptives.

The repeat-low dose model developed in the early 2000s closely resembles to the mucosal exposures of humans to HIV in the following ways. A physiologically relevant viral dose to what is seen in humans during exposure to seminal fluid is used, and repeated exposures mimic multiple sexual transmission events. Unlike the models which use a single high viral inoculum exposure, the repeat low-dose model [79, 151-153] allows the investigator to assess the efficacy of anti-HIV regimens in a repeated fashion that is closer to human use patterns.

Intravenous transmission - The intravenous transmission route in the SIV/SHIV non-human primate model has contributed to our understanding of HIV/AIDS associated disease pathogenesis and in the development of effective vaccines and anti-HIV therapies. Rhesus macaques infected intravenously with SIVmac251 or SHIV89.6P were analyzed for virological outcomes at peak, set-point and viral decline. A positive correlation was found to exist between peak and set point viral load among animals infected with both viruses. However, rhesus macaques infected with SIVmac251 had a greater variability for set point viral load and viral decline than among those that were positive with SHIV-89.6P [84]. The association between plasma viral kinetics and the development of AIDS and death in humans has been well characterized. A similar correlation can be found among rhesus macaques infected with SIV [154]. Rhesus macaques inoculated with chimeric SHIV showed variability in their disease progression. Intravenous inoculation of rhesus macaques with

SHIV-HxBc2 or SHIV-89.6 caused persistent viremia but no decline in their CD4 numbers. On the other hand, inoculation with SHIV-89.6 P, a biological isolate derived from in vivo passages of SHIV-89.6, and SHIV-KB9, a molecular clone of SHIV-89.6P, caused high viremia and rapid and profound loss of CD-4 T cells and immunodeficiency [155]. Intravenous infection of juvenile rhesus macaques with SIVmac251 led to development of AIDS like symptoms and the rapid progression to death as is seen in some patients with HIV. However it was also reported that 8 monkeys were persistently infected for prolonged periods of time. There was an effective correlation between the presence of a strong antibody response to SIV and the clinical outcome in these long-time survivors [156]. Pig-tailed macaques are also susceptible to intravenous inoculation with SIVmac251. Persistently high levels of viremia associated with a gradual decline of CD4+ T cells mimic closely the outcomes of HIV-1 infection in humans [72]. These examples illustrate the importance of choosing the most relevant virus/host combination when defining efficacy of anti-HIV strategies.

Although the intravenous route is used rarely in the NHP model today, the early proof of concept experiments using the intravenous route of infection in macaques helped to formulate the parameters of pathogenesis, disease progression and correlates of protection that are now being evaluated with mucosal routes of exposure. The NHP model has progressed more towards mucosal routes of transmission in both vaccine evaluation and PrEP studies in an effort to keep pace with the clinical strategies being developed.

Intrarectal transmission - The estimates of relative risk of HIV-1 acquisition for the different routes of sexual transmission has been determined to be the highest for rectal, followed by vaginal, and finally the urogenital route. The incidence of acquisition of HIV with unprotected anal intercourse was estimated to be 0.65%- 1.7% per act risk of transmission [157, 158]. Rectal intercourse is prevalent among men who have sex with men as well as within the heterosexual exposure group. It has been reported that among the heterosexual population surveyed for rectal intercourse, additional high risk behavior for HIV/STD such as the lack of condom use and multiple sex partners exist [159]. The per-act risk of HIV transmission associated with receptive anal intercourse is five times greater than that for receptive vaginal intercourse [160]. The presence of a single cell-layer of columnar epithelium along with increased expression of the CCR5 and CXCR4 receptors required for HIV entry augments the vulnerability of the rectal mucosa to infection with HIV [161]. An understanding of the rectal environment and mucosal mechanisms involved in rectal transmission of HIV through animal models will greatly facilitate the development of effective microbicides and vaccines.

A more appropriate model to mimic rectal transmission of HIV is achieved with a repeated low-dose exposure to virus. Consistent rectal infection can be achieved in rhesus macaques within the first four exposures with an inoculum of 10^5 RNA copies of SHIV162p3 which is within the range of HIV-1 RNA levels in semen (10^3–10^6 copies/ml). It was demonstrated that low-dose SIV infection of rhesus macaques, unlike high dose, gave rise to a longer eclipse phase (the time period between infection and first appearance of systemic viremia), and lowered activation of innate immunity [106]. No association of adaptive immune T-cell responses upon repeated rectal exposures and inherent resistance or delayed susceptibility to infection with SHIV162P3 among some rhesus macaques validates the use of this model as an effective approach to test various HIV prevention strategies .

Alternative models such as cynomolgus macaques have also been utilized for vaccine and PrEP studies with rectal SIV and SHIV exposures. Cynomolgus macaques of Philippine origin were infected intrarectally with multiple-low dose exposures to SIVmac239. However, there was a need for an escalating dose regimen to infect some of the macaques [162].Cynomolgus macaques are susceptible to infection by the rectal route with SIVsm, but have lower steady state plasma RNA concentrations than rhesus macaques [163]. Successful intrarectal inoculation of cynomolgus macaques with a single high dose of SIVmac239 and the ability to generate escape variants to CD8 T-cell responses has been demonstrated as well [164, 165]. Rectal transmission in cynomolgus macaques of hybrid SHIV viruses such as the pathogenic variant SHIV89.6P was achieved with a high dose of 1000 TCID50. These animals exhibited CD4+ cell depletion and a significant decline of their CD4+/CD8+ ratios [166].

Pig-tailed macaques, though highly utilized for intravaginal transmission studies, have been used sporadically for rectal transmission [167]. Intrarectal SIVmac251 infection of pig-tailed macaques led to persistently high levels of plasma viremia and continuous gradual decline of the CD4 cell counts [72]. The utilization of a pathogenic CCR5 variant clade C SHIV-1157ipd3N4 intrarectally in pig-tailed macaques results in an immunopathogenesis similar to SIV infection in rhesus macaques [168].

Intravaginal transmission - The lower transmission probability of vaginal infections with SIV/SHIV requires the administration of a higher inoculum of the virus vaginally compared to the rectal dose, or the use of Depo-Provera to thin the vaginal epithelium to increase the susceptibility of the macaques to vaginal SHIV/SIV transmission . The inherent resistance of the vaginal cavity to mucosal transmission and the need for the administration of high doses of SIV for successful transmission was established in the late 1980s [169]. Transient viremia and no seroconversion to SIVmac251 were achieved upon a single intravaginal inoculation [170]. Rhesus macaques of Chinese origin were equally susceptible as those of Indian origin to infection with high physiological doses of SIVmac251. Lower plasma viral loads than rhesus macaques of Indian origin were seen 6 weeks post infection among the Chinese rhesus macaques [171]. Intravaginal infection of pig-tailed macaques, the species that is widely sought after owing to its menstrual cycling similarity to humans, with 6x 10^3 TCID50 of the CCR5-tropic SHIVSF162P3 over 2 days infected all macaques with a moderate depletion of the CD4+ T cells. Although the mean peak viral load was similar to those infected intrarectally with SIVmac251, three of the eight macaques controlled their viremia to very low levels owing to their robust SHIV-specific cellular and humoral immune responses [72]. Rhesus macaques were also successfully infected intravaginally with chimeric SHIV89.6 in which the envelope glycoproteins were derived from HIV-1 89.6, a primary isolate that is CXCR4/CCR5, lymphotropic and monocytotropic, and not with SHIV (HxBC2) where the env fragment was derived from the CXCR4 T-tropic HIV-1 IIIB/LAI. Thus the ability of chimeric SHIVs to establish an infection mucosally is influenced by the properties provided by the cloned HIV-1 env fragments [172]. Unlike natural HIV infections that are primarily initiated by CCR5 tropic viruses, the chimeric SHIVs such as SHIV89.6 that produced successful vaginal infection in rhesus macaques are dual tropic (CCR5 and CXCR4). The above mentioned studies in rhesus macaques require the administration of high doses of virus to achieve mucosal infection in naïve control animals. A more relevant model with a repeated weekly exposure to a physiologically relevant dose of the SHIV162P3 in pig-tailed macaques is effective and more appropriate for preclinical evaluation of therapeutics targeted to early transmission events .

Pigtail macaques have a menstrual cycle very similar to women and have become a very important model for pre-exposure prophylaxis (PrEP) studies where inhibition of vaginal transmission is the primary endpoint. A low-dose titration in pig-tailed macaques showed that systemic infection can be achieved with 3 once-weekly intravaginal exposures to 10TCID50 of SHIV162P3 [152]. It was reported recently that the susceptibility to infection in normally cycling female pigtail macaques is substantially greater in the luteal phase when the challenge regimen used is the repeat low dose model [78]. This study has had great implications on study design for vaginal topical PrEP preclinical studies, and in the interpretation of clinical trial results. Currently, PrEP trials for vaginal transmission require that the enrolled participants must be on contraceptives . Given that we now know that contraceptive use can lead to a luteal-like state as observed with the Depo-Provera treated rhesus macaques, and susceptibility is increased in this state, the interpretation of protection in clinical trials is changing. It will be very important to model these different scenarios in the pigtail macaque for topical as well as systemic PrEP regimens. It is easy to treat all of the animals with Depo-Provera to mimic what is happening in clinical trials, but we must keep in mind that in a real world situation not all women will be taking hormonal contraceptives. Indeed, many women prefer non-hormonal forms of birth control, and it is imperative that we design our NHP studies to answer questions for this group as well [77].

Penile transmission - Men are infected through penile exposure to HIV in heterosexual and men who have sex with men (MSM) relationships . Limited preclinical research is available regarding the penile mode of transmission and an emphasis has been placed on vaginal and rectal transmission studies. The presence of foreskin has been associated with an approximately 50% increase in risk of acquisition of HIV [173-175]. The human penis, foreskin has potential HIV target cells such as CD4+ T cells, Langerhans cells, macrophages, and submucosal lymphoidal aggregates that are rich in CD3+ and CD4+ cells [176, 177]. Early penile transmission studies in rhesus macaques were limited to urethral exposures to SIVmac251 [169]. Successful infection of two adult and four juvenile rhesus macaques with urethral exposures to SIVmac251 was obtained in the above study. Recent epidemiologic evidence has prompted an increase in interest in establishing a penile transmission model. Infection of rhesus macaques with SIVmac251 through penile exposure has been recently reported [53, 178]. However, repeated exposure of macaques to a dose of 10 TCID50 (n=5) or 10^3 TCID50 (n=2) over 14 inoculations was insufficient to infect the animals Exposures to a high dose of SIVmac251 (10^5 TCID50) twice within the same day was needed to infect 3 of 5 animals. One of two macaques exposed twice within the same day to 10^5 TCID50 of SIVmac251 for a total of three-times over an 8 week period became systemically infected as well. The above rhesus macaque penile transmission study was used in an attempt to recapitulate the findings of the Merck Step trial which revealed enhanced HIV-1 infection in Ad5 seropositive individuals [179].

4. Vaccine research in NHP models

The high degree of variability among HIV-1 strains and the lack of defined correlates of immune protection in HIV-1 infected individuals or SIV/SHIV NHP models have collectively posed a considerable challenge for the development of a vaccine that confers sterilizing immunity. Vaccine design thus far has focused heavily on the induction of T-cell immunity, since HIV-1 neutralizing antibodies have been difficult to induce and do not play a dominant role in the control of viral load. Early vaccines employing recombinant HIV-1 envelope glycoprotein were efficient in neutralizing lab-adapted HIV-1 strains but not primary isolates . Furthermore, several in vivo studies in macaques have demonstrated that while certain humoral-based vaccine candidates conferred partial protection to animals challenged with SHIV strains, no protection was observed against challenges with more pathogenic SIVmac strains . However, this does not entirely rule out a role for humoral immunity, since a prime boost vaccination approach in a study involving SIVmne gp160 was shown to be effective in protecting cynomolgus macaques against intrarectal challenges with uncloned SIVmne and protection was associated with the development of SIV-specific neutralizing antibodies [180]. Similar approaches involving a recombinant vaccinia virus or baculovirus expressing SIVmac239 gp160 did not protect rhesus macaques against intravenous challenges with homologous SIVmac239 or heterologous SIVmac251 strains [181].

Although it is evident that a skewed focus on eliciting broad neutralizing antibodies will not suffice, it has also become clear that while HIV-1 gag vaccines can be strongly immunogenic, a potent T-cell response does not necessarily translate to protection. This was especially highlighted by the Merck STEP clinical trial which showed that following administration of a replication defective recombinant adenovirus 5 (rAd5) expressing HIV-1 subtype B Gag/Pol/Nef, those vaccine recipients who were already seropositive for Ad5 had a higher incidence of HIV-1 infection [182]. This is in contrast to preceding preclinical studies in which rhesus macaques exhibited a high level of both the magnitude and duration of virus-specific immune responses following a DNA prime- rAd5 boost regimen, and were protected against challenges with SHIV89.6 [183]. Subsequent studies demonstrated that the Ad5 vaccine did not protect against challenge with SIVmac239, and reduced viral loads only in animals with the protective MHC class I allele Mamu A*01 [184]. Furthermore, male rhesus macaques that were chronically infected with a host-range mutant Ad5 prior to immunization with an Ad5 vector expressing SIVmac239 Gag/Pol/Nef had a higher rate of infection following challenge with an escalating dose of SIVmac251 via penile exposure, recapitulating the outcome of the human clinical trial [179]. However unlike the Merck trial, the Ad5 immunized macaques showed a lower acute-phase viremia than the unimmunized animals.

The STEP Trial outcome led to a significant overhaul in the design and execution of vaccine studies. It was suggested that NHP models could not always be relied upon as a "gatekeeper" for determining go/no-go criteria. However NHP are the only animal models that best reflect many facets of HIV infection in humans, and therefore continue to a play a pivotal role in comparative and retrospective studies which can simultaneously inform vaccine strategies of both ongoing and future clinical trials.

Since the Merck STEP Trial, several NHP studies employing various types and combinations of HIV-1 antigen prime-boost vaccines have been conducted, with varying degrees of success. Rhesus macaques receiving a plasmid DNA prime and rAd5 vector expressing SIVmac239 env/gag/pol boost vaccine regimen, and challenged intrarectally for 12 weeks with either SIVmac251 or the heterogeneous SIVsmE660, exhibited 50% protection from infection with the latter virus strain [185]. In addition, among the SIVsmE660-infected animals, those expressing the Mamu-A*01 MHC class I allele were found to have a log lower plasma peak viremia. The vaccinated Mamu-A*01 negative animals in the SIVsmE660 group that were protected were also shown to express low levels of neutralizing antibodies and an envelope-specific CD4+ T cell response, highlighting roles for both humoral and cellular arms of the immune system. The presence of homozygous restrictive, allelic forms of the TRIM5alpha was shown to be associated with protection from infection [185]. The most recent, and perhaps most successful, vaccine study was the RV144 trial conducted in Thailand [186]. The vaccine candidates included a canarypox viral vector vaccine encoding clade B gag/pro and Clade E env as the prime (ALVAC-HIV vCP1521), and a boost with AIDSVAX gp120 B/E which is genetically engineered HIV-1 gp120 from both Clade B and E. Spanning over a six year period, this Phase IIb trial had an approximately 31% protection rate against HIV acquisition. While modest, this level of protection nonetheless re-energized the vaccine field, and several studies are underway in NHP models to recapitulate the results from the clinical trial, with the hope of identifying the specific immune response(s) that is responsible for protection.

The outcomes of HIV/SIV/SHIV vaccine trials thus far have made it apparent that the rate and level of virus acquisition and/or replication are at present, the only reliable factors when deciding the efficacy of a vaccine candidate, since the immune responses required for vaccine efficacy remain undefined. However, it is clear that NHP studies need to carefully account for the challenge virus as well as the genetic background of the macaque species, and perhaps standardize or implement more rigorous vaccine protocols to afford better predictive power and/or help in the identification and exclusion of confounding factors.

5. The role of the NHP model for Pre-exposure Prophylaxis

Microbicides are inhibitory compounds that when applied vaginally or rectally will prevent or reduce the likelihood of HIV transmission . PrEP is defined as the use of antiretroviral (ARV) drugs among HIV- negative individuals to prevent the acquisition of HIV. The successful use of ARVs in the treatment of HIV-infected individuals as post-exposure prophylaxis (PEP) and the associated knowledge gained on their safety have led the way for their use as PrEP agents. Various formulations of microbicides have been developed for rectal and vaginal application such as gels, films, suppositories (tablets) and intravaginal rings. It is necessary that a product that is destined for topical use is safe and widely acceptable, thereby promoting and enhancing adherence, cost effective and be able to deliver the drug at a high enough concentration locally to prevent the acquisition of HIV. The primary focus of microbicides has been placed on a coitally-dependent gel strategy, the method of choice for microbicide formulations, and intravaginal rings (IVR) that provide a sustained release of drugs over prolonged periods of time in a coitally-independent fashion.

Though Sub-Saharan Africa is home to only 10% of the world's population it contains every two of three people living with HIV. More than 60% of the people living with HIV in Sub-Saharan Africa are women, and of these 75% are between the ages of 15 and 24 [187]. The increasing risk associated with women and their inability to negotiate consistent condom use or monogamy emphasizes the need for the development of female-controlled methods of prevention of HIV acquisition. It was predicted that a vaginal microbicide that is 50% efficacious may prevent 33% of HIV infections in a period of 25 years upon 75% usage [188].

The effectiveness of PrEP in preventing mucosal infections with HIV will be influenced by the delivery of ARVs to a protective level at the mucosal site of transmission. The NHP model not only provides an experimentally controlled platform for the safety and pharmacokinetic evaluation of microbicides, but can also be used in the evaluation of efficacy in preventing mucosal transmission of HIV [189-192]. It is of utmost important for microbicides that are targeted for topical use in preventing sexually transmitted infections, such as HIV, to be tested in animal models prior to human trials. The sexual transmission of HIV involves a biologically complex milieu comprising initial infection among target cells at the port of entry (vaginal or rectal), the establishment of a small founder population, and local expansion to establish systemic infection . This poorly understood process cannot be properly evaluated in vitro. The recent failure and enhanced transmission observed in the first microbicide efficacy trials with nonoxynol-9 and Savvy [193, 194] warrant the need for controlled and careful investigation of topical products in animal models. A phase II/III trial with nonoxynol-9, an over the counter spermicide, in a vaginal gel formulation increased the risk of acquisition of HIV among users of the gel [195]. The detrimental effects associated with the multiple vaginal application of nonoxynol-9 such as epithelial disruption and inflammatory infiltration was also demonstrated in pig-tailed macaques [196].

The pharmacokinetic and pharmacodynamics evaluation of microbicides in animal models allows for the determination of not only the accumulation of ARVs in mucosal tissues , but also of the minimal effective dosing and the optimal timing with regards to the periods of virus exposure. The nonhuman primate model has been pivotal in producing preclinical data that can inform clinical trial design is this new and exciting field of prevention. There are several ARV PrEP candidates that have great potential for topical application and here we describe a few select ARVs and delivery methods that have progressed through initial preclinical evaluation in the NHP model. The implementation of ARVs for pre-exposure prophylaxis (PrEP) of HIV both as oral and topical applications is currently being investigated as outlined among the different trials in Table 4 [197-200].

Trial	Study population	Country	Route of Administration	Drug	Effect Size (95% CI)
Partners PrEP [197]	HIV serodiscordant couples	Kenya, Uganda	Oral	i.TDF/ Emtricitabine ii. TDF	73% (49-85) 62% (34-78)
CDC sponsored TDF2 [233]	Heterosexual men and women	Botswana	Oral	TDF/ emtricitabine	63% (22-83)
iPrEX [227]	MSM	South America, USA, South Africa, Thailand	Oral	TDF/ emtricitabine	44% (15-63)
CAPRISA-004 [198]	Sexually active HIV uninfected women	South Africa	Vaginal microbicide gel	1%TFV	39% (6-60)
VOICE [234, 235]	HIV-negative women	Uganda, South Africa, Zimbabwe	i. Oral ii. Vaginal microbicide gel	i. TFV ii. 1%TFV	Ineffective[a]
FEM-PrEP [200]	HIV uninfected women	Kenya, Tanzania, South Africa	Oral	TDF/ emtricitabine	0% (-69 -41)

TFV- Tenofovir, TDF-Tenofovir disproxil fumarate, [a]Both arms were halted for futility. Final data from VOICE trial has not been announced.

Table 4. ARV based oral and topical PrEP trials among different populations: Adapted from [197].

5.1. Antiretroviral inhibitors implemented in PrEP microbicide products

Several ARV based microbicides are currently under preclinical development in non-human primates to inhibit HIV replication at various stages of its lifecycle. The microbicides are classified based on the step that it inhibits in replication cycle of HIV such as entry, reverse transcription of its RNA genome, integration into the host chromosome, translation of new viral proteins, release and maturation of the progeny virions.

Entry inhibitors - Binding of HIV gp120 to CD4 on T helper cells and macrophages triggers conformational changes in gp120 that allows binding to the CCR5 or CXCR4 co-receptor. Next, the gp41 ectodomain forms a six- helix bundle that allows close proximity of the viral and cell membranes leading to fusion . Small molecule inhibitors that bind gp120 and prevent attachment to CD4 such as BMS-378806 have been shown to be effective as a vaginal microbicide in rhesus macaques upon a high dose challenge. BMS-378806 in combination with C52L, a bacterially expressed gp41-mediated fusion inhibitor peptide, protected macaques against vaginal challenge [201]. T1249, another fusion inhibitor, was also effective as a vaginal gel formulation against a variety of SHIV in macaques [202]. Cyanovirin, a cyanobacterial protein that binds non-competitively to gp120, was also effective in protecting pig-tailed macaques against vaginal infection [203]. CCR5 antagonists CMPD167 and maraviroc, and modified chemokines such as PSC-Rantes have shown protection in rhesus macaques against RLD vaginal challenge with SHIV [201, 204, 205].

Reverse transcriptase inhibitors - Nucleoside reverse transcriptase inhibitors (NRTIs) and non-nucleoside reverse transcriptase inhibitors (NNRTI) block reverse transcriptase activity. The NRTIs such as zidovudine, lamivudine, and Tenofovir (TFV) require phosphorylation by host cell enzymes to their pharmacologically active triphosphate (TP) anabolite [206-208]. The TPs are analogs of endogenous 2′-deoxynucleotides (dNTPs) and compete for incorporation into the growing HIV DNA chain by HIV reverse transcriptase leading to chain termination .

The potential of TFV for preventing acquisition of HIV derives from its capacity to prevent SIV infection in rhesus macaques. After four weeks subcutaneous administration of once daily TFV beginning 48 hours before and up to 24 hours after intravenous inoculation of SIV, macaques were protected against systemic infection. The macaques showed no evidence of virus in the plasma or PBMC for 56 weeks. Lymphoid tissues and major organs obtained from healthy euthanized animals 40 weeks post inoculation were also free of SIV. The efficacy of TFV and Truvada (TDF and emtricitabine) as PrEP agents was proven with repeated exposures to physiological equivalents of SHIV162P3 in rhesus macaques [153, 209, 210]. Intermittent dosing with an oral pre-exposure dose 1, 3 or 7 days before virus exposure followed by a dose of TDF/emtricitabine 2 hours after exposure was associated with a 16.7, 15.3, and 9.4 factor reduction respectively in comparison to the controls against rectal SHIV162P3 protection. No protection against rectal SHIV162P3 exposure was observed if the first dose was delayed up to 24 hours after exposure emphasizing the need for interdicting the initial replication events [211].

TFV alone (1%) or in combination with emtricitabine (5%) in a vaginal gel formulation was also effective in protecting pig-tailed macaques against a repeat low-dose exposure to SHIV162P3 [212]. The correlation of intracellular TFV-DP levels in vaginal tissue lymphocytes at the time of vaginal exposure and reduced efficacy in protecting pigtail macaques was demonstrated recently with intermittent application of a 1%TFV gel once per week and virus exposures occurring twice weekly. It was estimated that the median TFV-DP concentrations were 1810 fmol/10^6 cells at 4 hours and above 1000 fmol/10^6 cells in the vaginal lymphocytes that were obtained from animals necropsied at 1 and 2 days after gel application. However, the median TFV-DP concentrations dropped to 252 fmol/10^6 cells 3 days after gel application which correlated to 74% efficacy [213]. This study was therefore able to find a direct correlate between intracellular TFV-DP levels and efficacy in the nonhuman primate model.

NNRTIs differ from NRTIs in binding to the reverse transcriptase outside of the active site and have been shown to be efficacious in the vaginal SHIV challenge models in macaques.

Vaginal combination gels containing zinc acetate dehydrate and the NNRTI MIV-150 provided complete protection in rhesus macaques against RT-SHIV up to 24 hours following 2 weeks of daily gel application. Partial protection was seen with formulations containing zinc acetate or MIV alone [214]. MC 1220 in a gel formulation also provided partial protection against RT-SHIV in rhesus macaques [215].

Integrase inhibitors - HIV integrase is essential for incorporation of the viral genome into the host DNA and is an essential event for viral replication. Inhibitors that block this process are actively being developed for therapeutic applications and are just beginning to be investigated for PrEP. Because the integration step occurs later in the replication cycle than entry and reverse transcription, administration of integrase inhibitors may be effective when used as post-exposure prophylaxis (PEP). To address this question in the NHP model, topically applied L-870812 was evaluated for efficacy in preventing vaginal transmission of SHIV162P3 in a repeat low-dose macaque model. Pigtail macaques received 3 mL of a 0.2% L-870812 gel 30 minutes after intravaginal virus exposure with SHIV162P3 and partial efficacy was observed [216]. Further investigation of integrase inhibitors as sole PrEP agents and in combination with other PrEP agents is warranted given these encouraging results. A combination of ARVs that act at different stages of viral replication will theoretically provide broader protection.

5.2. Drug delivery vehicles

There are many different delivery platforms available for PrEP and these are being tested in NHP models. Many of the studies described above employ conventional gel formulations and are associated with problems such as leakage and the need to administer the gel shortly before every act of intercourse to prevent HIV acquisition. In addition there is also the lack of covertness with gel application which makes it difficult for women who need to use the microbicide without the knowledge of their partner. However, topical applications like gels, tablets, and films are administered directly to the site of transmission and very high local tissue levels can be achieved [217, 218]. Oral and injectable dosing is preferable in some settings, but the drug is delivered systemically, not locally, and therefore higher and more frequent dosing may be required for protection.

Alternative delivery platforms are being investigated in the NHP model to overcome some of the problems encountered with conventional dosing methods. For instance, intravaginal rings (IVR), such as those commercially available for contraception, can help overcome some of the barriers associated with conventional gel formulations and delivery. IVRs are torus shaped flexible drug delivery devices that are self –inserted and when placed is located close to the cervix in the upper two-thirds of the vagina and provide sustained release of one or more drugs for mucosal and possibly systemic effects. The advantageous properties of IVRs such as the capacity to provide sustained and controlled release of drugs over extended periods of time, non-coital dependency, and the need for a single application in women of only once a month or every few months, are beginning to be exploited in the field of microbicides [219-223].

The initial safety and size guidelines to develop ring devices that are suitable for use in pig-tailed and rhesus macaques came from the administration of different sized rings and the close monitoring of the safety of these devices. Non-medicated silicone elastomer vaginal rings of 3 different sizes were administered to pig-tailed and Chinese rhesus macaques for a 28 day period [224]. No signs of inflammation or irritation were observed on colposcopic examinations and the animals showed no behavioral changes or other problems following insertion of the rings. Mucosal proinflammatory cytokines were unchanged in the presence of the rings (for 4 weeks) or upon removal (4 weeks post removal). Safety analyses of macaque-sized elastomeric silicone and polyurethane intravaginal rings (IVRs) loaded with candidate ARV drugs were tested in pig-tailed macaques in four studies ranging in duration from 49 to 73 days with retention of the IVR being 28 days in each study. The presence of IVRs not only made of silicone but other polymers such as, polyurethane in pig-tailed macaques does not cause an alteration longitudinally in the levels of the proinflammatory cytokines locally or systemically and in the vaginal microbiological patterns [225, 226]. Efficacy studies in the NHP model with IVRs are just beginning, but preliminary pharmacokinetic studies are very promising [227-235].

6. Summary and outlook

As we move forward in our endeavors to prevent HIV infections, it is clear that having viable animal models are a vital component of a comprehensive approach to develop and test biomedical preventions. The field of HIV treatment and prevention has broadened to include not only vaccine discovery and treatment of infected individuals to PEP, PrEP, combination therapies, and discussions of eradication and cure. The pharmaceutical discoveries of recent years have increased our options for PEP and PrEP, and vaccine designs are becoming much more sophisticated. As the prevention field moves forward we are constantly modifying the macaque model to accommodate new combinations of interventions. The new SHIVs will have to incorporate the elements necessary to evaluate vaccines and other prevention modalities both singly and in combination. The likelihood that future clinical vaccine trials will be conducted in concert with PrEP trials is very high, and the recombinant viruses we use in the NHP models have to keep pace in evaluating promising candidates in the most rigorous way possible. The nonhuman primate model has adapted to aid researchers in answering ever more complex questions surrounding the interaction of the virus, host, and antiretroviral drugs. The coming years will be very interesting and fruitful as we move towards our common goal; to make HIV and AIDS a disease of our past, not of our future.

Disclaimer

The findings and conclusions are those of the author and do not necessarily represent the official position of the Centers for Disease Control and Prevention.

Author details

Lara E. Pereira
LRRI, Albuquerque, NM, USA

Priya Srinivasan and James M. Smith
Laboratory Branch, Division of HIV/AIDs Prevention, National Center for HIV/AIDS, Viral Hepatitis, STD, TB Prevention, Centers for Disease Control and Prevention, Atlanta, GA, USA

Acknowledgement

We would like to thank Dr. Michael Hendry and Dr. Janet McNicholl for valuable input. Work performed at the Centers for Disease Control and Prevention was supported in part with Federal funds from the National Institute of Allergy and Infectious Diseases, National Institutes of Health, Department of Health and Human Services, under Interagency Agreement no. Y1-AI-0681-01.

7. References

[1] Chen, Z., et al., Genetic characterization of new West African simian immunodeficiency virus SIVsm: geographic clustering of household-derived SIV strains with human immunodeficiency virus type 2 subtypes and genetically diverse viruses from a single feral sooty mangabey troop. J Virol, 1996. 70: p. 3617-3627.

[2] Gao, F., et al., Origin of HIV-1 in the chimpanzee *Pan troglodytes troglodytes*. Nature, 1999. 397: p. 436-441.

[3] Gao, F., et al., Genetic diversity of human immunodeficiency virus type 2: evidence for distinct sequence subtypes with differences in virus biology. J Virol, 1994. 68: p. 7433-7447.

[4] Gao, F., et al., Human infection by genetically diverse SIVSM-related HIV-2 in west Africa. Nature, 1992. 358: p. 495-499.

[5] Hirsch, V.M., et al., An African primate lentivirus (SIVsm) closely related to HIV-2. Nature, 1989. 339: p. 389-392.

[6] Huet, T., et al., Genetic organization of a chimpanzee lentivirus related to HIV-1. Nature, 1990. 345: p. 356-359.

[7] Peeters, M., et al., Isolation and partial characterization of an HIV-related virus occurring naturally in chimpanzees in Gabon. AIDS, 1989. 3: p. 625-630.

[8] Santiago, M.L., et al., Simian Immunodeficiency Virus Infection in Free-Ranging Sooty Mangabeys (*Cercocebus atys atys*) from the Taï Forest, Côte d'Ivoire: Implications for the Origin of Epidemic Human Immunodeficiency Virus Type 2. J Virol, 2005. 79: p. 12515-12527.

[9] Plantier, J.C., et al., A new human immunodeficiency virus derived from gorillas. Nat Med, 2009. 15(8): p. 871-2.

[10] Juompan, L.Y., et al., Analysis of the immune responses in chimpanzees infected with HIV type 1 isolates. AIDS Res Hum Retroviruses, 2008. 24: p. 573-586.

[11] Apetrei, C., et al., Immunovirological analyses of chronically simian immunodeficiency virus SIVmnd-1- and SIVmnd-2-infected mandrills (*Mandrillus sphinx*). J Virol, 2011. 85(24): p. 13077-87.

[12] Pandrea, I., et al., Simian immunodeficiency virus SIVagm.sab infection of Caribbean African green monkeys: a new model for the study of SIV pathogenesis in natural hosts. J Virol, 2006. 80(10): p. 4858-67.

[13] Estes, J.D., et al., Early resolution of acute immune activation and induction of PD-1 in SIV-Infected sooty mangabeys distinguishes nonpathogenic from pathogenic infection in rhesus macaques. J Immunol, 2008. 180: p. 6798-6807.

[14] Jacquelin, B., et al., Nonpathogenic SIV infection of African green monkeys induces a strong but rapidly controlled type I IFN response. J Clin Invest, 2009. 119: p. 3544-3555.

[15] Kaur, A., et al., Diverse host responses and outcomes following simian immunodeficiency virus SIVmac239 infection in sooty mangabeys and rhesus macaques. J Virol, 1998. 72: p. 9597-9611.

[16] Li, B., et al., Nonpathogenic simian immunodeficiency virus infection of sooty mangabeys is not associated with high levels of autologous neutralizing antibodies. J Virol, 2010. 84(12): p. 6248-53.

[17] Choudhary, S.K., et al., Low immune activation despite high levels of pathogenic human immunodeficiency virus Type 1 results in long-term asymptomatic disease. J Virol, 2007. 81: p. 8838-8842.

[18] Diop, O.M., et al., High levels of viral replication during primary simian immunodeficiency virus SIVagm infection are rapidly and strongly controlled in African green monkeys. J Virol, 2000. 74(16): p. 7538-47.

[19] Rey-Cuille, M.-A., et al., Simian immunodeficiency virus replicates to high levels in sooty mangabeys without inducing disease. J Virol, 1998. 72: p. 3872-3886.

[20] Beaumier, C.M., et al., CD4 downregulation by memory CD4+ T cells in vivo renders African green monkeys resistant to progressive SIVagm infection. Nat Med, 2009. 15: p. 879-885.

[21] Diop, O.M., et al., Plasmacytoid dendritic cell dynamics and alpha interferon production during Simian immunodeficiency virus infection with a nonpathogenic outcome. J Virol, 2008. 82: p. 5145-5152.

[22] Favre, D., et al., Critical loss of the balance between Th17 and T regulatory cell populations in pathogenic SIV infection. PLos Pathog, 2009. 5: p. e1000295.

[23] Jaroenpool, J., et al., Differences in the constitutive and SIV infection induced expression of Siglecs by hematopoietic cells from non-human primates. Cell Immunol, 2007. 250: p. 91-104.

[24] Kuhmann, S.E., et al., Frequent substitution polymorphisms in African green monkey CCR5 cluster at critical sites for infections by simian immunodeficiency virus SIVagm, implying ancient virus-host coevolution. J Virol, 2001. 75: p. 8449-8460.

[25] Kwa, S., et al., Plasmacytoid dendritic cells are recruited to the colorectum and contribute to immune activation during pathogenic SIV infection in rhesus macaques. Blood, 2011. 118: p. 2763-2773.
[26] Mandi, J.N., et al., Divergent TLR7 and TLR9 signaling and type I interferon production distinguish pathogenic and nonpathogenic AIDS virus infections. Nat Med, 2008. 14: p. 1077-1087.
[27] Nigam, P., et al., Loss of IL-17–producing CD8 T Cells during late chronic stage of pathogenic simian immunodeficiency virus infection. J Immunol, 2011. 186: p. 745-753.
[28] Paiardini, M., Th17 cells in natural SIV hosts. Curr Opin HIV AIDS, 2010. 5: p. 166-172.
[29] Paiardini, M., et al., Low levels of SIV infection in sooty mangabey central memory CD4+ T cells are associated with limited CCR5 expression. Nat Med, 2011. 17: p. 830-836.
[30] Pereira, L.E., P.R. Johnson, and A.A. Ansari, Sooty mangabeys and rhesus macaques exhibit significant divergent natural killer cell responses during both acute and chronic phases of SIV infection. Cell Immunol, 2008. 254: p. 10-19.
[31] Riddick, N.E., et al., A novel CCR5 mutation common in sooty mangabeys reveals SIVsmm infection of CCR5-null natural hosts and efficient alternative coreceptor use in vivo. PLos Pathog, 2010. 6: p. e1001064.
[32] Rout, N., et al., Paucity of CD4+ natural killer T (NKT) lymphocytes in sooty mangabeys is associated with lack of NKT cell depletion after SIV infection. PLos ONE, 2010. 5: p. e9787.
[33] Estes, J.D., et al., Damaged intestinal epithelial integrity linked to microbial translocation in pathogenic simian immunodeficiency virus infections. PLoS Pathog, 2010. 6(8): p. e1001052.
[34] Klatt, N.R., et al., Compromised gastrointestinal integrity in pigtail macaques is associated with increased microbial translocation, immune activation, and IL-17 production in the absence of SIV infection. Mucosal Immunol, 2010. 3(4): p. 387-98.
[35] Chan, M.L., et al., Limited CD4+ T cell proliferation leads to preservation of CD4+ T cell counts in SIV-infected sooty mangabeys. Proc Biol Sci, 2010. 277: p. 3773-3781.
[36] Gordon, S.N., et al., Short-lived infected cells support virus replication in sooty mangabeys naturally infected with simian immunodeficiency virus: implications for AIDS pathogenesis. J Virol, 2008. 82: p. 3725-3735.
[37] Milush, J.M., et al., Lack of clinical AIDS in SIV-infected sooty mangabeys with significant CD4+ T cell loss is associated with double-negative T cells. J Clin Invest, 2011. 121(3): p. 1102-10.
[38] Keele, B.F., et al., Increased mortality and AIDS-like immunopathology in wild chimpanzees infected with SIVcpz. Nature, 2009. 460: p. 515-519.
[39] Ling, B., et al., Classic AIDS in a sooty mangabey after an 18-year natural infection. J Virol, 2004. 78: p. 8902-8908.
[40] Barry, A.P., et al., Depletion of CD8+ cells in sooty mangabey monkeys naturally infected with simian immunodeficiency virus reveals limited role for immune control of virus replication in a natural host species. J Immunol, 2007. 178: p. 8002-8012.

[41] Gaufin, T., et al., Effect of B-cell depletion on viral replication and clinical outcome of simian immunodeficiency virus infection in a natural host. J Virol, 2009. 83: p. 10347-10357.

[42] Klatt, N.R., et al., Availability of activated CD4+ T cells dictates the level of viremia in naturally SIV-infected sooty mangabeys. J Clin Invest, 2008. 118: p. 2039-2049.

[43] Locher, C.P., et al., Baboons as an animal model for human immunodeficiency virus pathogenesis and vaccine development. Immunol Rev, 2001. 183: p. 127-140.

[44] Apetrei, C., et al., Molecular epidemiology of simian immunodeficiency virus SIVsm in U.S. primate centers unravels the origin of SIVmac and SIVstm. J. Virol., 2005. 79: p. 8991-9005.

[45] Johnson, P.R., et al., Molecular clones of SIVsm and SIVagm: Experimental infection of macaques and African green monkeys. J Med Primatol, 1990. 19: p. 279-286.

[46] Beer, B.E., et al., Immunodeficiency in the absence of high viral load in pig-tailed macaques infected with simian immunodeficiency virus SIVsun or SIVl'hoest. J Virol, 2005. 79: p. 14044-14056.

[47] Hirsch, V.M. and P.R. Johnson, Pathogenic diversity of simian immunodeficiency viruses. Virus Res, 1994. 32: p. 183-203.

[48] Karlsson, I., et al., Dynamics of T-cell responses and memory T cells during primary simian immunodeficiency virus infection in cynomolgus macaques. J Virol, 2007. 81(24): p. 13456-68.

[49] Cohen, J., Did Merck's failed HIV vaccine cause harm? Science, 2007. 318: p. 1048-1049.

[50] Bolton, D.L., et al., Comparison of systemic and mucosal vaccination: impact on intravenous and rectal SIV challenge. Mucosal Immunol, 2012. 5: p. 41-52.

[51] Marx, P.A., et al., Progesterone implants enhance SIV vaginal transmission and early virus load. Nat Med, 1996. 2: p. 1084-1089.

[52] Miller, C.J., Mucosal transmission of simian immunodeficiency virus. Curr Top Microbiol Immunol, 1994. 188: p. 107-22.

[53] Ma, Z.M., et al., SIVmac251 is inefficiently transmitted to rhesus macaques by penile inoculation with a single SIVenv variant found in ramp-up phase plasma. AIDS Res Hum Retroviruses, 2011. 27: p. 1259-1269.

[54] Qureshi, H., et al., Low-Dose Penile SIVmac251 Exposure of Rhesus Macaques Infected with Adenovirus Type 5 (Ad5) and Then Immunized with a Replication-Defective Ad5-Based SIV gag/pol/nef Vaccine Recapitulates the Results of the Phase IIb Step Trial of a Similar HIV-1 Vaccine. J Virol, 2012. 86(4): p. 2239-50.

[55] Shen, Y., et al., Induction of an AIDS virus-related tuberculosis-like disease in macaques: a model of simian immunodeficiency virus- mycobacterium coinfection. Infect Immun, 2002. 70: p. 869-877.

[56] Gottlieb, G.S., et al., Dual HIV-1 infection associated with rapid disease progression. Lancet, 2004. 363: p. 619-622.

[57] Carrington, M., et al., HLA and HIV-1: heterozygote advantage and B*35-Cw*04 disadvantage. Science, 1999. 283(5408): p. 1748-52.

[58] Fellay, J., et al., A whole-genome association study of major determinants for host control of HIV-1. Science, 2007. 317(5840): p. 944-7.

[59] Smith, M.W., et al., Contrasting genetic influence of CCR2 and CCR5 variants on HIV-1 infection and disease progression. Hemophilia Growth and Development Study (HGDS), Multicenter AIDS Cohort Study (MACS), Multicenter Hemophilia Cohort Study (MHCS), San Francisco City Cohort (SFCC), ALIVE Study. Science, 1997. 277(5328): p. 959-65.

[60] Ling, B., et al., SIV(mac) pathogenesis in rhesus macaques of Chinese and Indian origin compared with primary HIV infections in humans. AIDS, 2002. 16(11): p. 1489-96.

[61] Maness, N.J., et al., Chinese origin rhesus macaque major histocompatibility complex class I molecules promiscuously present epitopes from SIV associated with molecules of Indian origin; implications for immunodominance and viral escape. Immunogenetics, 2011. 63(9): p. 587-97.

[62] Southwood, S., et al., Functional analysis of frequently expressed Chinese rhesus macaque MHC class I molecules Mamu-A1*02601 and Mamu-B*08301 reveals HLA-A2 and HLA-A3 supertypic specificities. Immunogenetics, 2011. 63(5): p. 275-90.

[63] Muhl, T., et al., MHC class I alleles influence set-point viral load and survival time in simian immunodeficiency virus-infected rhesus monkeys. J Immunol, 2002. 169(6): p. 3438-46.

[64] Otting, N., et al., Unparalleled complexity of the MHC class I region in rhesus macaques. Proc Natl Acad Sci U S A, 2005. 102(5): p. 1626-31.

[65] Sauermann, U., Making the animal model for AIDS research more precise: the impact of major histocompatibility complex (MHC) genes on pathogenesis and disease progression in SIV-infected monkeys. Curr Mol Med, 2001. 1(4): p. 515-22.

[66] Wambua, D., et al., SIV-infected Chinese-origin rhesus macaques express specific MHC class I alleles in either elite controllers or normal progressors. J Med Primatol, 2011. 40(4): p. 244-7.

[67] Knapp, L.A., et al., A high frequency of Mamu-A*01 in the rhesus macaque detected by polymerase chain reaction with sequence-specific primers and direct sequencing. Tissue Antigens, 1997. 50(6): p. 657-61.

[68] Pal, R., et al., ALVAC-SIV-gag-pol-env-based vaccination and macaque major histocompatibility complex class I (A*01) delay simian immunodeficiency virus SIVmac-induced immunodeficiency. J Virol, 2002. 76(1): p. 292-302.

[69] Lim, S.Y., et al., Contributions of Mamu-A*01 status and TRIM5 allele expression, but not CCL3L copy number variation, to the control of SIVmac251 replication in Indian-origin rhesus monkeys. PLoS Genet, 2010. 6(6): p. e1000997.

[70] Yant, L.J., et al., The high-frequency major histocompatibility complex class I allele Mamu-B*17 is associated with control of simian immunodeficiency virus SIVmac239 replication. J Virol, 2006. 80(10): p. 5074-7.

[71] Du, Y., et al., Seasonal changes in the reproductive physiology of female rhesus macaques (*Macaca mulatta*). J Am Assoc Lab Anim Sci, 2010. 49(3): p. 289-93.

[72] Batten, C.J., et al., Comparative evaluation of simian, simian-human, and human immunodeficiency virus infections in the pigtail macaque (*Macaca nemestrina*) model. AIDS Res Hum Retroviruses, 2006. 22(6): p. 580-8.

[73] Klatt, N.R., et al., Dynamics of simian immunodeficiency virus SIVmac239 infection in pigtail macaques. J Virol, 2012. 86(2): p. 1203-13.

[74] Fernandez, C.S., et al., Screening and confirmatory testing of MHC class I alleles in pig-tailed macaques. Immunogenetics, 2011. 63(8): p. 511-21.

[75] Moore, C., et al., Identification of the peptide-binding motif recognized by the pigtail macaque class I MHC molecule Mane-A1*082:01 (Mane A*0301). Immunogenetics, 2012.

[76] Blakley, G.B., T.W. Beamer, and W.R. Dukelow, Characteristics of the menstrual cycle in nonhuman primates. IV. Timed mating in *Macaca nemestrina*. Lab Anim, 1981. 15(4): p. 351-3.

[77] Heffron, R., et al., Use of hormonal contraceptives and risk of HIV-1 transmission: a prospective cohort study. Lancet Infect Dis, 2012. 12(1): p. 19-26.

[78] Vishwanathan, S.A., et al., High susceptibility to repeated, low-dose, vaginal SHIV exposure late in the luteal phase of the menstrual cycle of pigtail macaques. J Acquir Immune Defic Syndr, 2011. 57(4): p. 261-4.

[79] Kim, C.N., et al., Repetitive exposures with simian/human immunodeficiency viruses: strategy to study HIV pre-clinical interventions in non-human primates. J Med Primatol, 2006. 35(4-5): p. 210-6.

[80] Henning, T., et al., Development of a pigtail macaque model of sexually transmitted infection/HIV coinfection using *Chlamydia trachomatis, Trichomonas vaginalis,* and SHIV(SF162P3). J Med Primatol, 2011. 40(4): p. 214-23.

[81] Kuang, Y.Q., et al., Genotyping of TRIM5 locus in northern pig-tailed macaques (*Macaca leonina*), a primate species susceptible to Human Immunodeficiency Virus type 1 infection. Retrovirology, 2009. 6: p. 58.

[82] Liao, C.H., et al., A novel fusion gene, TRIM5-Cyclophilin A in the pig-tailed macaque determines its susceptibility to HIV-1 infection. AIDS, 2007. 21 Suppl 8: p. S19-26.

[83] Virgen, C.A., et al., Independent genesis of chimeric TRIM5-cyclophilin proteins in two primate species. Proc Natl Acad Sci U S A, 2008. 105(9): p. 3563-8.

[84] Reimann, K.A., et al., Pathogenicity of simian-human immunodeficiency virus SHIV-89.6P and SIVmac is attenuated in cynomolgus macaques and associated with early T-lymphocyte responses. J Virol, 2005. 79(14): p. 8878-85.

[85] Burwitz, B.J., et al., Mauritian cynomolgus macaques share two exceptionally common major histocompatibility complex class I alleles that restrict simian immunodeficiency virus-specific CD8+ T cells. J Virol, 2009. 83(12): p. 6011-9.

[86] Krebs, K.C., et al., Unusually high frequency MHC class I alleles in Mauritian origin cynomolgus macaques. J Immunol, 2005. 175(8): p. 5230-9.

[87] Lin, P.L., et al., Quantitative comparison of active and latent tuberculosis in the cynomolgus macaque model. Infect Immun, 2009. 77(10): p. 4631-42.

[88] Allan, J.S., et al., Species-specific diversity among simian immunodeficiency viruses from African green monkeys. J Virol, 1991. 65(6): p. 2816-28.

[89] Beer, B.E., et al., Patterns of genomic sequence diversity among their simian immunodeficiency viruses suggest that L'Hoest monkeys (*Cercopithecus lhoesti*) are a natural lentivirus reservoir. J Virol, 2000. 74(8): p. 3892-8.

[90] Beer, B.E., et al., Characterization of novel simian immunodeficiency viruses from red-capped mangabeys from Nigeria (SIVrcmNG409 and -NG411). J Virol, 2001. 75(24): p. 12014-27.

[91] Courgnaud, V., et al., Characterization of a novel simian immunodeficiency virus from guereza colobus monkeys (*Colobus guereza*) in Cameroon: a new lineage in the nonhuman primate lentivirus family. J Virol, 2001. 75(2): p. 857-66.

[92] Courgnaud, V., et al., Characterization of a novel simian immunodeficiency virus with a vpu gene from greater spot-nosed monkeys (*Cercopithecus nictitans*) provides new insights into simian/human immunodeficiency virus phylogeny. J Virol, 2002. 76(16): p. 8298-309.

[93] Hu, J., et al., Characterization and comparison of recombinant simian immunodeficiency virus from drill (*Mandrillus leucophaeus*) and mandrill (*Mandrillus sphinx*) isolates. J Virol, 2003. 77(8): p. 4867-80.

[94] Keele, B.F., et al., Chimpanzee reservoirs of pandemic and nonpandemic HIV-1. Science, 2006. 313(5786): p. 523-6.

[95] Daniel, M.D., et al., Isolation of T-cell tropic HTLV-III-like retrovirus from macaques. Science, 1985. 228(4704): p. 1201-4.

[96] Kestler, H., et al., Induction of AIDS in rhesus monkeys by molecularly cloned simian immunodeficiency virus. Science, 1990. 248(4959): p. 1109-12.

[97] Letvin, N.L., et al., Induction of AIDS-like disease in macaque monkeys with T-cell tropic retrovirus STLV-III. Science, 1985. 230(4721): p. 71-3.

[98] Luciw, P.A., et al., Genetic and biological comparisons of pathogenic and nonpathogenic molecular clones of simian immunodeficiency virus (SIVmac). AIDS Res Hum Retroviruses, 1992. 8(3): p. 395-402.

[99] Mori, K., et al., Complex determinants of macrophage tropism in env of simian immunodeficiency virus. J Virol, 1992. 66(4): p. 2067-75.

[100] Koff, W.C., et al., HIV vaccine design: insights from live attenuated SIV vaccines. Nat Immunol, 2006. 7(1): p. 19-23.

[101] Haaland, R.E., et al., Inflammatory genital infections mitigate a severe genetic bottleneck in heterosexual transmission of subtype A and C HIV-1. PLoS Pathog, 2009. 5(1): p. e1000274.

[102] Salazar-Gonzalez, J.F., et al., Genetic identity, biological phenotype, and evolutionary pathways of transmitted/founder viruses in acute and early HIV-1 infection. J Exp Med, 2009. 206(6): p. 1273-89.

[103] Long, E.M., et al., Gender differences in HIV-1 diversity at time of infection. Nat Med, 2000. 6(1): p. 71-5.

[104] Ritola, K., et al., Multiple V1/V2 env variants are frequently present during primary infection with human immunodeficiency virus type 1. J Virol, 2004. 78(20): p. 11208-18.

[105] Sagar, M., et al., Human immunodeficiency virus type 1 (HIV-1) diversity at time of infection is not restricted to certain risk groups or specific HIV-1 subtypes. J Virol, 2004. 78(13): p. 7279-83.

[106] Liu, J., et al., Low-dose mucosal simian immunodeficiency virus infection restricts early replication kinetics and transmitted virus variants in rhesus monkeys. J Virol, 2010. 84(19): p. 10406-12.
[107] Stone, M., et al., A limited number of simian immunodeficiency virus (SIV) env variants are transmitted to rhesus macaques vaginally inoculated with SIVmac251. J Virol, 2010. 84(14): p. 7083-95.
[108] Whitney, J.B., et al., Genital tract sequestration of SIV following acute infection. PLoS Pathog, 2011. 7(2): p. e1001293.
[109] Bixby, J.G., et al., Diversity of envelope genes from an uncloned stock of SIVmac251. AIDS Res Hum Retroviruses, 2010. 26(10): p. 1115-31.
[110] Gicheru, M.M., et al., Neutralizing antibody responses in Africa green monkeys naturally infected with simian immunodeficiency virus (SIVagm). J Med Primatol, 1999. 28(3): p. 97-104.
[111] Glamann, J. and V.M. Hirsch, Characterization of a macaque recombinant monoclonal antibody that binds to a CD4-induced epitope and neutralizes simian immunodeficiency virus. J Virol, 2000. 74(15): p. 7158-63.
[112] Hirsch, V., et al., A molecularly cloned, pathogenic, neutralization-resistant simian immunodeficiency virus, SIVsmE543-3. J Virol, 1997. 71(2): p. 1608-20.
[113] Kimata, J.T., et al., Emerging cytopathic and antigenic simian immunodeficiency virus variants influence AIDS progression. Nat Med, 1999. 5(5): p. 535-41.
[114] Sugimoto, C., et al., Protection of macaques with diverse MHC genotypes against a heterologous SIV by vaccination with a deglycosylated live-attenuated SIV. PLoS One, 2010. 5(7): p. e11678.
[115] Seaman, M.S., et al., Tiered categorization of a diverse panel of HIV-1 Env pseudoviruses for assessment of neutralizing antibodies. J Virol, 2010. 84(3): p. 1439-52.
[116] Siddappa, N.B., et al., Development of a tier 1 R5 clade C simian-human immunodeficiency virus as a tool to test neutralizing antibody-based immunoprophylaxis. J Med Primatol, 2011. 40(2): p. 120-128.
[117] Edinger, A.L., et al., Differential utilization of CCR5 by macrophage and T cell tropic simian immunodeficiency virus strains. Proc Natl Acad Sci U S A, 1997. 94(8): p. 4005-10.
[118] Edinger, A.L., et al., Use of GPR1, GPR15, and STRL33 as coreceptors by diverse human immunodeficiency virus type 1 and simian immunodeficiency virus envelope proteins. Virology, 1998. 249(2): p. 367-78.
[119] Arasteh, K. and H. Stocker, Tropism switch in patients infected with HIV-1 and its clinical implications for the treatment with CCR5-receptor inhibitors. Eur J Med Res, 2007. 12(9): p. 397-402.
[120] Chu, C. and P.A. Selwyn, Complications of HIV infection: a systems-based approach. Am Fam Physician, 2011. 83(4): p. 395-406.
[121] Stephens, E.B., et al., Significance of macrophage tropism of SIV in the macaque model of HIV disease. J Leukoc Biol, 1997. 62(1): p. 12-9.

[122] Reimann, K.A., et al., A chimeric simian/human immunodeficiency virus expressing a primary patient human immunodeficiency virus type 1 isolate env causes an AIDS-like disease after in vivo passage in rhesus monkeys. J Virol, 1996. 70(10): p. 6922-8.
[123] Harouse, J.M., et al., Distinct pathogenic sequela in rhesus macaques infected with CCR5 or CXCR4 utilizing SHIVs. Science, 1999. 284(5415): p. 816-819.
[124] Luciw, P.A., et al., Persistent infection of rhesus macaques with T-cell-line-tropic and macrophage-tropic clones of simian/human immunodeficiency viruses (SHIV). Proc Natl Acad Sci U S A, 1995. 92(16): p. 7490-4.
[125] Narayan, S.V., et al., Characterization of a neutralization-escape variant of SHIVKU-1, a virus that causes acquired immune deficiency syndrome in pig-tailed macaques. Virology, 1999. 256(1): p. 54-63.
[126] Buch, S.J., et al., Innate differences between simian-human immunodeficiency virus (SHIV)(KU-2)-infected rhesus and pig-tailed macaques in development of neurological disease. Virology, 2002. 295(1): p. 54-62.
[127] Stephens, E.B., et al., Simian-human immunodeficiency virus-associated nephropathy in macaques. AIDS Res Hum Retroviruses, 2000. 16(13): p. 1295-306.
[128] Harouse, J.M., et al., Mucosal transmission of pathogenic CXCR4-utilizing SHIVSF33A variants in rhesus macaques. Virology, 1998. 248(1): p. 95-107.
[129] Joag, S.V., et al., Animal model of mucosally transmitted human immunodeficiency virus type 1 disease: intravaginal and oral deposition of simian/human immunodeficiency virus in macaques results in systemic infection, elimination of CD4+ T cells, and AIDS. J Virol, 1997. 71(5): p. 4016-23.
[130] Lu, Y., et al., Rhesus macaques that become systemically infected with pathogenic SHIV 89.6-PD after intravenous, rectal, or vaginal inoculation and fail to make an antiviral antibody response rapidly develop AIDS. J Acquir Immune Defic Syndr Hum Retrovirol, 1998. 19(1): p. 6-18.
[131] Harouse, J.M., et al., Mucosal transmission and induction of simian AIDS by CCR5-specific simian/human immunodeficiency virus SHIVSF162P3. J Virol, 2001. 75(4): p. 1990-1995.
[132] Pal, R., et al., Characterization of a simian human immunodeficiency virus encoding the envelope gene from the CCR5-tropic HIV-1 Ba-L. J Acquir Immune Defic Syndr, 2003. 33(3): p. 300-7.
[133] Igarashi, T., et al., Emergence of a highly pathogenic simian/human immunodeficiency virus in a rhesus macaque treated with anti-CD8 mAb during a primary infection with a nonpathogenic virus. Proc Natl Acad Sci U S A, 1999. 96(24): p. 14049-54.
[134] Humbert, M., et al., SHIV-1157i and passaged progeny viruses encoding R5 HIV-1 clade C env cause AIDS in rhesus monkeys. Retrovirology, 2008. 5: p. 94.
[135] Song, R.J., et al., Molecularly cloned SHIV-1157ipd3N4: a highly replication-competent, mucosally transmissible R5 simian-human immunodeficiency virus encoding HIV clade C Env. J Virol, 2006. 80(17): p. 8729-38.
[136] Siddappa, N.B., et al., R5 clade C SHIV strains with tier 1 or 2 neutralization sensitivity: tools to dissect env evolution and to develop AIDS vaccines in primate models. PLoS One, 2010. 5(7): p. e11689.

[137] Chen, Z., et al., Enhanced infectivity of an R5-tropic simian/human immunodeficiency virus carrying human immunodeficiency virus type 1 subtype C envelope after serial passages in pig-tailed macaques (*Macaca nemestrina*). J Virol, 2000. 74(14): p. 6501-10.
[138] Balzarini, J., E. De Clercq, and K. Uberla, SIV/HIV-1 hybrid virus expressing the reverse transcriptase gene of HIV-1 remains sensitive to HIV-1-specific reverse transcriptase inhibitors after passage in rhesus macaques. J Acquir Immune Defic Syndr Hum Retrovirol, 1997. 15(1): p. 1-4.
[139] Soderberg, K., et al., A nucleotide substitution in the tRNA(Lys) primer binding site dramatically increases replication of recombinant simian immunodeficiency virus containing a human immunodeficiency virus type 1 reverse transcriptase. J Virol, 2002. 76(11): p. 5803-6.
[140] Ambrose, Z., et al., In vitro characterization of a simian immunodeficiency virus-human immunodeficiency virus (HIV) chimera expressing HIV type 1 reverse transcriptase to study antiviral resistance in pigtail macaques. J Virol, 2004. 78(24): p. 13553-61.
[141] Hofman, M.J., et al., Efavirenz therapy in rhesus macaques infected with a chimera of simian immunodeficiency virus containing reverse transcriptase from human immunodeficiency virus type 1. Antimicrob Agents Chemother, 2004. 48(9): p. 3483-90.
[142] Kearney, M., et al., Genetic diversity of simian immunodeficiency virus encoding HIV-1 reverse transcriptase persists in macaques despite antiretroviral therapy. J Virol, 2011. 85(2): p. 1067-76.
[143] Shao, W., et al., RT-SHIV subpopulation dynamics in infected macaques during anti-HIV therapy. Retrovirology, 2009. 6: p. 101.
[144] Smith, J.M., et al., Generation of a dual RT Env SHIV that is infectious in rhesus macaques. J Med Primatol, 2010. 39(4): p. 213-23.
[145] Pal, R., et al., Virological and molecular characterization of a simian human immunodeficiency virus (SHIV) encoding the envelope and reverse transcriptase genes from HIV-1. Virology, 2012. 432: p. 173-183.
[146] Ishimatsu, M., et al., Construction of a novel SHIV having an HIV-1-derived protease gene and its infection to rhesus macaques: a useful tool for in vivo efficacy tests of protease inhibitors. Microbes Infect, 2007. 9(4): p. 475-82.
[147] Hatziioannou, T., et al., A macaque model of HIV-1 infection. Proc Natl Acad Sci U S A, 2009. 106(11): p. 4425-9.
[148] Hatziioannou, T., et al., Generation of simian-tropic HIV-1 by restriction factor evasion. Science, 2006. 314(5796): p. 95.
[149] Humes, D. and J. Overbaugh, Adaptation of subtype a human immunodeficiency virus type 1 envelope to pig-tailed macaque cells. J Virol, 2011. 85(9): p. 4409-20.
[150] Sanders-Beer, B., et al., Depo-Provera does not alter disease progression in SIVmac-infected female Chinese rhesus macaques. AIDS Res Hum Retroviruses, 2010. 26(4): p. 433-43.
[151] Kersh, E.N., et al., Repeated rectal SHIVSF162P3 exposures do not consistently induce sustained T cell responses prior to systemic infection in the repeat-low dose preclinical macaque model. AIDS Res Hum Retroviruses, 2009. 25(9): p. 905-17.

[152] Otten, R.A., et al., Multiple vaginal exposures to low doses of R5 simian-human immunodeficiency virus: strategy to study HIV preclinical interventions in nonhuman primates. J Infect Dis, 2005. 191(2): p. 164-73.
[153] Subbarao, S., et al., Direct stringency comparison of two macaque models (single-high vs. repeat-low) for mucosal HIV transmission using an identical anti-HIV chemoprophylaxis intervention. J Med Primatol, 2007. 36(4-5): p. 238-43.
[154] Chakrabarti, L., et al., Variable course of primary simian immundeficiency virus infection in lymph nodes: relation to disease progression. J Virol, 1994. 68: p. 6634-6643.
[155] Reimann, K.A., et al., Viral burden and disease progression in rhesus monkeys infected with chimeric simian-human immunodeficiency viruses. Virology, 1999. 256(1): p. 15-21.
[156] Daniel, M.D., et al., Long-term persistent infection of macaque monkeys with the simian immunodeficiency virus. J Gen Virol, 1987. 68 (Pt 12): p. 3183-9.
[157] Boily, M.C., et al., Heterosexual risk of HIV-1 infection per sexual act: systematic review and meta-analysis of observational studies. Lancet Infect Dis, 2009. 9(2): p. 118-29.
[158] Jin, F., et al., Per-contact probability of HIV transmission in homosexual men in Sydney in the era of HAART. AIDS, 2010. 24(6): p. 907-13.
[159] Leichliter, J.S., Heterosexual anal sex: part of an expanding sexual repertoire? Sex Transm Dis, 2008. 35(11): p. 910-1.
[160] Varghese, B., et al., Reducing the risk of sexual HIV transmission: quantifying the per-act risk for HIV on the basis of choice of partner, sex act, and condom use. Sex Transm Dis, 2002. 29(1): p. 38-43.
[161] Anton, P.A., et al., Enhanced levels of functional HIV-1 co-receptors on human mucosal T cells demonstrated using intestinal biopsy tissue. AIDS, 2000. 14(12): p. 1761-5.
[162] Willer, D.O., et al., Multi-low-dose mucosal simian immunodeficiency virus SIVmac239 challenge of cynomolgus macaques immunized with "hyperattenuated" SIV constructs. J Virol, 2010. 84(5): p. 2304-17.
[163] ten Haaft, P., et al., Comparison of early plasma RNA loads in different macaque species and the impact of different routes of exposure on SIV/SHIV infection. J Med Primatol, 2001. 30(4): p. 207-14.
[164] Bimber, B.N., et al., Ultradeep pyrosequencing detects complex patterns of CD8+ T-lymphocyte escape in simian immunodeficiency virus-infected macaques. J Virol, 2009. 83(16): p. 8247-53.
[165] Wiseman, R.W., et al., Simian immunodeficiency virus SIVmac239 infection of major histocompatibility complex-identical cynomolgus macaques from Mauritius. J Virol, 2007. 81(1): p. 349-61.
[166] Tsai, C.C., et al., Cyanovirin-N gel as a topical microbicide prevents rectal transmission of SHIV89.6P in macaques. AIDS Res Hum Retroviruses, 2003. 19(7): p. 535-41.

[167] Patton, D.L., et al., Preclinical safety assessments of UC781 anti-human immunodeficiency virus topical microbicide formulations. Antimicrob Agents Chemother, 2007. 51(5): p. 1608-15.

[168] Ho, O., et al., Pathogenic infection of *Macaca nemestrina* with a CCR5-tropic subtype-C simian-human immunodeficiency virus. Retrovirology, 2009. 6: p. 65.

[169] Miller, C.J., et al., Genital mucosal transmission of simian immunodeficiency virus: animal model for heterosexual transmission of human immunodeficiency virus. J Virol, 1989. 63(10): p. 4277-84.

[170] Miller, C.J., et al., Intravaginal inoculation of rhesus macaques with cell-free simian immunodeficiency virus results in persistent or transient viremia. J Virol, 1994. 68: p. 6391-6400.

[171] Marthas, M.L., et al., Titration of an SIVmac251 stock by vaginal inoculation of Indian and Chinese origin rhesus macaques: transmission efficiency, viral loads, and antibody responses. AIDS Res Hum Retroviruses, 2001. 17(15): p. 1455-66.

[172] Lu, Y., et al., Vaginal transmission of chimeric simian/human immunodeficiency viruses in rhesus macaques. J Virol, 1996. 70(5): p. 3045-50.

[173] Auvert, B., et al., Randomized, controlled intervention trial of male circumcision for reduction of HIV infection risk: the ANRS 1265 Trial. PLoS Med, 2005. 2(11): p. e298.

[174] Lissouba, P., et al., Adult male circumcision as an intervention against HIV: an operational study of uptake in a South African community (ANRS 12126). BMC Infect Dis, 2011. 11: p. 253.

[175] Mahiane, S.G., et al., Transmission probabilities of HIV and herpes simplex virus type 2, effect of male circumcision and interaction: a longitudinal study in a township of South Africa. AIDS, 2009. 23(3): p. 377-383.

[176] Hirbod, T., et al., Abundant expression of HIV target cells and C-type lectin receptors in the foreskin tissue of young Kenyan men. Am J Pathol, 2010. 176(6): p. 2798-805.

[177] McCoombe, S.G. and R.V. Short, Potential HIV-1 target cells in the human penis. AIDS, 2006. 20(11): p. 1491-5.

[178] Yeh, W.W., et al., The TRIM5 gene modulates penile mucosal acquisition of simian immunodeficiency virus in rhesus monkeys. J Virol, 2011. 85(19): p. 10389-98.

[179] Qureshi, H., et al., Low-dose penile SIVmac251 exposure of rhesus macaques infected with adenovirus type 5 (Ad5) and then immunized with a replication-defective Ad5-based SIV gag/pol/nef vaccine recapitulates the results of the phase IIb step trial of a similar HIV-1 vaccine. J Virol, 2012. 86: p. 2239-2250.

[180] Polacino, P., et al., Protection of macaques against intrarectal infection by a combination immunization regimen with recombinant simian immunodeficiency virus SIVmne gp160 vaccines. J Virol, 1999. 73(4): p. 3134-46.

[181] Ahmad, S., et al., Reduced virus load in rhesus macaques immunized with recombinant gp160 and challenged with simian immunodeficiency virus. AIDS Res Hum Retroviruses, 1994. 10(2): p. 195-204.

[182] Buchbinder, S.P., et al., Efficacy assessment of a cell-mediated immunity HIV-1 vaccine (the Step Study): a double-blind, randomised, placebo-controlled, test-of-concept trial. Lancet, 2008. 372(9653): p. 1881-93.

[183] S, S., et al., Replication-defective adenovirus serotype 5 vectors elicit durable cellular and humoral immune responses in nonhuman primates. J Virol, 2005. 79: p. 6516-6522.

[184] Casimiro, D.R., et al., Attenuation of simian immunodeficiency virus SIVmac239 infection by prophylactic immunization with dna and recombinant adenoviral vaccine vectors expressing Gag. J Virol, 2005. 79(24): p. 15547-55.

[185] Letvin, N.L., et al., Immune and Genetic Correlates of Vaccine Protection Against Mucosal Infection by SIV in Monkeys. Sci Transl Med, 2011. 3(81): p. 81ra36.

[186] Plotkin, S.A., The RV144 Thai HIV vaccine trial. Hum Vaccin, 2010. 6(2): p. Epub.

[187] Quinn, T.C. and J. Overbaugh, HIV/AIDS in women: an expanding epidemic. Science, 2005. 308(5728): p. 1582-3.

[188] Boily, M.C., et al., The future role of rectal and vaginal microbicides to prevent HIV infection in heterosexual populations: implications for product development and prevention. Sexually Transmitted Infections, 2011. 87(7): p. 646-653.

[189] Dias, A.S., et al., Animal models used for the evaluation of antiretroviral therapies. Curr Hiv Res, 2006. 4: p. 431-436.

[190] Hendrix, C.W., Y.J. Cao, and E.J. Fuchs, Topical microbicides to prevent HIV: clinical drug development challenges. Annu Rev Pharmacol Toxicol, 2009. 49: p. 349-375.

[191] Van Rompay, K.K., Evaluation of antiretrovirals in animal models of HIV infection. Antiviral Res, 2010. 85: p. 159-175.

[192] Van Rompay, K.K., The use of nonhuman primate models of HIV infection for the evaluation of antiviral strategies. AIDS Res Hum Retroviruses, 2012. 28: p. 16-35.

[193] Feldblum, P., et al., SAVVY vaginal gel (C31G) for prevention of HIV infection: a randomized controlled trial in Nigeria. PLos ONE, 2008. 3: p. e1474.

[194] Peterson, L., et al., SAVVY (C31G) gel for prevention of HIV infection in women: a Phase 3, double-blind, randomized, placebo-controlled trial in Ghana. PLos ONE, 2007. 2: p. e1312.

[195] Van Damme, L., et al., Effectiveness of COL-1492, a nonoxynol-9 vaginal gel, on HIV-1 transmission in female sex workers: a randomised controlled trial. Lancet, 2002. 360(9338): p. 971-977.

[196] Patton, D.L., et al., Effects of multiple applications of benzalkonium chloride and nonoxynol 9 on the vaginal epithelium in the pigtailed macaque (Macaca nemestrina). American Journal of Obstetrics and Gynecology, 1999. 180(5): p. 1080-1087.

[197] Celum, C. and J.M. Baeten, Tenofovir-based pre-exposure prophylaxis for HIV prevention: evolving evidence. Curr Opin Infect Dis, 2012. 25(1): p. 51-7.

[198] Karim, Q.A., et al., Effectiveness and Safety of Tenofovir Gel, an Antiretroviral Microbicide, for the Prevention of HIV Infection in Women. Science, 2010. 329(5996): p. 1168-1174.

[199] Karim, S.S. and Q.A. Karim, Antiretroviral prophylaxis: a defining moment in HIV control. Lancet, 2011. 378(9809): p. e23-5.

[200] Van Damme, L., Corneli, A., Ahmed, K., Agot, K., Lombaard, J., Kapiga, S., Grant, R., Kashuba, A., Crucitti, T., Taylor, D., and FEM-PrEP Study group. The FEM-PrEP Trial of Emtricitabine/Tenofovir Disoproxil Fumarate (Truvada) among African Women. in 19th Conference on Retroviruses and Opportunistic Infections. 2012. Seattle, WA, USA.

[201] Veazey, R.S., et al., Protection of macaques from vaginal SHIV challenge by vaginally delivered inhibitors of virus-cell fusion. Nature, 2005. 438(7064): p. 99-102.

[202] Veazey, R.S., et al., Tropism-independent protection of macaques against vaginal transmission of three SHIVs by the HIV-1 fusion inhibitor T-1249. Proc Natl Acad Sci U S A, 2008. 105(30): p. 10531-10536.

[203] Tsai, C.C., et al., Cyanovirin-N inhibits AIDS virus infections in vaginal transmission models. AIDS Res Hum Retroviruses, 2004. 20(1): p. 11-18.

[204] Lederman, M.M., et al., Prevention of vaginal SHIV transmission in rhesus macaques through inhibition of CCR5. Science, 2004. 306(5695): p. 485-487.

[205] Veazey, R.S., et al., Protection of Rhesus Macaques from Vaginal Infection by Vaginally Delivered Maraviroc, an Inhibitor of HIV-1 Entry via the CCR5 Co-Receptor. Journal of Infectious Diseases, 2010. 202(5): p. 739-744.

[206] Anderson, P.L. and J.E. Rower, Zidovudine and Lamivudine for HIV Infection. Clin Med Rev Ther, 2010. 2: p. a2004.

[207] Robbins, B.L., et al., Anti-human immunodeficiency virus activity and cellular metabolism of a potential prodrug of the acyclic nucleoside phosphonate 9-R-(2-phosphonomethoxypropyl)adenine (PMPA), bis(isopropyloxymethylcarbonyl)PMPA. Antimicrob Agents Chemother, 1998. 42(3): p. 612-617.

[208] Rower, J.E., et al., The effect of HIV-1 infection and sex on the cellular pharmacology of the antiretroviral drugs zidovudine and lamivudine. Antimicrob Agents Chemother, 2012.

[209] Garcia-Lerma, J.G., et al., Prevention of rectal SHIV transmission in macaques by daily or intermittent prophylaxis with emtricitabine and tenofovir. PLoS Med, 2008. 5(2): p. e28.

[210] Subbarao, S., et al., Chemoprophylaxis with tenofovir disoproxil fumarate provided partial protection against infection with simian human immunodeficiency virus in macaques given multiple virus challenges. J Infect Dis, 2006. 194(7): p. 904-11.

[211] Garcia-Lerma, J.G., et al., Intermittent prophylaxis with oral truvada protects macaques from rectal SHIV infection. Sci Transl Med, 2010. 2(14): p. 14ra4.

[212] Parikh, U.M., et al., Complete protection from repeated vaginal simian-human immunodeficiency virus exposures in macaques by a topical gel containing tenofovir alone or with emtricitabine. J Virol, 2009. 83(20): p. 10358-65.

[213] Dobard, C., et al., Durable protection from vaginal simian-human immunodeficiency virus infection in macaques by tenofovir gel and its relationship to drug levels in tissue. J Virol, 2012. 86(2): p. 718-25.

[214] Kenney, J., et al., An Antiretroviral/Zinc Combination Gel Provides 24 Hours of Complete Protection against Vaginal SHIV Infection in Macaques. PLoS One, 2011. 6(1).

[215] Stolte-Leeb, N., et al., Topical Nonnucleoside Reverse Transcriptase Inhibitor MC 1220 Partially Prevents Vaginal RT-SHIV Infection of Macaques. AIDS Res Hum Retroviruses, 2011. 27(9): p. 933-943.

[216] Dobard, C., Sharma,S., Martin, A., Hazuda, D., Hanson, D., Smith, J., Otten, R.A., Novembre, F., Garcia-Lerma, G., Heneine, W. Protection Against Repeated Vaginal

SHIV Exposures in Macaques by a Topical Gel with an Integrase Inhibitor. in Microbicides 2010. 2010. Pittsburgh, PA, USA.

[217] Bunge, K., et al., The Safety, Persistence, and Acceptability of an Antiretroviral Microbicide Candidate UC781. J Acquir Immune Defic Syndr, 2012. 60(4): p. 337-43.

[218] Karim, S.S., et al., Drug concentrations after topical and oral antiretroviral pre-exposure prophylaxis: implications for HIV prevention in women. Lancet, 2011. 378(9787): p. 279-81.

[219] Clark, M.R., et al., A hot-melt extruded intravaginal ring for the sustained delivery of the antiretroviral microbicide UC781. Journal of Pharmaceutical Sciences, 2012. 101(2): p. 576-587.

[220] Gupta, K.M., et al., Polyurethane intravaginal ring for controlled delivery of dapivirine, a nonnucleoside reverse transcriptase inhibitor of HIV-1 (vol 97, pg 4228, 2008). Journal of Pharmaceutical Sciences, 2009. 98(3): p. 1199-1199.

[221] Johnson, T.J., et al., Segmented polyurethane intravaginal rings for the sustained combined delivery of antiretroviral agents dapivirine and tenofovir. European Journal of Pharmaceutical Sciences, 2010. 39(4): p. 203-212.

[222] Malcolm, R.K., et al., Long-term, controlled release of the HIV microbicide TMC120 from silicone elastomer vaginal rings. Journal of Antimicrobial Chemotherapy, 2005. 56(5): p. 954-956.

[223] Woolfson, A.D., et al., Intravaginal ring delivery of the reverse transcriptase inhibitor TMC 120 as an HIV microbicide. International Journal of Pharmaceutics, 2006. 325(1-2): p. 82-89.

[224] Promadej-Lanier, N., et al., Development and evaluation of a vaginal ring device for sustained delivery of HIV microbicides to non-human primates. J Med Primatol, 2009. 38(4): p. 263-271.

[225] Gunawardana, M., et al., Microbial biofilms on the surface of intravaginal rings worn in non-human primates. Journal of Medical Microbiology, 2011. 60(6): p. 828-837.

[226] Srinivasan, P., Rabe, L., Ellenberger, D., Mitchell, J., Hendry, M., McNicholl, J., Malcolm, K., Kiser, P., Otten, R., Smith, J. Multi-Study Assessment of Vaginal Cytokines and Microflora in the Safety Evaluation of Intravaginal Rings in Pig-Tailed Macaques. in Microbicides 2010. 2010. Pittsburgh, PA, USA.

[227] Grant, R.M., et al., Preexposure chemoprophylaxis for HIV prevention in men who have sex with men. N Engl J Med, 2010. 363(27): p. 2587-99.

[228] Himathongkham, S., et al., Simian-human immunodeficiency virus containing a human immunodeficiency virus type 1 subtype-E envelope gene: persistent infection, CD4(+) T-cell depletion, and mucosal membrane transmission in macaques. J Virol, 2000. 74(17): p. 7851-60.

[229] Li, J., et al., Infection of cynomolgus monkeys with a chimeric HIV-1/SIVmac virus that expresses the HIV-1 envelope glycoproteins. J Acquir Immune Defic Syndr, 1992. 5(7): p. 639-46.

[230] Morton, W.R., et al., Transmission of the simian immunodeficiency virus SIVmne in macaques and baboons. J Med Primatol, 1989. 18(3-4): p. 237-45.

[231] Overbaugh, J., et al., Variation in simian immunodeficiency virus env is confined to V1 and V4 during progression to simian AIDS. J Virol, 1991. 65(12): p. 7025-31.

[232] Shibata, R., et al., Infection and pathogenicity of chimeric simian-human immunodeficiency viruses in macaques: determinants of high virus loads and CD4 cell killing. J Infect Dis, 1997. 176(2): p. 362-73.

[233] Thigpen, M.C., Kebaabetswe, P.M., Smith, D.K., Segolodi,T.M. , Soud, F.A., Chillag, K., Chirwa, L.I., Kasonde, M., Mutanhaurwa, R., Henderson, F.L., Pathak, S., Gvetadze, R., Rose,C.E., Paxton, L.A., for the TDF2 Study Group. Daily oral antiretroviral use for the prevention of HIV infection in heterosexually active young adults in Botswana: results from the TDF2 study. in 6th IAS Conference on HIV Pathogenesis, Treatment and Prevention 2011. Rome, Italy.

[234] Microbicide Trials Network Statement on Decision to Discontinue Use of Tenofovir Gel in VOICE, a Major HIV Prevention Study in Women 2011.

[235] MTN Statement on Decision to Discontinue Use of Oral Tenofovir Tablets in VOICE, a Major HIV Prevention Study in Women, 2011.

[236] Hirsch, V.M., et al., Simian immunodeficiency virus infection of macaques: end-stage disease is characterized by widespread distribution of proviral DNA in tissues. J Infect Dis, 1991. 163(5): p. 976-88.

[237] Dewhurst, S., et al., Sequence analysis and acute pathogenicity of molecularly cloned SIVSMM-PBj14. Nature, 1990. 345(6276): p. 636-40.

[238] Dewhurst, S., et al., Molecular clones from a non-acutely pathogenic derivative of SIVsmmPBj14: characterization and comparison to acutely pathogenic clones. AIDS Res Hum Retroviruses, 1992. 8(6): p. 1179-87.

[239] Benveniste, R.E., et al., Isolation of a lentivirus from a macaque with lymphoma: comparison with HTLV-III/LAV and other lentiviruses. J Virol, 1986. 60(2): p. 483-90.

[240] Benveniste, R.E., et al., Characterization of clones of HIV-1 infected HuT 78 cells defective in gag gene processing and of SIV clones producing large amounts of envelope glycoprotein. J Med Primatol, 1990. 19(3-4): p. 351-66.

[241] Benveniste, R.E., et al., Inoculation of baboons and macaques with simian immunodeficiency virus/Mne, a primate lentivirus closely related to human immunodeficiency virus type 2. J Virol, 1988. 62(6): p. 2091-101.

[242] Kimata, J.T., A. Mozaffarian, and J. Overbaugh, A lymph node-derived cytopathic simian immunodeficiency virus Mne variant replicates in nonstimulated peripheral blood mononuclear cells. J Virol, 1998. 72(1): p. 245-56.

[243] Kimata, J.T. and J. Overbaugh, The cytopathicity of a simian immunodeficiency virus Mne variant is determined by mutations in Gag and Env. J Virol, 1997. 71(10): p. 7629-39.

Chapter 17

Feline Immunodeficiency Virus (FIV) Infection in Cats: A Possible Cause of Renal Pathological Changes

Natasa Tozon, Mauro Pistello and Alessandro Poli

Additional information is available at the end of the chapter

1. Introduction

The feline immunodeficiency virus (FIV) is a lentivirus isolated from domestic cats with an acquired immunodeficiency syndrome-like condition, named feline AIDS (F-AIDS). The major immunological abnormalities observed in FIV-infected cats included a profound decline in the absolute number of the CD4+ T cells that caused the inversion of the CD4+/CD8+ T cell ratio and increased susceptibility to opportunistic infections and various clinic-pathological conditions [1]. FIV viruses encompass a large group of strains classified in subgroups from A to E, which are unevenly distributed geographically and have an inter-subtype diversity > 26% [2]. The isolates used in our study were Petaluma, of group A, and Pisa-M2, a local isolate belonging to group B, which encloses all isolates hitherto sequenced and circulating in Italy [3 4]. Serological screenings performed in the past demonstrated that the virus is distributed worldwide and incidence varies from 1 – 14% in healthy cats and up to 44% in sick cats. As other lentiviruses, FIV is a complex retrovirus with structural genes *gag, pol* and *env*, and a few accessory genes [5]; *gag* encodes the capsid protein p24, used in most diagnostic tests, and other inner structural proteins, *pol* encodes the enzymes necessary for viral replication and therefore targeted by most anti-lentiviral drugs, and *env* encode the outer glycoprotein (gp95) and trans-membrane protein (gp36) serving as viral receptor and, being constantly under immunological pressure, the less conserved proteins among the different subtypes. Like the human immunodeficiency virus (HIV), the gp95 is comprised of variable and conserved regions and binds the CD134 molecule, the FIV primary receptor [6]. Studies on HIV have shown that some conserved epitopes are accessible for neutralizing antibodies, while the co-receptor binding site is composed by interspersed domains. The binding site remains largely hidden and is therefore inaccessible for mentioned antibody. Whereas overall HIV and FIV Env structure is maintained [7], HIV uses various co-receptors, including a range transmembrane domain G-protein-coupled receptors. In contrast,, all FIV strains tested so far use CXCR4 as a co-receptor [7]. Cats, once infected with FIV, remain infected life-long and in the face of strong humoral and cell-mediated immune responses that appear shortly after the initial viremic phase [2].

The acute phase of infection lasts a few days to a few weeks and is asymptomatic in a large proportion of cats. If clinically overt, it manifests with fever, lethargy and peripheral lymphadenomegaly with possible neutropenia. The acute phase eventually subsides and the infected cat enters in asymptomatic period that typically lasts 4 to 6 years or is life-long in some cats. In 30% cats and with percentages that greatly depend on cofactors and cat life-style [2], the infection proceeds to the last stage, the F-AIDS, that is characterized by profound immunodeficiency and, consequently, the presence of secondary infections sustained by viruses, bacteria, fungi, or protozoa, and various neoplastic diseases. Like HIV, FIV also infects and may damage the central nervous system as demonstrated in the past in experimental conditions [8-11]. As mentioned, clinical presentation and outcome of disease depend upon a combination of secondary factors and host immune responses. Immunodeficiency combined with immunostimulation by various factors most frequently results in the emergence of severe forms of gingivostomatitis, chronic rhinitis, lymphadenopathy, weight loss and immune-mediated glomerulonephritis [2]. Weaver and co-workers reported reproductive failure in FIV-infected cats. Viral DNA in placental and fetal tissues in affected cats was confirmed by PCR [12].

Despite detailed knowledge of most clinicopathological features during FIV infection, information on renal involvement is limited. Unspecified renal abnormalities were reported in some infected cats living in Australia [13] and in 5.5% of those living in New Zealand [14]. Ishida et al found that 9.3% of 700 Japanese FIV-infected cats presented clinical signs of renal diseases [15]. Most pathological findings observed in the kidney of naturally FIV-infected cats resemble those described in HIV-infected patients [16], but it is not clear whether FIV has a direct role in the induction of the renal damage or accelerates a phenomenon triggered by other factors. The fact that renal damage is mostly found in natural FIV infection supports the latter hypothesis [17]. However, since there are no detailed descriptions of the renal lesions found in experimentally FIV-infected cats this issue is still open. The aim of our study was to investigate the histological renal alterations caused by FIV in animals experimentally inoculated with FIV strains of different pathogenicity and at different times post-infection. Here, specific pathogen free (SPF) cats singly or doubly infected with Petaluma and Pisa-M2 were housed in germ-free conditions to exclude the influence of other pathogens. The pathological findings in these animals were compared with those found in naturally infected cats. These results were also compared to those found in HIV patients.

2. Material and methods

2.1. Cats

Ninety-nine naturally infected cats were collected from 1990 to 1993 and after diagnosis of FIV infection performed by western blot. Animals were referred to the Department of

Animal Pathology of the University of Pisa by veterinarian practitioners and owners from different part of Tuscany, Italy. All the subjects were submitted to an accurate clinical examination and classified according to a previously proposed classification [18]. Thirty-six of these subjects were sacrificed and immediately necropsied. There was no investigator bias in this sampling as the only criterion used was the owner's consent to post-mortem examination. Fifteen cats who tested positive for leukemia virus p27 antigen (CiteCombo FIV_FeLV, Agritech Systems, Portland, Me, USA) and feline infectious peritonitis antibodies (Diasystems Celisa FIP, Tech America, Omaha, NE, USA) were excluded from the study, as these viruses are known to be associated with renal alterations. The 21 selected cats were 16 males and 5 females, with a mean age of 96.0 months ± 40.3 months, 10 cats were in the symptomatic phase of infection phase, while 11 had full-blown F-AIDS.

Fifty-six specific pathogen free SPF cats, infected with Petaluma and/or Pisa-M2 isolates at six-ten months of age, were included in the study. All subjects were females that at time of analyses aged between 2 and 6 years (mean age of 47.8 months ± 14.4 months). Seven-teen animals were inoculated with Petaluma (group 1), 28 with Pisa-M2 isolate (group 2), and 11 were first inoculated with Petaluma and, one year later, superinfected with Pisa-M2 (group 3). Petaluma isolate was obtained from supernatant of persistently infected FL4 cells [19], while Pisa-M2 was a local isolate propagated in vivo by monthly passages in SPF cats and never passaged in vitro [20]. Animals were inoculated intravenously with either 2 ml of freshly collected blood (Pisa-M2) or 20 cat infectious dose 50% of FL-4 supernatant (Petaluma). All cats seroconverted in 4-6 weeks and were characterized for a steady reduction in the number of circulating CD4+ lymphocyte that approximately halved in 1 year. Four FIV-negative,SPF cats were used as negative controls (group C). Infected and control cats were housed in biosafety hazard level 3 conditions at the Retrovirus Center of the University of Pisa, and were daily monitored for clinical conditions throughout the observation period. Physical examination was performed weekly for the first two months postinfection (pi) and then monthly. At 12, 24, 30, 36 and 48 months pi, randomly selected animals were deeply anesthesized, and euthanized for necropsy.

2.2. Biochemistry and urine analysis

Urine specimens were obtained by cystocentesis. After centrifugation, supernatants were used to determine protein and creatinine concentration using two commercial assays (BioRad, Richmond, Calif., USA, and Creatinine - Jaffe method, Verbena, Milano, Italy, respectively). In cats with marked proteinuria (>2 g/L), urine protein/urine creatinin ratio (UPC) was calculated using the following formula: P(g/L) x 100 / (Cr mmol/L / 0.0885). Protein qualitative analysis was performed with sodium dodecyl sulfate-polyacrylamide gel (SDS-PAGE) according to Leamlli [21].

Blood samples for determination of biochemical profile were collected into serum separator tubes (Vacuette, Greiner Bio-One, Kremsmunster, Austria) and stood for 30 min at 4°C to clot, then centrifuged (1300 g for 10 min) to separate the serum. Serum samples were assayed for selected biochemical parameters including urea, creatinine, total protein, albumin, using an automated analysis on a spectrophotometer (LKB Biochrom Ltd., Cambridge, UK). Serum albumin/globulin ratio was calculated.

2.3. FIV serology

All cats were screened for FIV antibodies and feline leukaemia virus antigen by a commercial ELISA (CITE COMBO FIV-FeLV;Agritech Systems, Portland, Maine) according to manufacturer's instructions.

FIV antibodies, detected with above rapid test, were confirmed by Western blot (WB). FIV antigen for WB analysis was produced from persistently FIV-infected FL4 T-cells. The virus was pelleted from tissue cultures medium, purified throughout a 10 to 50% continuous sucrose gradient and then disrupted by sonication followed by treatment with Triton X-100. Viral proteins were separated by electrophoresis with 12% SDS-PAGE and blotted onto nitrocellulose by standard methods. The nitrocellulose sheets were then blocked with 1% bovine serum albumin, cut into 0.5 cm wide strips, dried, and stored in the cold until use. Individual strips were incubated for two hours with serum samples diluted 1:100 in PBS-Tween 20 (0.05%), washed thoroughly, incubated with horseradish peroxidase-conjugated rabbit anti-cat immunoglobulin G (Bethyl Laboratories, Montgomery, Texas) for one hour. The strips were washed and incubated with 0.05% diaminobenzidine and 0.01% of H O (what is this?) in 0.1M Tris pH 7.4 to visualize antigen-antibody binding. Strips were read by densitometric scanning (BioRad) immediately after the reaction was stopped with distilled water. The molecular weights of the reactive proteins were established by comparison with prestained low-molecular-weight markers (BioRad). Each WB contained positive and negative control sera. The sample was scored positively when at least two of p25, p31, gp40, gp65, and gp95 FIV-specific bands were clearly detectable.

2.4. PCR

Buffy coat of 2 ml whole blood samples was used to detect FIV DNA. FIV DNA extraction and amplification was performed as described [22]. All precautions were taken to avoid possible contamination and samples were examined at least twice in separate experiments. DNA from peripheral blood mononuclear cells (PBMC) of uninfected cats and from Petaluma-infected FL-4 cells were used as negative and positive controls, respectively.

2.5. Flow citometry

T lymphocyte subsets were examined by flow cytometric analysis as described [23]. Flow cytometry analysis was performed by using fluorescein conjugated murine monoclonal antibodies to feline CD4 and CD8 T-cells surface markers (Southern, Biotech, Birmingham, AL,USA) and an Epics Elite cell analyzer (Coulter Electronics, Hialeah, Fla.).

2.6. Histology

Renal tissue samples were fixed in 10% buffered formalin solution and embedded in paraffin. 3μm thick sections from each specimen were stained with hematoxylin and eosin, periodic-acidic Schiff and Jones periodic acid-silver methenamine. Sections with inflammatory lesions were stained with Ziehl-Neelsen acid-fast and Gram to exclude bacterial infections. Amyloid was demonstrated by the alkaline Congo red staining with polarization on 8 μm sections [24]. Differentiation between primary and secondary amyloidosis was based on staining by a modified Romhanyi method with pre treatment with potassium permanganate [25] and on immunohistochemistry (IHC) with antibodies against amyloid A protein.

2.7. Immunohistochemistry

The localization of IgG, IgA, IgM and C3 deposits was investigated by both indirect immunofluorescence method (IF) and streptavidin-biotin peroxidase method. IF was performed using as primary antibodies primary sheep monospecific antibodies to cat IgG, IgM, IgA and C3 (binding Site, Birmingham, UK) and a rabbit fluorescein anti-sheep IgG (vector Laboratorie, Burlingame, CA, USA), as previously described [16]. Control sections were incubated with normal sheep serum (Dako, Golstrup, Denmark) before treatment with the secondary antiserum. For IHC, sections were de-waxed in xylene, passed through a graded series of alcohols, and rehydrated in deionised water. For Ig and C3 localization, the tissues were digested with 0.5% protease (Protease XXIV; Sigma, Saint Louis, Mo, USA) in 0.05 M Tris-Hcl, pH 7.6. Endogenous peroxidases were exhausted with 0.5% hydrogen peroxide for 30 minutes and after that, three washes were performed in 0.05% Tween Tris Buffered Saline solution (TBST) at pH 7.6. Normal serum from the host species of the secondary antibody diluted 1/10 in TBST was added to the sections and incubated for 30 minutes at room temperature. After three washes, the primary antibodies diluted in TBST were applied and incubated for 1 hour at RT. The antisera used included unlabeled sheep anti cat IgG, IgA, IgM and C3, an anti-AA (murine monoclonal mc4 against human AA protein, culture supernatant and anti-cat AA and AL (polyclonal antibody of rabbit origin; kind gift of R. P. Link, University of Munich, Germany). After three washes, secondary biotinylated antibody (Vectastain®, Vector Labs Inc., Burlingame, CA, USA) was added and incubated for 30 minutes at RT. Peroxidase reaction was developed for 10 minutes using diaminobenzidine (DAB) (Impact DAB® ,Vector Labs inc., Burlingame, CA, USA) and blocked with deionised water. Negative controls were performed omitting the primary antibody and replacing the antibody with normal sheep or rabbit serum or murine subclass matched (IgG_1) unrelated primary monoclonal antibody.

2.8. Statistics

Statistical analysis was performed using the statistical package SPSS Advanced Statistics 13.0 (SPSS Inc., Chicago, IL, USA). Chi-square test was used to investigate the significance of the relationship between protein expression and individual variables. Statistical significance was based on a 5% (0.05) significance level.

3. Results

3.1. Immunological data

All FIV-seropositive cats, as determined by rapid test and then WB analysis, also scored positive for FIV DNA in whole blood samples (data not shown). The experimentally infected cats included in the study were routinely examined for CD4+ and CD8+ T lymphocyte subsets by flow cytometry and respective CD4+/CD8+ T cell ratio calculated. Inversion of the CD4+/CD8+ T cell ratio due to a selective decline in the absolute number of the CD4+ T cells was confirmed in 71.4% cats infected with FIV-Pisa M2, 76.5% of FIV-Petaluma infected cats and in all cats infected with both virus strains (Table 1). Although diminution of CD4+ T-cells and inversion CD4+/CD8+ correlated positively with duration of infection, no significant relationships were found between immunological data and renal alteration.

3.2. Clinical data

Total serum protein, albumin and globulins concentration values in experimentally infected cats were in the reference range, regardless infecting virus isolate and time post inoculation. None of the 56 SPF cats included in our study presented clinical signs of azotemia.

Serum creatinine concentration was measured in 37 experimentally infected cats and only one cat, infected with FIV isolate Pisa M2 had slightly increased concentration of serum creatinine (144 μmol/L), mild proteinuria (3.9 g/L), and UPC ratio of 0.43, which is classified as stage 2 of chronic renal failure (CRF) [26].

Urine protein concentration was measured in all 56 experimentally and 21 naturally infected cats. Eighteen naturally infected cats (82%) had mild to sever proteinuria, mean value 26.46±22.41 (range 3.5 – 62 g/L). In experimentally infected cats, proteinuria (> 2mg/L) ranged from 18% in cats infected with both virus strains with mean value 14.3±22.73 (2.7-60 g/L), 32% in cats infected with strain Pisa M2 (mean value 11.78±22.80, ranging 2.2 – 100) and 58% in cats infected with Petaluma strain, in which the mean value of urine proteins concentration was the lowest 4.25±2.81 (2 - 8.25 g/L) (meaning not clear to me). UPC in proteinuric cats was calculated in order to confirm the renal proteinuria. UPC values were the highest in cats infected with Pisa M2 (mean 3.27±6.34; ranged 0.53-17.63), slightly lower in cats infected with both virus strains (mean 3.0±4.39; ranged 0.55-13.01) and the lowest in cats infected with Petaluma strain (mean 2.56±3.03; ranged 0.31 – 7.02).

In addition, electrophoresis of urine proteins was performed in an attempt to establish the localization and severity of renal alteration. 10/21 naturally infected cats had glomerulo non-selective proteinuria, 8/21 glomerulo non-selective and tubular, and only 3 of 21 cats had glomerulo selective proteinuria. Glomerulo selective proteinuria was confirmed only in 3 proteinuric cats, infected with Petaluma strain. In the others experimentally infected cats proteinuria glomerulo non-selective was most frequently found: 7/10, 7/9 and 1/2 cats infected with Petaluma, Pisa-M2 and both strains respectively. Remaining 2/9 (infected with

Pisa-M2) and 1/2 cats (infected with both strains) had glomerulo non-selective and tubular proteinuria (Table 1).

No clinical and selected laboratory parameters in SPF cats enclosed in the control group were found.

IRIS staging		Naturally FIV-infected cats	Experimentally FIV-infected cats		
			Petaluma	Pisa M2	Petaluma + Pisa M2
$CD4^+/CD8^+$	< 2.0	ND	13/17	20/28	11/11
serum creatinine (stage 1 - 4)	1 (< 140)	9/13	5/5	20/21	11/11
	2 (140-249)	3/13	0/5	1/21	0/11
	3 (250-439)	0/13	0/5	0/21	0/11
	4 (> 440)	1/13	0/5	0/21	0/11
urine protein concentration	< 2 g/L	3/21	5/17	10/28	5/11
	> 2 g/L	**18/21**	**12/17**	**18/28**	**6/11**
UPC (substaging)	< 0.2 (non proteinuric)	ND	0/12	0/18	0/6
	0.2-0.4 (borderline proteinuric)	ND	2/12	9/18	4/6
	> 0.4 (proteinuric)	ND	**10/12**	**9/18**	**2/6**
SDS-PAGE	GS	0/21	3/10	0/9	0/2
	GNS	10/21	7/10	7/9	1/2
	GNS+T	8/21	0/10	2/9	1/2

Legend: ND - not done; GS - glomerulo selective; GNS - glomerulo non-selective; GNS+T - glomerulo non-selective and tubular.

Table 1. Inversion of the CD4+/CD8+ T cell ratio, serum creatinine value, proteinuria, and urine protein/creatinine (UPC) ratio according to the IRIS classification.

3.3. Light microscopy

Table 2 summarizes the main histological glomerular alterations observed in naturally and experimentally FIV-infected cats. Glomerular changes were detected in 18 of 21 naturally infected subjects. Mild mesangial matrix increase with occasional segmental glomerulosclerosis was observed in 9 subjects (Figure 1A), while immune mediated glomerulonephritis of mesangioproliferative type was detected in 3 animals. In eight naturally FIV-infected cats, amyloid deposition was also detected (Figure 1E). These were segmental and focal in six cases and diffuse in two. In all cases the amyloid deposits were KMnO4 sensitive. In experimentally FIV-infected animals, glomerular changes were detected in 9 of 17 Petaluma-infected cats, in 12 of 28 Pisa-M2-infected cats and in six of the 11 cats infected with both strain. In Petaluma-infected cats mesangial widening was observed in six subjects, while 3 showed a mesangioproliferative glomerulonephritis. In Pisa-M2-infected cats mesangial widening was detected in six subjects, five showed a mesangioproliferative glomerulonephritis (Figure 1B), and one cats a membranoproliferative glomerulonephritis (Figure 1D). The exam of the kidneys from the eleven cats infected with both Petaluma and Pisa-M2 strains demonstrated the presence of mesangial widening in three subjects and mesangioproliferative glomerulonephritis in other three cats. Ten of the 16 SPF cats, sacrificed at 12 months post-infection showed no renal alteration (three and seven subjects infected with Petaluma and Pisa-M2, respectively), while 4 presented mesangial widening (two cats each infected with Petaluma and Pisa-M2) and two glomerulonephritis (one each infected with Petaluma and Pisa-M2). Of the 13 subjects sacrificed at 24 months post-infection, eight showed no alterations (4 each infected with Petaluma and Pisa-M2), while mesangial widening was observed in two cats (one each infected with Petaluma and Pisa-M2) and glomeruloneprhitis was detected in remaining three cats (two infected with Petaluma and one with Pisa-M2). Finally, 9 of the 27 cats sacrificed after 30 months post-infection, nine had mesangial widening (three each infected with Petaluma, Pisa-M2, and both Petaluma and Pisa-M2), while glomerulonephritis was detected in seven cats (four infected with Pisa-M2 and 3 with both Petaluma and Pisa-M2). Eleven of these cats, i.e. those sacrificed after 30 months post-infection, had no renal changes. In affected glomeruli of naturally and experimentally infected cats, dilatation of the Bowman's space was a frequent finding and, occasionally, protein droplets were present in prominent epithelial cells, particularly in subjects with an heavy proteinuria. The presence of mesangial widening and glomerulonephritis was detected both in experimentally (15/56 and 12/56, respectively) and naturally infected cats (8/21 and 3/21, respectively). Of note, naturally infected cats presented glomerular amyloid deposits that were never detected in the experimentally infected ones ($P<0.001$).

Histopathological alterations	Control cats	Naturally FIV-infected cats	Experimentally FIV-infected cats		
			Petaluma	Pisa M2	Petaluma + Pisa M2
Glomerular					
Bowman's space dilatation	0/4	8/21	3/17	6/28	3/11
Mesangial widening	0/4	8/21	6/17	6/28	3/11
Mesangioproliferative glomerulonephritis	0/4	3/21	3/17	5/28	3/11
Membranoproliferative glomerulonephritis	0/4	0/21	0/17	1/28	0/11
Segmental glomerulosclerosis	0/4	1/21	0/17	0/28	0/11
Glomerular amyloidosis	0/4	8/21	0/17	0/28	0/11
No alterations	4/4	3/21	8/17	16/28	5/11

Table 2. Main histological glomerular findings in naturally and experimentally FIV-infected cats and uninfected controls.

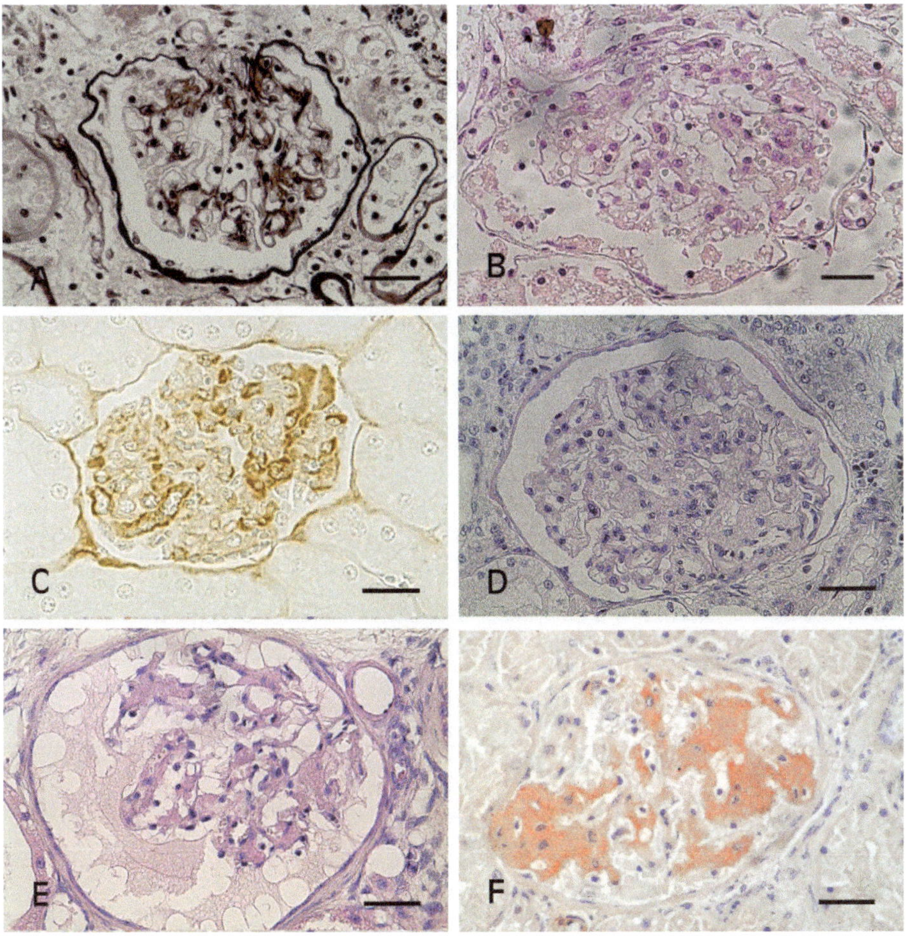

Figure 1. A. Naturally FIV-infected cat. Mesangial widening. Mild increase in mesangial matrix with a minimal increase in intraglomerular dellularity. Jones' periodic acid-silver methenamine stain. (Bar = 80 μm) B. Experimentally Pisa-M2-infected cat. Mesangioproliferative glomerulonephritis. Focal mild proliferation of mesangial cells. Hematoxylin-Eosin stain. (Bar = 80 μm) C. Experimentally Pisa-M2-infected cat. Mesangioproliferative glomerulonephritis. Segmental deposition of IgG. Strepavidin biotin peroxidise complex method, Mayer's hematoxylin counterstain. (Bar = 80 μm) D. Experimentally Pisa-M2-infected cat. Membranoproliferative glomerulonephritis. Mesangial enlargement and thickening of capillary walls. Hematoxylin-Eosin stain. (Bar = 80 μm) E. Naturally FIV-infected cat. Mild amyloid deposition (pale structurless material), occupaing the slightly expanded mesangial areas. H-E stain. (Bar = 80 μm) F. Naturally FIV-infected cat. The amyloid is immunoreactive with the antiserum to feline AA amyloid. Strepavidin biotin peroxidise complex method, Mayer's hematoxylin counterstain. (Bar = 80 μm).

Tubulointerstitial alterations were frequently detected in naturally and experimentally infected cats. In the former, degeneration of tubular epithelial cells was observed in ten cats, tubular microcysts in eight, and giant protein tubular casts in four subjects (Table 3). Only six Petaluma-infected cats showed degenerative changes of tubular epithelial cells, while no alteration were detected in the other eleven animals. In Pisa-M2-infected cats, degenerative changes were observed in eleven subjects, tubular microcysts in two and giant protein casts in only one subject, while 17 cats presented no tubular alterations. In cats infected with both strains, degenerative changes of tubular epithelial cells was detected in three cats, tubular microcysts in two and giant protein tubular casts in one subjects. Eight cats showed no alterations. Interstitial alterations were commonly observed in naturally infected cats (Table 4) and consisted of interstitial infiltration by lymphocytes and plasmacells. This was scanty periglomerular (eight subjects), diffuse without fibrosis (six subjects) and diffuse with interstitial fibrosis (three subjects). Interstitial amyloidosis was detected in seven subjects, while no interstitial alterations were detected in four naturally infected cats. Also in these cases the amyloid deposits were $KMnO_4$ sensitive. Experimentally infected cats had seldom interstitial alterations. Scanty periglomerular infiltrates were detected in 1/12 Petaluma-infected subjects sacrificed at 24 months post-infection, 3/17 cats infected with Pisa-M2 (one sacrificed at 24 months and two sacrificed ≥ 30 months post-infection) and 2/6 cats infected with both viruses and sacrificed ≥ 30 months post-infection.

Histopathological alterations	Control cats	Naturally FIV-infected cats	Experimentally FIV -infected cats		
			Petaluma	Pisa M2	Petaluma + Pisa M2
Tubular					
Degeneration of tubular epithelial cells	0/4	10/21	6/17	11/28	3/11
Tubular microcysts	0/4	8/21	0/17	2/28	2/11
Giant protein tubular casts	0/4	4/21	0/17	1/28	1/11
No alterations	4/4	3/21	11/17	17/28	8/11
Interstitial					
Scanty periglomeral infiltrates	0/4	8/21	1/17	3/28	2/11
Diffuse interstitial infiltrates without fibrosis	0/4	6/21	0/17	0/28	0/11
Diffuse interstitial infiltrates with fibrosis	0/4	3/21	0/17	0/28	0/11
Interstitial amyloidosis	0/4	7/21	0/17	0/28	0/11
No alterations	4/4	4/21	16/17	25/28	9/11

Table 3. Main histological tubular and interstitial findings in naturally and experimentally FIV-infected cats and uninfected controls.

Tubular alterations were more frequently detected in naturally infected cats (18/21) than in experimentally ones (22/56). Particularly, the presence of giant protein tubular cats (4/21 *vs* 2/56; P<0.=5) and tubular microcysts (8/21 vs 4/56; P<0.05) was more frequently detected in naturally than experimentally infected subjects. Interstitial alterations were also markedly more frequently in naturally infected cats (17/21) compared to experimentally infected cats (6/56; P<0.001), particularly the presence of diffuse interstitial infiltrates and interstitial amyloidosis was never detected in the latter group.

In Table 4, the renal alterations according virus strain inoculated and time post-inoculation are presented. 14/29 cats without any histological renal alteration observed had the lowest mean value of urine protein concentration (uP) 3.95±1.37 g/L (2.5 – 7.05) and expected the lowest UPC mean value of 0.45±0.12 (0.25-0.67). The mean values of uP and UPC in 10 proteinuric cats with mesangial widening was slightly higher: 3.54±1.52 g/L (2.0 – 5.4) and 0.81±0.44 (0.53 – 1.94), respectively. Five cats with similar mesangial alteration had uP concentration lowest then 2.0 g/L. Significantly higher mean values were established in 12 cats with glomerular alteration. Mean value of uP in this group was 21.53±29.39 g/L (2.8 – 100.0) and UPC ration was 4.8±5.77 (0.90 – 17.63). All 20 cats with tubular alteration had gloerulonephritis (9/20) or mensangial widening (11/20) too. Three of them were un-proteinuric. Only four of six cats with interstitial infiltrates were proteinuric, two 24 months pi and 4 after more then 30 months pi.

Lasting	Virus inoculated	Renal changes				
		No alterations	Mesangial widening	Glomerulonephritis	Tubular alterations	Interstitial infiltrates
12 months pi	Petaluma (n=6)	3	2	1	2	0
	Pisa M2 (n=10)	7	2	1	2	0
24 months pi	Petaluma (n=7)	4	1	2	1	1
	Pisa M2 (n=6)	4	1	1	2	1
> 30 months pi	Petaluma (n=4)	1	3	0	3	0
	Pisa M2 (n=12)	5	3	4	7	2
	Petaluma + Pisa M2 (n=11)	5	3	3	3	2

Table 4. Renal alterations detected in FIV experimentally infected cats sacrificed with different lasting.

3.4. Immunohistochemistry

The results of immunohistochemical investigations are summarized in table 5. By IF and IHC positive specimens showed segmental, predominantly granular mesangial deposits of IgG, IgM and C3, while rarely scattered granular deposits were detected along the capillary loops (Figure 1C). IgA staining was never observed. Cellular infiltrates were characterized by the presence of IgG secreting plasma cells and scattered IgM. Large proteinaceous casts were positive for IgG and weakly for IgA. Amyloid deposits were always positive for the mouse monoclonal anti-human AA and the rabbit polyclonal against the feline AA amyloid (Figure 1F), while were always negative for the rabbit polyclonal anti-AL amyloid.

Immunohistochemistry	Control cats	Naturally FIV-infected cats	Experimentally FIV-infected cats		
			Petaluma	Pisa M2	Petaluma + Pisa M2
IgG deposits in mesangium	0/4	3/21	3/17	5/28	3/11
IgG deposits in capilalry loops	0/4	1/21	1/17	2/28	2/11
IgM deposits	0/4	14/21	6/17	6/28	3/11
IgA deposits	0/4	0/21	0/17	0/28	0/11
C3 deposits	0/4	14/21	6/17	6/28	3/11

Table 5. Main immunohistochemical findings in naturally and experimentally FIV-infected cats and uninfected controls.

4. Discussion

The results of our investigation clearly demonstrate that FIV infection induce tissue alterations in kidneys. The study on naturally infected subjects confirmed the presence of renal alterations in a high percentage of the examined animals (18/21). Eleven cases presented glomerular changes (three glomerulonephritis and 8 glomerular amyloidosis) and tubulointerstitial lesions, and were therefore considered severe alterations. The other seven subjects presented milder glomerular changes that consisted in mesangial-matrix expansion with or without segmental glomerulosclerosis.

Previous studies with naturally FIV-infected cats suggested significantly higher rates of renal dysfunction and histological changes compared to FIV seronegative ones. Examinations of 326 sick cats from Australia demonstrated a significant association between FIV infection and azotemia and palpably small kidneys [27]. Concerning small kidneys, as noted by abdominal palpation, they were also reported by Brown and colleagues [28]. Nonspecific renal abnormalities were also reported by several studies [13,29]. The percentage of FIV infected cats with similar renal alteration ranged from 5.5% in New Zealand [14] to 9.3% (from a survey of 700 cats) in Japan [15]. In 76 cats from three regions in Italy (Piemonte, Liguria and Val d'Aosta) 9% were affected by renal disease [30]. Previous histopathological and ultrastructural investigations described kidney abnormalities in 12 of 15 cats [16] and 10 of 14 cats [17] with naturally acquired FIV infection. Six of the twelve subjects of the first study presented lesions that caused a marked increase in serum BUN and creatinine concentration and heavy glomerular non-selective proteinuria; the other nine cats with renal abnormalities, the urine protein content was higher than normal range (>0,2g/l) [16]. Results obtained in the present study showed similar findings. 18 of 21 (82%) of naturally infected cats had mild to sever proteinuria (mean value of 26.46±22.41 (ranging from 3.5 – 62 g/L). 10/21 cats had glomerulo non-selective proteinuria, 8/21 of them combined with tubular proteinuria.

The investigations carried out on experimentally FIV-infected SPF cats demonstrated renal alterations partially similar to those detected in naturally FIV-infected ones. Particularly, mesangial widening with or without segmental glomerulosclerosis and immune mediated glomerulonephritis were observed in these subjects, no matter that they were infected with different FIV isolates, maintained in isolation units, and sacrificed at different times post-infection.

Mesangial widening with segmental to diffuse glomerulosclerosis [16], nephrosclerosis [29] and thickened Bowman's membrane [28] have been previously described in naturally FIV-infected cats. These alterations represent glomerular reactions common to many apparently unrelated, clinical entities that are currently believed to result from intraglomerular hemodynamic alterations [31]. In FIV-infected cats hemodynamic alterations might be mediated by sustained production of lymphokines and/or factors of mesangial proliferation with activity on glomerular capillary permeability as a consequence of the chronic systemic viral infection. Although controversial, increasing evidence supports a direct effect of the virus on renal cells either as a result of exposure to viral proteins or direct renal parenchyma infection. The use of a HIV-1 transgenic mouse model demonstrated a direct etiologic link between HIV- 1 expression in kidney and the development of segmental glomerulosclerosis in HIV associated nephropathy (HIVAN) with unique viral-host interactions, which depends on inherent features of the virus and, at the same time, host response [32]. In FIV infection the direct role of the virus in the pathogenesis of renal alterations is postulated by the presence of p24 viral antigen in tubular epithelial cells as well as scattered interstitial inflammatory and glomerular cells and by detection of FIV *gag* DNA and RNA sequences in these subjects [17,33].

Even if FIV-infected cats often present hypergammaglobulinemia, which is believed to be triggered by chronic polyclonal B cell activation [34], which, in turn, can lead to the production of immune complexes [34,35] and auto-antibodies [36], immune complex glomerulonephritis are infrequent. In a previous study on 15 naturally FIV-infected cats only one subjects showed IgG deposits in mesangial areas [16). In this study IgG deposits were detected in 3/21 naturally and in 11/56 experimentally FIV-infected cats, associated with segmental and focal mesangioproliferative glomerulonephritis in 13 cases and only with a membranoproliferative glomerulonephritis. Even if, as mentioned, immune mediated glomerulonephritis seem uncommon in FIV-infected cats, previous studies demonstrated that the mean concentration of circulating IgG immune complex (CIC) in FIV-infected cats were significantly higher than in control cats, while IgM levels increased only slightly. The immunoglobulin fractions from 10/15 renal tissue samples were analysed, found to be polyclonal, and only partly specific for FIV antigens. All these results, including hypergammaglobulinemia and high levels of CIC, together suggest that IC might play a role in the pathogenesis of the renal alteration observed in FIV-infected animals [34]. The evidence of focal and granular deposits of IgM and C3 in mesangium and sclerotic loops of the other subjects is likely the result from nonspecific trapping of serum proteins rather than from immune complex deposition [16].

Tubulo-interstitial lesions consisting of interstitial infiltration by lymphocytes and plasma cells, as well as fibrosis and tubular degenerative changes have been detected in a high proportion of naturally FIV-infected cats [16,28,29,37], but rarely in experimentally infected ones (17/21 vs 6/56, respectively).

Our study confirmed that glomerular and interstitial amyloidosis can be observed in the kidney of naturally FIV-infected animals as previously reported [17,37,38], but amyloid deposits were no detected in the renal tissues of the 56 experimentally infected cats examined. Histochemical and immunohistochemical studies demonstrated that amyloid deposits were consistent with secondary amyloidosis, associated with chronic infections. Previous unpublished data, demonstrated that naturally FIV-infected cats had a higher prevalence of renal amyloidosis compared to uninfected subjects, 12/34 naturally FIV-infected cats vs 1/30 age-matched control cats. The data of this study show that FIV infection alone is not sufficient for the development of amyloid deposition, as demonstrated by the absence of amyloidosis the 56 experimentally FIV-infected cats and that other concurrent factors are needed.

In cats naturally and experimentally infected with FIV have been reported the presence of renal lymphoid tumours [39,40]. In our series we have no cases of lymphosarcoma, but the lack of these neoplastic alterations could be related to the reduced number of subjects examined.

Clinicopathological studies revealed the relatively high possibility of mild to sever renal proteinuria without clinical signs of azotemia. None of 56 SPF cats included in our study presented any clinical signs of azotemia except one cat that was infected by Pisa-M2, sacrificed one year post-infection and that showed serum creatinine concentration (144 μmol/L) with mild proteinuria (3.9 g/L and UPC 0.43) (CRF stage 2) [26]. Renal proteinuria, established by UPC was present in 10 of 17 cats infected with Petaluma, 9 of 28 cats, infected with Pisa-M2 and 2 of 11 in cats infected with both virus isolates, regardless the time from infection. However, the most severe renal proteinuria was observed in cats infected with Pisa-M2 (mean 3.27±6.34; ranged 0.53-17.63), slightly milder in cats infected with both virus strains (mean 3.0±4.39; ranged 0.55-13.01) and the less severe in cats infected with Petaluma (mean 2.56±3.03; ranged 0.31 – 7.02). Fourteen of 29 cats without any histological renal alteration observed had the lowest mean value of urine protein concentration (uP) 3.95±1.37 g/L (2.5 – 7.05) and the lowest UPC mean value of 0.45±0.12 (0.25-0.67). The mean values of uP and UPC in 10 proteinuric cats with mesangial widening was slightly higher 3.54±1.52 g/L (2.0 – 5.4) and 0.81±0.44 (0.53 – 1.94), respectively. Five cats with similar mesangial alteration were aproteinuric. (>2.0 g/L). Significantly higher mean values were established in 12 cats with glomerular alteration; mean value of uP in this group was 21.53±29.39 g/L (2.8 – 100.0) and UPC ration was 4.8±5.77 (0.90 – 17.63). All 20 cats with tubular alteration had glomerulonephritis (9/20) or mensangial widening (11/20). Three of them were aproteinuric. Only four of six cats, with interstitial infiltrates were proteinuric, two 24 months post-infection and 4 after over 30 months post inoculation. In addition, electrophoresis of urine proteins confirmed the correlation between proteins excreted in the urine and the histological alterations found in observed cats; three of 21 cats had glomerulo selective proteinura, 15 glomerulo non-selective, three glomerulo non-selective and tubular proteinuria.

The overwhelming majority of experimentally infected cats (71.4 to 100%) had inverted CD4+/CD8+ T cell ratio that depended on infecting viral isolate and, albeit with low or no statistical significance, time of infection. Furthermore, no correlation between CD4+/CD8+ T cell ratio and renal alteration was found. As well as clinical and laboratory findings, as azotemia and proteinuria, renal disease in HIV positive patients seem to be similar in FIV infected, which do not correlate with CD4+ T-cell count or CD4+/CD8+ T cell ratio [28].

There are many reports about various organ system involvements, including renal in HIV-infected people [41]. Patient with HIVAN may develop a spectrum of renal pathology that most likely manifests with an acute rapidly progressive loss of renal function, characterised by proteinuria, nephrotic syndrome and azotemia [27]. Typical histological features consist of focal sclerosing glomerulopathy and microcystic tubular dilatation. Some of the patients have mesengial proliferation [27,41,42]. The pathogenesis of HIVAN is still unclear, although presence of viral proteins in glomerular and tubular epithelium cells suggested an important role of HIV in the initiation or progression of HIVAN [27]. Glomerular manifestations include antigen-antibody complex and nonimmune-complex-mediated pathology [43,44].

5. Conclusion

In conclusion, our study confirmed that renal involvement occurs in a high proportion of naturally FIV-infected cats and that these alterations can, in part, be detected in experimentally infected subjects. In all, these results suggest a causative relationship between FIV infection and renal abnormalities. This damage seems to consist of mesangial increase, sometimes accompanied by mesangial cell proliferation and glomerulosclerosis, a lower percentage of immune mediate glomerulonephritis and, in naturally infected subjects' glomerular and interstitial amyloidosis. Besides, these alteration are partially similar to those detected in HIV-infected patients, FIV-infected cats might represent an interesting natural animal model for the study of the pathogenesis of HIV-associated nephropathy and renal alterations associated with chronic viral infection.

Author details

Natasa Tozon
Clinic for Small Animal Medicine and Surgery, Veterinary Faculty, University of Ljubljana, Ljubljana, Slovenia

Mauro Pistello
Department of Experimental Pathology, Medical Biotechnologies, Infectious Diseases and Epidemiology, University of Pisa, Pisa, Italy

Alessandro Poli
Department of Animal Pathology, Prophylaxis and Food Hygiene, Veterinary Faculty, University of Pisa, Pisa, Italy

Acknowledgement

This work was supported by Ministero della Salute – Istituto Superiore di Sanità, "IV° Programma Nazionale di Ricerca sull'AIDS" "Progetto Nazionale AIDS – Italian Concerted AIDS Vaccine".

6. References

[1] Ackley CD, Yamamoto JK, Levy N (1990) Immunologic abnormalities in pathogen-free cats experimentally infected with feline immunodeficiency virus. J. virol. 64: 5652-5655.
[2] Hosie MJ, Addie D, Belak S (2009) Feline immunodeficiency ABCD guideline on prevention and management. J. fel. med. and surg. 11: 575-584.
[3] Hayward JJ, Rodrigo AG (2010) Molecular epidemiology of feline immunodeficiency virus in the domestic cat (felis catus). Vet. immunol. immunopathol. 134: 68-74.
[4] Pistello M, Cammarota G, Nicoletti E (1997) Analysis of the genetic and phylogenetic relationship of Italian isolates of feline immunodeficiency virus indicates a high prevalence and heterogeneity of subtype B. j. gen. virol. 9: 2247-2257.
[5] Kenyon JC, Lever AM (2011) The molecular biology of feline immunodeficiency virus (FIV). Viruses 11: 2192-2213.
[6] Shimoima M, Miyazawa T, Ikeda Y (2004) Use of CD134 as a primary receptor by the feline immunodeficiency virus. Science 303: 1192-1195.
[7] Hosie MJ, Pajek D, Samman A (2011) Feline immunodeficiency Virus (FIV) Neutralization: A Review. Viruses 3: 1879-1890.
[8] Phillips TR, Prospero Garcia O, Wheeler DW (1996) Neurologic dysfunctions caused by a molecular clone of feline immunodefecience virus, FIV-PPR. J. neurovirol. 2: 388-396.
[9] Poli A, Abramo F, Di Iorio C (1997) Neuropathology in cats experimentally infected with feline immunodeficiency virus: a morphological, immunocytochemical and morphometric study. J. Neurovirol. 3: 361-368.
[10] Kennedy JM, Hoke A, Zhu Y (2004) Peripheral neuropathy in lentivirus infection: evidence of inflammation and axonal injury. AIDS 18: 1241-1250.
[11] Ryan G, Grimes T, Brakin B (2005) Neuropathology associated with feline immunodeficiency virus infection highlights prominent lymphocyte trafficking through both the blood-brain and blood-choroid plexus barriers. J. neurovirol. 11: 337-345.

[12] Weaver CC, Burgess SC, Nelson PD (2005) Placental immunopathology and pregnancy failure in the FIV-infected cat. Placenta 26: 138-147.

[13] Belford CJ, Miller RI, Mitchell G (1989) Evidence of feline immunodeficiency virus in Queensland cats: preliminary observations. Aust. vet. pract. 19: 4-6.

[14] Swinney GR, Pauli JV, Jones BR (1989) Feline T-lyphotropic virus (FTLV) (feline immunodeficiency virus infection) in cats in New Zealand. N. Z. vet. j. 37: 41-43.

[15] Ishida T, Washizu T, Toriyabe K (1989) Feline immunodeficiency virus infection in cats of Japan. J. am. vet. med. assoc. 194: 221-225.

[16] Poli A, Abramo F, Taccini E (1993) Renal involvement in feline immunodeficiency virus infection: a clinicopathological study. Nephron 64: 282-288.

[17] Poli A, Abramo F, Mateucci D (1995) Renal involvement in feline immunodeficiency virus: p24 antigen detection, virus isolation and PCR analysis. Vet. immunol. Immunopathol. 46: 13-20.

[18] Pedersen, NC (1993) Feline immunodeficiency virus infection. In: Levy JA, editor, The Retroviruses. New York: Plenum Press, Vol. 2, pp 181-222.

[19] Yamamoto JK, Ackley CD, Zochlinski H (1991) Development of IL-2 independent feline lymphoid cell ciles chronically infected with feline immunodeficiency virus: importance for diagnostic reagents and vaccines. Intervirol. 32: 361-375.

[20] Pistello M, Matteucci D, Bonci F (2003) AIDS vaccination studies using an ex vivo feline immunodeficiency virus model: protection from a highly heterogeneous virulent intraclade challenge administered systemically or mucosally by an attenuated vaccine. J. virol. 77: 10740-10750.

[21] Laemmli UK (1970) Cleavage of Structural Proteins during the Assembly of the Head of Bacteriophage T4. Nature 227: 680- 685.

[22] Matteucci D, Baldinotti F, Mazzetti P (1993) Detection of feline immunodeficiency virus in saliva and plasma by cultivation and polymerase chain reaction. J. clin. microbiol. 31: 494-501.

[23] Torten M, Franchini M, Barlough JE (1991) Progressive immune dysfunction in cats experimentally infected with feline immunodeficiency virus. J. virol. 5: 2225-2230.

[24] Puchtler H, Waldrop FS, Meloan SN (1985) A review of light, polarization, and fluorescence microscopic methods for amyloid. Appl. pathol. 3: 5-17.

[25] Whright JR, Colkins E, Humphrey RL (1977) Potassium permanganate reaction in amyloidosis. A histologic method to assist in differntiating forms of this disease. Lab. invest. 36: 274-275.

[26] International Renal Interest Society (IRIS) (2009) IRIS Staging of CKD. Available: http://www.iris-kidney.com/guidelines/en/index.shtml. Accessed 2012 Apr 10.

[27] Thomas JB, Robinson F, Chadwick GJ (1993) Association of renal disease indicators with feline immunodeficiency virus infection. J. am. anim. hosp. assoc. 29: 320-326.

[28] Levy J (1996) FIV causes nephropathy in cats. Proceedings of the 14th Annual ACVIM forum. San Antonio, 1996: 56.

[29] Brown PJ, Cherida D, Hopper D (1991) Pathological features of lymphoid tissues in cats with natural feline immunodeficiency virus infection. J. comp. path. 104: 345-355.

[30] Bo S, Garetto M, Latti D (1992) Indagine epidemiologica e quadri clinici di FIV e FeLV nell'Italia nord-occidentale in una popolazione di 850 gatti. Veterinaria 4: 105-112.
[31] Marin R, Gorostidi M, Fernandez-Vega F (2005) Systemic and glomerular hypertension and progression of chronic renal disease: the dilemma of nephrosclerosis. Kidney. int. suppl.2005: 52–56.
[32] Avila-Casado C, Fortoul TI, Chugh SS (2011) HIV associated nephropathy: experimentals models. Contrib. Nephrol. 169: 270-285.
[33] Beebe AM, Duan N, Faith TG (1994) Primary stage of feline immunodeficiency virus infection: viral dissemination and cellular targets. J. virol. 68: 3080-3091.
[34] Poli A, Falcone L, Bigalli L (1995) Circulating immune complex and analysis of renal immune deposits in feline immunodeficiency virus-infected cats. Clin. exp. immunol. 101: 254-258.
[35] Matsumoto H, Takemura N, Sako T (1997) Serum concentration circulating immune complexes in cats infected with feline immunodeficiency virus detected by immune adherence hemagglutination method. J. vet. med. sci. 59: 395-396.
[36] Pennisi MG, Masucci M, De Majo M (1994) Presenza di anticorpi anti-nucleo in gatti FIV positivi. Proceedings of SCIVAC 48: 973-976.
[37] Ishida T, Taniguchi A, Matsumura S (1992) Long-term clinical observations on feline immunodeficiency virus infected asymptomatic carries. Vet. immunol. immunopathol. 1-2: 15-22.
[38] Shibata T, Sawashima Y, Sawashima K, (1995) Two cases of systemic amyloidosis in FIV-infected cats. J. Japan vet. med. assoc. 48: 268-270.
[39] Feder BM. (1993) Feline immundeficiency virus: association with cancer. Proceedings of 11th Annual ACVIM forum 1993: 832-4.
[40] Callanan JJ, Thomson H, Toth SR (1992) Clinical and pathological findings in feline immunodeficiency virus experimental infection. Vet. immunol. immunopathol. 1-2: 3-13.
[41] Rao TK. (1991) Human Immunodeficiency virus (HIV) associated nephropathy. Annu. rev. med. 42: 391-401.
[42] Kopp JB, Klotman ME, Adler SH (1992) Progressive glomerulosclerosis and enhanced renal accumulation of basement membrane components in mice transgenic for human immunodeficiency virus type 1 genes. Proc. natl. acad. sci. 89: 1577-1581.
[43] Naicker S, Fabian J, Naidoo S (2007) Infection and gloerulonephritis. Semin. immunopaathol. 29: 397-414.
[44] Pakasa NM, Binda PM (2011) HIV-associated immune complex glomerulonephritis with "lupus-like" features. Saudi. j. kidney. dis. transpl. 4:769-773.

Permissions

The contributors of this book come from diverse backgrounds, making this book a truly international effort. This book will bring forth new frontiers with its revolutionizing research information and detailed analysis of the nascent developments around the world.

We would like to thank Prof. Dr. Krassimir Metodiev, for lending his expertise to make the book truly unique. He has played a crucial role in the development of this book. Without his invaluable contribution this book wouldn't have been possible. He has made vital efforts to compile up to date information on the varied aspects of this subject to make this book a valuable addition to the collection of many professionals and students.

This book was conceptualized with the vision of imparting up-to-date information and advanced data in this field. To ensure the same, a matchless editorial board was set up. Every individual on the board went through rigorous rounds of assessment to prove their worth. After which they invested a large part of their time researching and compiling the most relevant data for our readers. Conferences and sessions were held from time to time between the editorial board and the contributing authors to present the data in the most comprehensible form. The editorial team has worked tirelessly to provide valuable and valid information to help people across the globe.

Every chapter published in this book has been scrutinized by our experts. Their significance has been extensively debated. The topics covered herein carry significant findings which will fuel the growth of the discipline. They may even be implemented as practical applications or may be referred to as a beginning point for another development. Chapters in this book were first published by InTech; hereby published with permission under the Creative Commons Attribution License or equivalent.

The editorial board has been involved in producing this book since its inception. They have spent rigorous hours researching and exploring the diverse topics which have resulted in the successful publishing of this book. They have passed on their knowledge of decades through this book. To expedite this challenging task, the publisher supported the team at every step. A small team of assistant editors was also appointed to further simplify the editing procedure and attain best results for the readers.

Our editorial team has been hand-picked from every corner of the world. Their multi-ethnicity adds dynamic inputs to the discussions which result in innovative outcomes. These outcomes are then further discussed with the researchers and contributors who give their valuable feedback and opinion regarding the same. The feedback is then collaborated with the researches and they are edited in a comprehensive manner to aid the understanding of the subject.

Apart from the editorial board, the designing team has also invested a significant amount of their time in understanding the subject and creating the most relevant covers. They scrutinized every image to scout for the most suitable representation of the subject and create an appropriate cover for the book.

The publishing team has been involved in this book since its early stages. They were actively engaged in every process, be it collecting the data, connecting with the contributors or procuring relevant information. The team has been an ardent support to the editorial, designing and production team. Their endless efforts to recruit the best for this project, has resulted in the accomplishment of this book. They are a veteran in the field of academics and their pool of knowledge is as vast as their experience in printing. Their expertise and guidance has proved useful at every step. Their uncompromising quality standards have made this book an exceptional effort. Their encouragement from time to time has been an inspiration for everyone.

The publisher and the editorial board hope that this book will prove to be a valuable piece of knowledge for researchers, students, practitioners and scholars across the globe.

List of Contributors

Yıldız Camcıoğlu
Istanbul University Cerrahpasa Medical School, Department of Pediatrics, Infectious Diseases, Clinical Immunology and Allergy Division, Cerrahpasa, Istanbul

Mary A. Slatter and Andrew R. Gennery
The Institute for Cellular Medicine, Newcastle upon Tyne University, Newcastle upon Tyne, UK

Winni De Haes
Institute of Tropical Medicine of Antwerp, Department of Biomedical Sciences, Virology Unit, Antwerp, Belgium

Charlotte Pollard
Institute of Tropical Medicine of Antwerp, Department of Biomedical Sciences, Virology Unit, Antwerp, Belgium
Laboratory of Molecular Immunology, Ghent University, Belgium

Guido Vanham
Institute of Tropical Medicine of Antwerp, Department of Biomedical Sciences, Virology Unit, Antwerp, Belgium
Faculty of Pharmaceutical, Veterinary and Biomedical Sciences, University of Antwerp, Belgium
Faculty of Medicine and Pharmacology, Vrije Universiteit Brussel, Belgium

Joanna Rejman
Laboratory of General Biochemistry and Physical Pharmacy, Ghent University, Belgium

Paula Lazarova
Dept. Cellular Therapy, University Rikshospital-Radiumhospital, Oslo, Norway
Clinical laboratory, District Hospital "St. Anna", Varna, Bulgaria

Krassimir Metodiev
Dept. Preclinical & Clinical Sciences, Medical University, Varna, Bulgaria

Gunnar Kvalheim
Dept. Cellular Therapy, University Rikshospital-Radiumhospital, Oslo, Norway

Luis Enrique Jerez Puebla
Parasitology Department, Institute Pedro Kourí (IPK), Havana, Cuba

Umezurike Hughes Okafor
Enugu State University Teaching Hospital, Parklane, Enugu, Nigeria

Cleo G. Anastassopoulou
Division of Genetics, Cell and Developmental Biology, Department of Biology, University of Patras, Patras, Greece

Ricardo U. Sorensen
Department of Pediatrics, New Orleans, Louisiana, USA

Tammy Harvey
Jeffrey Modell Center for Immunodeficiencies, New Orleans, Louisiana, USA

Lily E. Leiva
Louisiana State University Health Science Center, New Orleans, Louisiana, USA

Marco Rossi and Pierosandro Tagliaferri
Translational Medical Oncology Unit, Department of Experimental and Clinical Medicine, Magna Græcia University and Tommaso Campanella Cancer Center, Catanzaro, Italy

Pierfrancesco Tassone
Translational Medical Oncology Unit, Department of Experimental and Clinical Medicine, Magna Græcia University and Tommaso Campanella Cancer Center, Catanzaro, Italy
Temple University's College of Science & Technology, Philadelphia, PA, USA

Kerina Duri
University of Zimbabwe, College of Health Sciences, Department of Immunology, Harare, Zimbabwe

Hortensia Álvarez Díaz, Ana Mariño Callejo and José Francisco García Rodríguez
Infectious Diseases Unit, Department of Internal Medicine, Hospital Arquitecto Marcide-Profesor Novoa Santos, Sanitary Area of Ferrol, A Coruña, Spain

Deepak Joshi and Kosh Agarwal
Institute of Liver Studies, King's College Hospital, Denmark Hill, London, UK

Moosa Patel
Clinical Haematology Unit, Department of Medicine, Chris Hani Baragwanath Academic Hospital and Faculty of Health Sciences, University of the Witwatersrand, Johannesburg, South Africa

Teresa Whitaker
Hallows College, Dublin, Ireland

Paul Ryan
Department of Sociology, NUI Maynooth, Co. Kildare, Ireland

Gemma Cox
Young Ballymun, Dublin, Ireland

Fabiana Alves and Jenner Karlisson Pimenta dos Reis
Universidade Federal de Minas Gerais, Brazil

Lara E. Pereira
LRRI, Albuquerque, NM, USA

Priya Srinivasan and James M. Smith
Laboratory Branch, Division of HIV/AIDs Prevention, National Center for HIV/AIDS, Viral Hepatitis, STD, TB Prevention, Centers for Disease Control and Prevention, Atlanta, GA, USA

Natasa Tozon
Clinic for Small Animal Medicine and Surgery, Veterinary Faculty, University of Ljubljana, Ljubljana, Slovenia

Mauro Pistello
Department of Experimental Pathology, Medical Biotechnologies, Infectious Diseases and Epidemiology, University of Pisa, Pisa, Italy

Alessandro Poli
Department of Animal Pathology, Prophylaxis and Food Hygiene, Veterinary Faculty, University of Pisa, Pisa, Italy